Fibroids

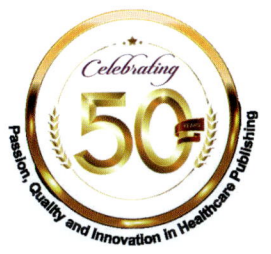

Fibroids

Editors

Narendra Malhotra
MD FICOG FICMCH FICS FRCOG FMAS FIAP
Management Director
Global Rainbow Healthcare
Agra, Uttar Pradesh, India
Vice President
World Association of Perinatal Medicine
Past President, FOGSI

Poonam Goyal MBBS MD FICOG
ART Specialist and Ultrasonologist
Department of IVF and Infertility
Max Superspecialty Hospital
New Delhi, India

Co-Editors

Jaideep Malhotra MD
Management Director
Rainbow IVF
Agra, Uttar Pradesh, India
President, FOGSI
President Elect, ISAR, ISPAT, SAFOG

Bhavana Mittal
DNB FNB MNAMS
Director
Shivam IVF and Infertility Centre
New Delhi, India

Foreword

Alka Kriplani (Padma Shri)

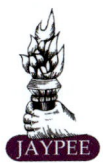

JAYPEE BROTHERS MEDICAL PUBLISHERS
The Health Sciences Publisher
New Delhi | London

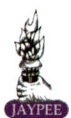
Jaypee Brothers Medical Publishers (P) Ltd

Headquarters
Jaypee Brothers Medical Publishers (P) Ltd
4838/24, Ansari Road, Daryaganj
New Delhi 110 002, India
Phone: +91-11-43574357
Fax: +91-11-43574314
E-mail: jaypee@jaypeebrothers.com

Overseas Offices
J P Medical Ltd
83 Victoria Street, London
SW1H 0HW (UK)
Phone: +44 20 3170 8910
Fax: +44 (0)20 3008 6180
E-mail: info@jpmedpub.com

Website: www.jaypeebrothers.com
Website: www.jaypeedigital.com

© 2019, Jaypee Brothers Medical Publishers

The views and opinions expressed in this book are solely those of the original contributor(s)/author(s) and do not necessarily represent those of editor(s) of the book.

All rights reserved. No part of this publication may be reproduced, stored or transmitted in any form or by any means, electronic, mechanical, photocopying, recording or otherwise, without the prior permission in writing of the publishers.

All brand names and product names used in this book are trade names, service marks, trademarks or registered trademarks of their respective owners. The publisher is not associated with any product or vendor mentioned in this book.

Medical knowledge and practice change constantly. This book is designed to provide accurate, authoritative information about the subject matter in question. However, readers are advised to check the most current information available on procedures included and check information from the manufacturer of each product to be administered, to verify the recommended dose, formula, method and duration of administration, adverse effects and contraindications. It is the responsibility of the practitioner to take all appropriate safety precautions. Neither the publisher nor the author(s)/editor(s) assume any liability for any injury and/or damage to persons or property arising from or related to use of material in this book.

This book is sold on the understanding that the publisher is not engaged in providing professional medical services. If such advice or services are required, the services of a competent medical professional should be sought.

Every effort has been made where necessary to contact holders of copyright to obtain permission to reproduce copyright material. If any have been inadvertently overlooked, the publisher will be pleased to make the necessary arrangements at the first opportunity. The **CD/DVD-ROM** (if any) provided in the sealed envelope with this book is complimentary and free of cost. **Not meant for sale.**

Inquiries for bulk sales may be solicited at: jaypee@jaypeebrothers.com

Fibroids

First Edition: **2019**
ISBN: 978-93-5270-549-8
Print and bound in India.

Dedication

The debilitating disease, uterine fibroid is affecting a lot number of women.
This book is a small effort to create a better world for women by imparting the
knowledge to clinicians taking care of women's health.
I am thankful to my better half Dr Jaideep Malhotra for her
continuous unconditional support.
I am grateful to my parents for their blessings.

Narendra Malhotra

This book is dedicated to all patients, who blindly trusted me to treat them
and in the process, they taught and made me what I am today.
I am thankful to my parents for their blessings. I am grateful to
my spouse and children for their love.

Poonam Goyal

We as a clinician should be always updated
with recent advances in medical science.
This is an effort towards that
I am thankful to my spouse Dr Narendra Malhotra and
my kids for their 24/7 support in all my endeavors.
I am grateful to my FOGSI family for their faith in me.

Jaideep Malhotra

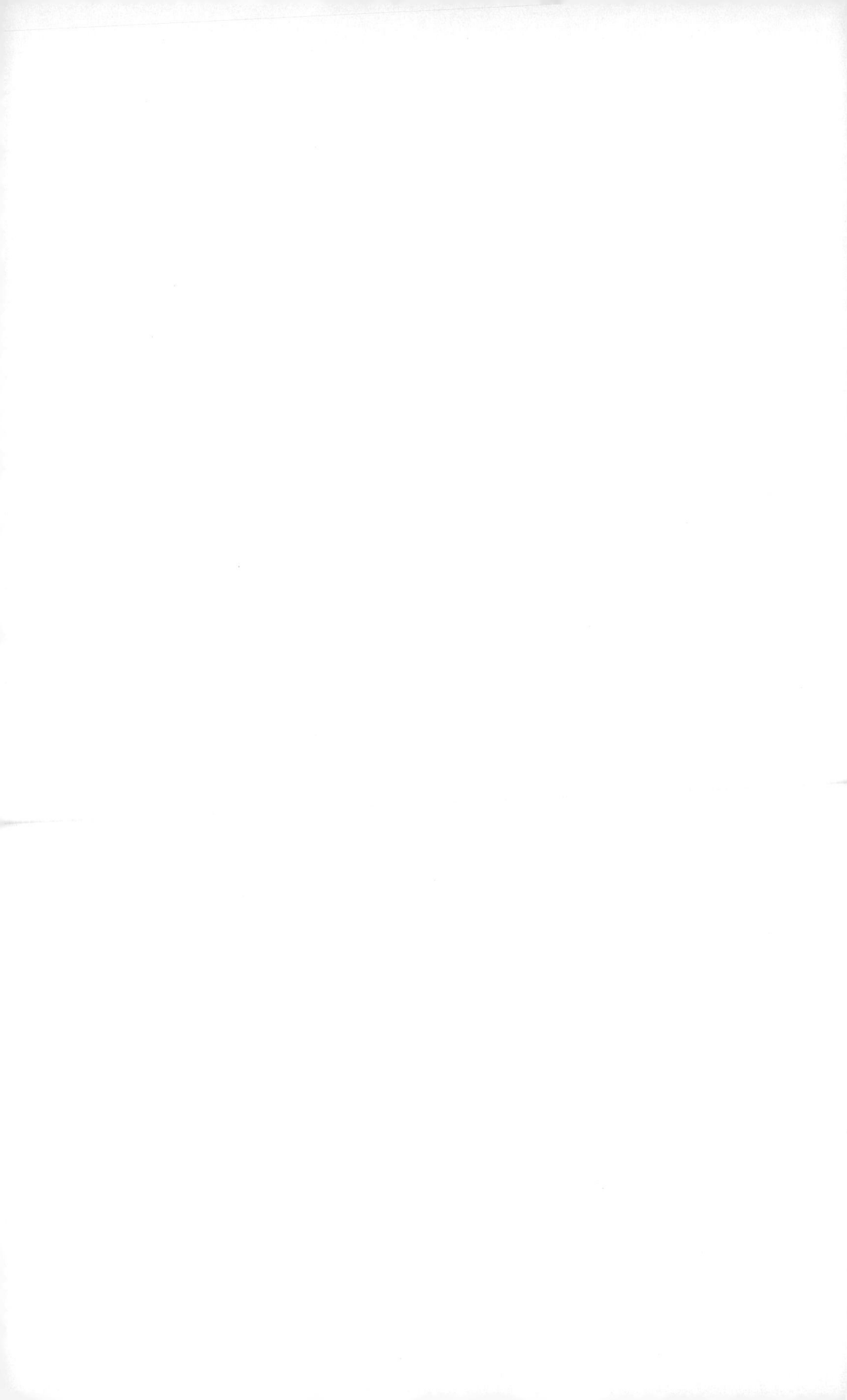

Contributors

Kavita Agarwal DGO DNB MICOG
Assistant Professor
Vardhman Mahavir Medical College and
Safdarjung Hospital
New Delhi, India

Shemi Bansal Dip GO
Consultant
Department of Obstetrics and Gynecology
Global Rainbow Hospital
Agra, Uttar Pradesh, India

Dhaval A Baxi DGO DNB
Gynecological Endoscopic Surgeon
Sri Aurobindo Medical College and
Postgraduate Institute
Indore, Madhya Pradesh, India

Sonam D Baxi MBBS MS
Obstetrician and Gynecologist
Disha Fertility and Surgical Centre
Indore, Madhya Pradesh, India

Vimee Bindra MBBS MS MHA
Consultant Gynecologist
Laparoscopic Surgeon and Infertility
Specialist
Apollo Hospitals and Apollo Cradle
Hyderabad, Telangana, India

Sunita Chandra MBBS MD
Director
Rajendra Nagar Hospital and IVF Center
Morpheus Lucknow Fertility Center
Lucknow, Uttar Pradesh, India

Rutvij Dalal MBBS DNB DGO (Gold Medalist)
FNB Consultant IVF
Ahmedabad, Gujarat, India

Venus Dalal MD MRCOG
Ex-Senior Resident
All India Institute of Medical Sciences
New Delhi, India

Shaik Meera Esha MS (Obs & Gyne)
Consultant
Aster Ramesh Hospitals
Guntur, Andhra Pradesh, India

Ruchika Garg MRCOGI CIMP FICMCH FMAS
Assistant Professor
SN Medical College
Agra, Uttar Pradesh, India

Kavitha Gautham MS (OG) FICOG
Lead Clinician and Founder Director
Bloom Fertility Centre
Chennai, Tamil Nadu, India

Poonam Goyal MBBS MD
ART Specialist and Ultrasonologist
Department of Obstetrics and Gynecology
Max Superspecialty Hospital
New Delhi, India

Gunjan Gupta
MD MRCOG (London) EUDGES (France)
Infertility Specialist and
Laparoscopy Specialist
Gunjans IVF World
Ghaziabad, Uttar Pradesh, India

Shalu Gupta
MS DNB (OBGYN) MNAMS Fellow National Board
(FNB)—Reproductive Medicine
Senior Consultant (Fertility)
Cloudnine
Gurugram, Haryana, India

Meenu Handa MS DNB
Fellow Reproductive Medicine
Senior IVF Consultant
Fortis Bloom Hospital
Gurugram, Haryana, India

Kundan Ingale MBBS DGO DNB MICOG
Director
Nirmiti Clinic
A Centre for Assisted Reproduction
Pune, Maharashtra, India

Ashish Kale MBBS MD DNB MNAMS MICOG FICS
Director
Ashakiran Hospital and Asha IVF Centre
Pune, Maharashtra, India

Anita Kant MD MICOG FICOG FICS PGDMLS
Director and Head
Department of Obstetrics and Gynecology
Asian Institute of Medical Sciences
Faridabad, Haryana, India

Anuradha Khar MD FIRM
Director
Nurture IVF
Bengaluru, Karnataka, India

Poonam Loomba MD (Obs and Gyne)
Consultant
Loomba Hospital and IVF Centre
Ambala Cantt, Haryana, India

Arti Luthra MS FICOG FICMCH
Director and Senior Consultant
Luthra Maternity and Infertility Centre
Dehradun, Uttarakhand, India

Reeta Mahey MD DNB
Associate Professor (ART)
All India Institute of Medical Sciences
New Delhi, India

Jaideep Malhotra MD
Management Director
Rainbow IVF
Agra, Uttar Pradesh, India
President, FOGSI
President Elect, ISAR, ISPAT, SAFOG

Narendra Malhotra
MD FICOG FICMCH FICS FRCOG FMAS FIAP
Management Director
Global Rainbow Healthcare
Agra, Uttar Pradesh, India
Vice President
World Association of Perinatal Medicine
Past President, FOGSI

Bhavana Mittal DNB FNB MNAMS
Director
Shivam IVF and Infertility Centre
New Delhi, India

Apoorva Pallam Reddy
MBBS MS DNB (Obs & Gyne)
Fellowship in Reproductive Gyne
Consultant
Reproductive Medicine and Endoscopy
Mathrutva Fertility Centre
Bengaluru, Karnataka, India

Seema Pandey MD FICOG FRM
Chief Consultant and Infertility Specialist
Seema Hospital and Eva Fertility Clinic and IVF Centre
Azamgarh, Uttar Pradesh, India

Sandeep Patil DNB FMAS MBBS
Consultant and Endoscopic Surgeon
Yashadaa Hospital
Mumbai, Maharashtra, India

Neha Priyadarshini MD
Fellow in Reproductive Medicine
Satvik IVF
Dhanbad, Jharkhand, India

Divya Sahetya MBBS MS FICOG
Fellowship in Reproductive Medicine
Consultant and Infertility Specialist
Pushpaa Hospital
Mumbai, Maharashtra, India

Ankesh R Sahetya DNB DGO MBBS MNAMS
Assistant Honorary
Oshiwara Maternity Home
Mumbai, Maharashtra, India

Mohit Rajendra Saraogi
MD DNB DGO MNAMS FCPS (Gold Medal) ICOG (Fellow) (Gold Medal)
Director
Saraogi Hospital and Iris IVF Centre
Mumbai, Maharashtra, India

Selvapriya Saravanan MD OG DRM (Kiel)
Fellow Fetal Medicine
Director, Spring Fertility and Fetocare
Kanyakumari, Kerala, India

Esha Sharma MS DNB
Consultant and Fertility Specialist
Motherhood Fertility Centre
Siliguri, West Bengal, India
Fellowship in Reproductive Medicine (ICOG)

Diksha Goswami Sharma
MD DNB MRCOG FNB (Reproductive Medicine)
IVF Consultant
Rainbow IVF
Agra, Uttar Pradesh, India

Manpreet Sharma MS (Obs & Gyne)
Consultant
Department of Obstetrics and Gynecology
Global Rainbow Hospitals
Agra, Uttar Pradesh, India

Garima Sharma MD DGO MBBS
Fellow Reproductive Medicine and IVF
Sir Ganga Ram Hospital
New Delhi, India

Rakhi Singh
DGO DRM (Kiel) DPE (Kiel) FICOG FIAOG
Director and Senior Fertility Specialist
Abalone Clinic and IVF Centre
Noida, Uttar Pradesh, India

Prakash Trivedi MD DNB FCPS DGO
Director
Dr Trivedi's Total Health Care Centre and
Aakar IVF Centre
Head
Department of Obstetrics and Gynecology
Rajawadi Municipal General Hospital
Mumbai, Maharashtra, India

Soumil Trivedi DNB FMAS MBBS
Co-Director and Consultant
Endoscopic Surgeon
Dr Trivedi's Total Health Care Centre
Speciality Consultant
Rajawadi Municipal General Hospital
Mumbai, Maharashtra, India

Rajalaxmi Walavalkar
MRCOG DNB FCPS FRMDGO DFP
Consultant
Department of Reproductive
Medicine and Surgery
Cocoon Fertility
Mumbai, Maharashtra, India

Foreword

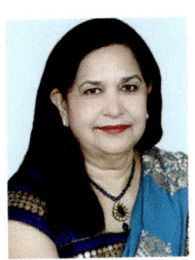

Fibroids is a book containing comprehensive encyclopedic insightful and in-depth information about the fibroid disease. It is amazing to see how the book unfolds step-by-step covering each and every aspect related to fibroids. The goal behind is to provide clinical guidance to busy practitioners. In recent decades, there has been significant change for the good in medical knowledge and experience. Loads and loads of information are just a click away but still there is no match for concise, practical and well-written book. It provides evidence-based management, according to the guidelines for specific condition related to fibroids. The text gives detailed knowledge supported by flowcharts.

As a physician, caring for women with fibroid disease, it is painful to witness frustration, pain and angst caused by uterine fibroids. The issue is further aggravated by the prevalence of uterine fibroids in women. Every third woman is affected by the disease and suffers from the adverse impact of fibroids in their lives. I myself have tackled so many nuisance creating fibroids at AIIMS. I realize sometimes the treating physicians is in dilemma to decide between the two treatment options. In such cases, this handy book can act as a guide. It covers a whole lot of spectrum of treatment, which is currently available. It will help in better understanding of these enigmatic tumors having infinite presentations with varied location, size and number. Currently, there is no preventive therapy available, so we have to fight fibroids head on. Dr Jaideep Malhotra is dear friend, very hard working and she has command on the subject. Her contribution makes this book special.

I greatly appreciate the efforts of the editors in bringing out such book. Dr Narendra Malhotra is a visionary and has a laser-like focus. He has contributed a lot towards our gyne fraternity. Dr Poonam Goyal is a hard-working person with good knowledge of the subject. I admire her continuous efforts in spite of being a busy practitioner.

At the end, I would say, this book will be of great help to the practicing doctors and post-graduate students in providing precise guidance. I wish good luck to Dr Narendra Malhotra, Poonam Goyal, Jaideep Malhotra and Bhavana Mittal and also to the budding authors who have really contributed the best. Dr Prakash Trivedi's chapter is a wonderful contribution.

Alka Kriplani (Padma Shri)
MD FRCOG FAMS FICOG FIMSA FICMCH FCLS
Director and Head
Department of Gynecology, Obstetrics and ART
Paras Hospitals, Gurugram, Haryana, India
Ex-Professor and Head
Department of Obstetrics and Gynecology
All India Institute of Medical Sciences
New Delhi, India

Preface

Uterine fibroid is a common gynecological pathology. This debilitating yet abstruse disease affects over 40% women worldwide. In fact, statistics show that 1 out of every 3 women in India are suffering from uterine fibroids. The disease may be asymptomatic or patient may present with severe symptoms of pain and bleeding.

Medical experts have been trying to conquer the disease since the earliest times to provide better service to the patients. Till date, there is a rapid innovation in the field of fibroid management to improve the quality of life of the suffering patients. Focus now has shifted to medical and conservative approaches rather than surgical approach.

We are highly thankful to M/s Jaypee Brothers Medical Publishers (P) Ltd, New Delhi, India, for publishing the book on a very interesting topic. We also express our gratitude to the contributors of the book who have provided pearls of knowledge from their expertise. We must also mention the unconditional support of our family members.

We whole heartedly dedicate this book to our patients who had confidence in us.

May God forever cherish the desire of every medical professional to gain knowledge.

Narendra Malhotra
Poonam Goyal

Acknowledgments

When Dr Narendra Malhotra floated the idea of a book on *Fibroids*, it seemed to be a Herculean task. But the concept came alive with extended hands of many to give a push. Dr Narendra Malhotra was always there 24×7 for guidance. We also extend special thanks to Dr Jaideep Malhotra for being a critic as well as guide.

We express our gratitude to Dr Alka Kriplani, who in spite of her packed schedule agreed to write foreword for the book. We sincerely thank Dr Prakash Trivedi for his contribution.

We express our heartfelt thanks and acknowledge the help of advocate Ms Aditee Goyal, Dr Pallaavi Goel, Dr VK Goyal, Dr AK Mittal, Dr Manju Mittal and Dr Tarun Mittal.

Contributors/Authors who all are best in their fields have worked hard and have done full justice to the chapters.

We especially appreciate the constant support and encouragement of Shri Jitendar P Vij (Group Chairman) and Mr Ankit Vij (Managing Director), M/s Jaypee Brothers Medical Publishers (P) Ltd, New Delhi, India, in helping to publish this textbook and also their associates particularly Ms Chetna Malhotra Vohra (Associate Director—Content Strategy) and Ms Prerna Bajaj (Development Editor), who have been prompt, efficient and most helpful.

Now waiting for the response of our readers.

Poonam Goyal
Bhavana Mittal

Contents

1. **Understanding Fibroids** 1
   Arti Luthra, Narendra Malhotra, Jaideep Malhotra

2. **Diagnosis of Fibroids** 13
   Ankesh R Sahetya, Divya Sahetya

3. **Clinical Rainbow of Fibroids** 24
   Poonam Goyal

4. **Management of Fibroids in Adolescent Girl** 31
   Vimee Bindra, Shaik Meera Esha

5. **Fibroids and Infertility** 36
   Bhavana Mittal

6. **Fibroids in Pregnancy** 41
   Dhaval A Baxi, Sonam D Baxi

7. **Management of AUB with Fibroid** 49
   Kundan Ingale, Ashish Kale

8. **Management of Fibroids in Perimenopausal Women** 61
   Esha Sharma

9. **Management of Fibroids in a Menopausal Woman** 69
   Selvapriya Saravanan

10. **Can We Leave Fibroids Alone?** 74
    Anuradha Khar

11. **Surgical Management of Fibroids** 79
    Rajalaxmi Walavalkar, Garima Sharma, Vimee Bindra

12. **Controversies Regarding Fibroid Morcellation** 96
    Prakash Trivedi, Soumil Trivedi, Sandeep Patil

13. **Medical Management of Fibroids** 106
    Poonam Loomba, Poonam Goyal

14. **Newer Nonsurgical Treatment Options for Fibroids** 117
    Shalu Gupta, Meenu Handa

15. **Fibroids and Malignancy** 126
    Reeta Mahey, Venus Dalal

16. **Recurrence and Treatment Outcomes in Fibroids** 130
    Kavitha Gautham

17. **Fibroids and Sexual Dysfunction** 139
    Mohit Rajendra Saraogi

18. Fibroids and Gastrointestinal Symptoms 143
    Sunita Chandra, Poonam Goyal

19. Genitourinary Dysfunction in Uterine Fibroids 146
    Rutvij Dalal

20. Infrequent or Atypical Fibroid Syndrome 152
    Neha Priyadarshini

21. What's New in the World of Fibroids? 161
    Apoorva Pallam Reddy

22. How Much Should She Worry? Reassuring Patients with Fibroids 172
    Rakhi Singh, Seema Pandey

23. Holistic Approach to Fibroids 179
    Gunjan Gupta

24. Uterine Fibroid in a Nutshell 185
    Ruchika Garg

25. Case Scenarios 191
    Diksha Goswami Sharma, Anita Kant

26. Perplexing Situations with Fibroids 207
    Poonam Goyal

27. Counseling in a Patient of Fibroid 209
    Poonam Goyal

28. Emerging and Hopeful Strategies toward Nonsurgical
    Management of Fibroids 211
    *Narendra Malhotra, Manpreet Sharma, Shemi Dunsui, Poonam Goyal,
    Jaideep Malhotra*

29. Ulipristal: Experience in Few Cases 216
    Poonam Goyal

30. Fibroid Management Guidelines 222
    Kavita Agarwal

Index 227

Understanding Fibroids

Arti Luthra, Narendra Malhotra, Jaideep Malhotra

INTRODUCTION

Uterine fibroids (leiomyomata) are benign tumors of the uterus primarily composed of smooth muscle and fibrous connective tissue. They range in size from seedlings to large uterine tumors. They may or may not be symptomatic.

DIFFERENT TERMS

The different terms are fibromyoma, myofibroma, myoma, fibroma, leiomyofibroma, fibroleiomyoma, and fibroid.
- Fibroid is the least accurate term to be used. Leiomyoma is a reasonably accurate term. It emphasizes the origin from smooth muscle cells and predominance of smooth muscle component.
- Leiomyomas are the most common tumors of female pelvis (Fig. 1.1) thus the most common indication for hysterectomy.

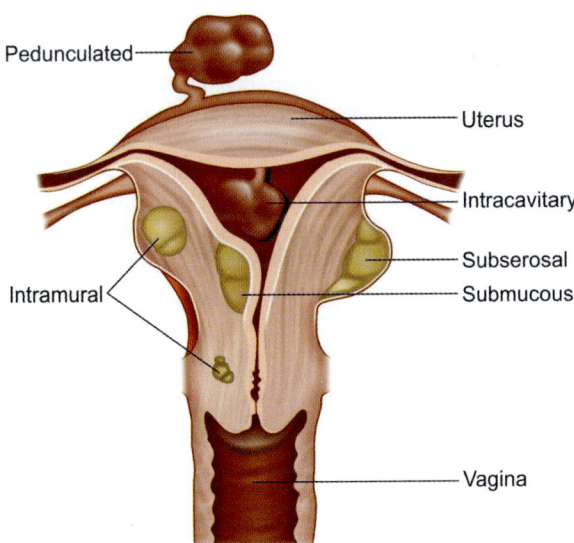

Fig. 1.1: Leiomyomas: various sites.

EPIDEMIOLOGY

The true *incidence* and prevalence of uterine fibroids in the general female population are unknown because the condition is frequently asymptomatic and therefore not identified.

Incidence increases with age during the reproductive years such that cases occur in 20-50% of women older than 30 years.

ETIOLOGY

These are benign tumors mainly composed of smooth muscles along with varying amount of fibrous connective tissue. They are well circumscribed but not capsulated.
- *Racial predominance*: More common in black women than in white. There is no explanation for this racial difference. Leiomyomata also are larger and occur at a younger age in black women.
- *Genetic predisposition*: Patients with leiomyomata often have a positive family history of leiomyoma.
    - There is possibility of gene coding in development of leiomyomata.
    - The true genetic contribution to the development of leiomyomas still needs to be defined.
- *Estrogen dependence*: Continuous estrogen secretion is the most important underlying risk factor in the development of leiomyoma.
    - The evidence in support of estrogen and progesterone is impressive.
    - Myomas are rarely found before puberty.
    - The growth of leiomyoma usually ceases after menopause. Actual regression in the tumor size may occur.
    - New myomas rarely appear after menopause. Possibility of malignant change should be ruled out in a leiomyoma, which enlarges after menopause.
    - Association of leiomyomas with endometrial hyperplasia, abnormal uterine bleeding, and endometrial hyperplasia.
    - Myomas increase in size during pregnancy and with combined contraceptive pills. Myomas tend to shrink after delivery. Mifepristone, a progesterone receptor inhibitor and gonadotropin releasing hormone (GnRH) agonist cause reduction in the size of leiomyomas.
    - Less common in smokers because of associated hypoestrogenic state.
- *Parity*: Higher risk in older nulliparous women. Relative risk decreases with each pregnancy.
- *Obesity*: Conversion of androgens to estrogens by fat aromatase increases the risk in obese women.
- *Effect of pregnancy*: Significant enlargement of leiomyoma during pregnancy proves relation of estrogen and progesterone to the growth of leiomyoma. The fibroids are often associated with adenomyosis, pelvic endometriosis, and pelvic inflammatory disease.
- A pseudocapsule is seen on ultrasonography (USG) scan, which differentiates it from normal myometrium.

ANATOMY

- A typical myoma is well-circumscribed tumor with a pseudocapsule.
- It is firm in consistency. The cut surface is pinkish white and has a whorled appearance. The capsule consists of connective tissue, which fixes the tumor to the myometrium (Fig. 1.2).
- The blood vessels lie in the capsule and send radial branches into the myoma (Fig. 1.2).
- Degeneration is noticeable early and most frequently in the central part of the tumor due to least blood supply (Figs. 1.3A and B).
- Calcification begins at the periphery and spreads inwards along the vessels.

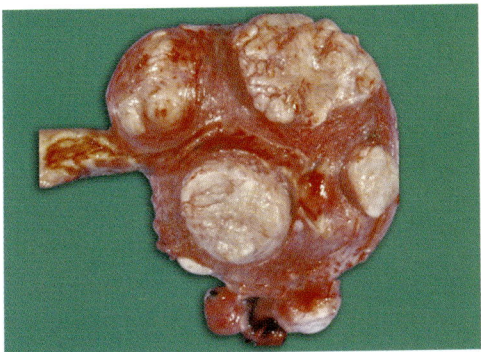

Fig. 1.2: Capsule around fibroid.

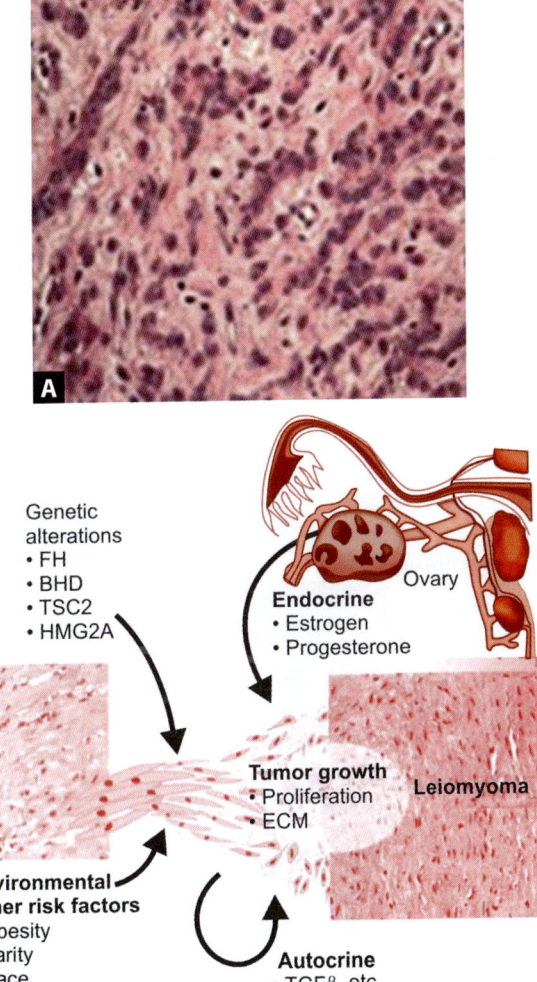

Figs. 1.3A and B: Degeneration in the central part of the tumor.

4 *Fibroids*

Distribution of Myomas in the Body of Uterus (Figs. 1.4 and 1.5)

- Intramural (interstitial) 75%
- Submucous 15%
- Subserous 10%.

They may also arise from:
- Round ligament
- Utero-ovarian ligament
- Uterosacral ligaments
- Cervical, submucous, and broad ligament fibroids are usually single (Flowchart 1.1).

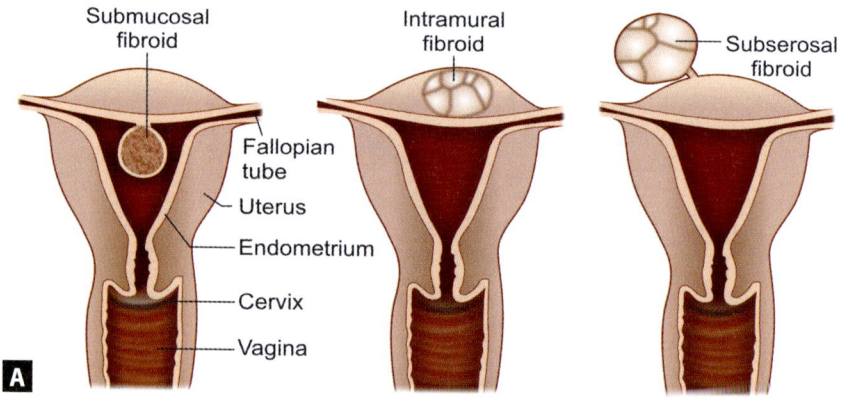

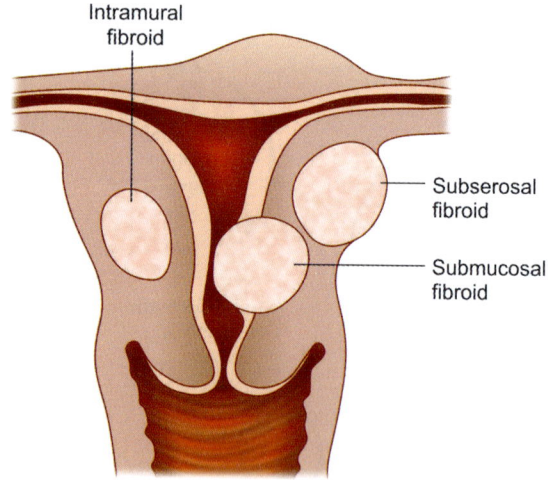

Figs. 1.4A and B

Understanding Fibroids **5**

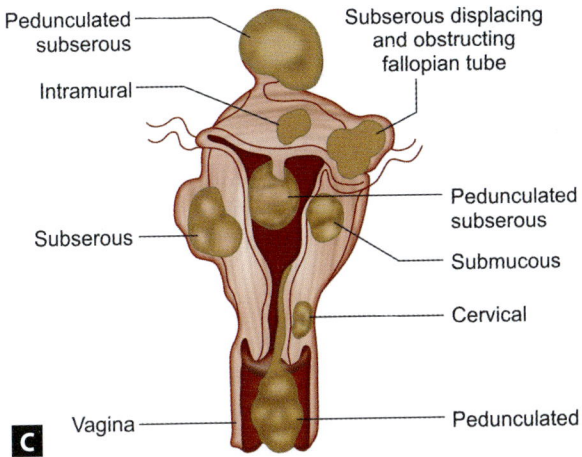

Figs. 1.4A to C: Distribution of myomas.

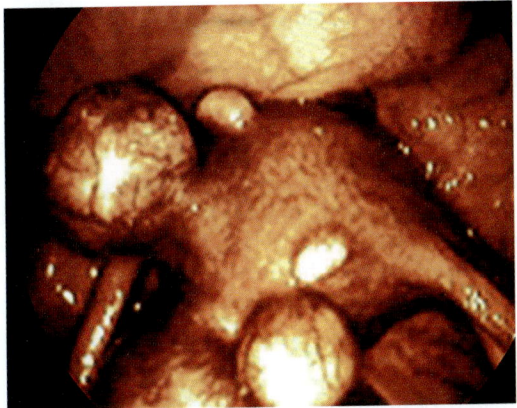

Fig. 1.5: Subserosal fibroids on laparoscopy.

Flowchart 1.1: Distribution of uterine fibroids.

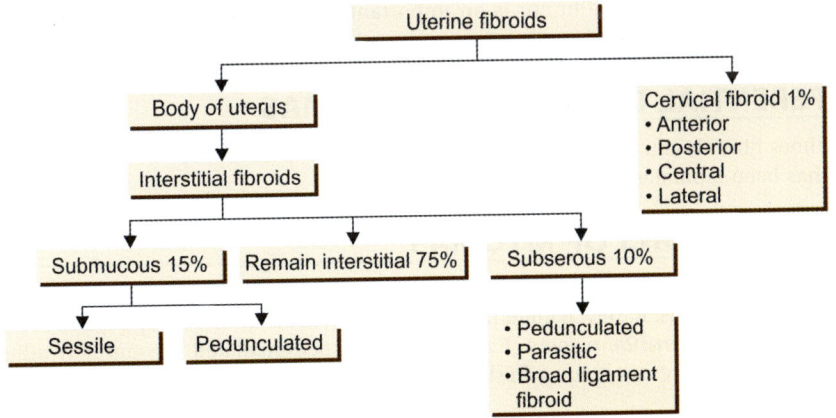

CLINICAL FEATURES

Secondary Changes in Fibroid

Atrophy
- Atrophic changes occur due to diminished vascularity after menopause.
- After childbirth, the tumor also gets much smaller in size.
- GnRH agonists can cause up to 50% reduction in size, which regrows after stopping the therapy.

Calcareous Degeneration
Phosphates and carbonates are deposited in the periphery along the course of vessels.
  In old patients with long-standing myomas, they are like womb stones in graveyard.

Red Degeneration
- Most often seen in pregnant patients with leiomyomas.
- It is not uncommon to see it in painful myomas in women over the age of 40.
- The lady may present with severe abdominal pain.

Hyaline Degeneration
- It is the most common type of degeneration affecting fibroids of all sizes except the tiny ones.
- It is common in myomas having more connective tissues.
- The least vascular central part of the tumor is the most common site.
- The consistency changes to soft elastic as compared to firm consistency of fibroid.
- Cut surface shows areas of irregular homogeneous tissue with loss of whorl pattern.
- On microscopic examination, both the muscle and fibrous tissue show hyaline changes.

Sarcomatous Change
- Incidence is less than 0.5% of all myomas.
- Intramural and submucous tumors have a higher potential for sarcomatous change than subserous change. It is rare for the malignant change to develop in women under 40 years.
- If a tumor grows rapidly in a postmenopausal woman along with bleeding per vaginam (PV).
- The consistency is soft and friable and not firm like a simple myoma.
- Nonencapsulation of the tumor is an important sign. Sarcoma is highly malignant and spreads by bloodstream.

DIFFERENTIAL DIAGNOSIS OF MYOMAS
Sometimes fibroids can be confused with other lesions in pelvis. A detailed differential diagnosis has been tabulated in Table 1.1.

COMPLICATIONS OF MYOMAS
- *Torsion*: A pedunculated subserous myoma may undergo rotation at the site of its attachment to the uterus. Rarely, patient may present with acute abdominal pain due to torsion.
- *Wandering or parasitic myoma*: Rarely, a rotated pedunculated myoma may adhere to the adjacent viscera, obtain a fresh blood supply from it, and be detached completely from the uterus.

Table 1.1: Differential diagnosis in fibroids.

Disease	Differentiating signs/symptoms	Diagnostic tests
Adenomyosis (Fig. 1.6)	Congestive dysmenorrhea	• Distinguished by histopathological examination • Imaging with pelvic ultrasonography and MRI
Endometrial polyp (Fig. 1.7)	Spasmodic dysmenorrhea Intermenstrual spotting	• Sonohysterography (SHG) shows a well-circumscribed isoechoic polypoid mass with stalk contained within the endometrial stripe • T2-weighted MRI images may show decreased signal intensity compared with endometrium
Endometrial hyperplasia (Fig. 1.8)	Heavy and irregular bleeding PV with passage of clots	• Hysteroscopic-guided endometrial biopsy and curettage followed by histopathology
Endometrial carcinoma (Fig. 1.9)	Because of the high prevalence of uterine fibroids in the general female population, a substantial number of patients with endometrial carcinoma will present with abnormal vaginal bleeding or discharge in association with uterine fibroids	• *Endometrial sampling*: An abnormal endometrial biopsy would show either precursor histology for endometrial carcinoma (simple/complex hyperplasia or simple atypical/complex atypical hyperplasia) or frank endometrial carcinoma • *Dilatation and curettage*: Persistence of irregular vaginal bleeding despite a negative endometrial biopsy should be pursued by dilatation and curettage
Uterine sarcoma (leiomyosarcoma, endometrial stromal sarcoma, and mixed mesodermal tumor) (Fig. 1.10)	Rapid growth of the tumor may be present in uterine sarcomas	• No test can reliably diagnose uterine sarcoma • Serial MRI can identify rapid uterine growth and show characteristics associated with sarcomas such as indistinct borders and invasion into contiguous organs
Pregnancy (Fig. 1.11)	Symptoms of pregnancy (e.g. morning sickness) and missed menstrual period are associated with abdominal expansion over a few weeks	• Pelvic ultrasonography visualizes the pregnancy sac • The urine or blood beta-hCG pregnancy test is positive
Ovarian cancer (Figs. 1.12A to C)	Ovarian cancer is differentiated by rapid tumor growth associated with atypical age for leiomyoma (e.g. postmeno-pausal women not on hormone replacement therapy), rapid weight loss, or ascites	• Pelvic ultrasonography and MRI are useful first-line investigations. MRI may show characteristic low-signal intensity on T2-weighted images seen with uterine fibroids, may show surrounding tissue invasion, and can more exactly define the origin of pelvic masses
Tumors of the GI tract and urinary system, lymphomas, and bone tumors (Figs. 1.13A to C)	These serious conditions are differentiated by rapid tumor growth associated with atypical age for leiomyoma (e.g. postmenopausal women not on hormone replacement therapy), surrounding tissue invasion, rapid weight loss, or ascites	• Pelvic ultrasonography and MRI are useful first-line investigations • Surgery and histopathological examination

(GI: Gastrointestinal: hCG: Human chorionic gonadotropin; MRI: Magnetic resonance imaging: PV: Per vaginam)

- *Inversion of uterus* can occur due to fundal submucous myoma.
- *Capsular hemorrhage*: If one of the large veins overlying a subserous myoma ruptures and profuse intraperitoneal hemorrhage may occur leading to hemorrhagic shock.
- *Infection*: Blood stained foul-smelling discharge may occur in submucous myoma and myomatous polyp. Infection is common in puerperium and can cause puerperal sepsis too. Infected myomatous polyp can cause delayed postpartum hemorrhage (PPH) or sepsis.
- *Associated endometrial carcinoma*: In women over 40 years of age, associated endometrial carcinoma can occur in 3% cases. Associated hyperestrogenism is the predisposing factor in both the cases.

CLINICAL SYMPTOMATOLOGY

Menstrual Disturbances
- Menorrhagia
- Polymenorrhagia
- Intermenstrual bleeding
- Continuous bleeding PV
- Postmenopausal disorders.
- Pain
  - Abdominal pain
  - Spasmodic dysmenorrhea
  - Backache
- Lump in abdomen
- Mass protruding into the vagina
- Pressure symptoms on adjacent viscera—bladder, ureters, and rectum
- Miscarriage, early labor, and PPH
- Uterine inversion
- Excessive discharge PV
- About 50% of fibroids are asymptomatic detected on routine check-up and USG.

ACUTE CLINICAL CONDITIONS

Acute clinical conditions associated with leiomyomata are:
- Acute retention of urine
- Acute abdominal pain due to red degeneration in fibroid due to associated pregnancy
- Torsion of a pedunculated polyp
- Hemorrhage
- Infection
- Sarcomatous change
- Rare entity of thromboembolism in labor.

PHYSICAL SIGNS

- Pallor—due to low hemoglobin caused by heavy periods.
- Abdominal lump—a mass arising out of pelvis with smooth margins, firm in consistency, with well-defined margins, smooth or bossy surface.
- The mass is mobile from side to side unless it is too big in size.
- The mobility may be limited due to adhesions, associated endometriosis or in broad-ligament myomas.

Understanding Fibroids 9

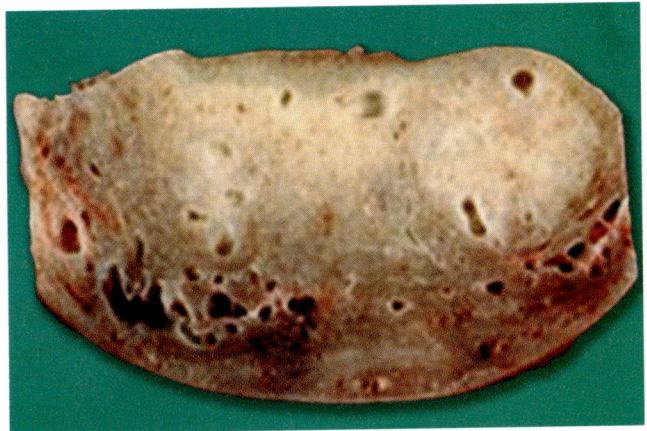

Fig. 1.6: Adenomyosis.

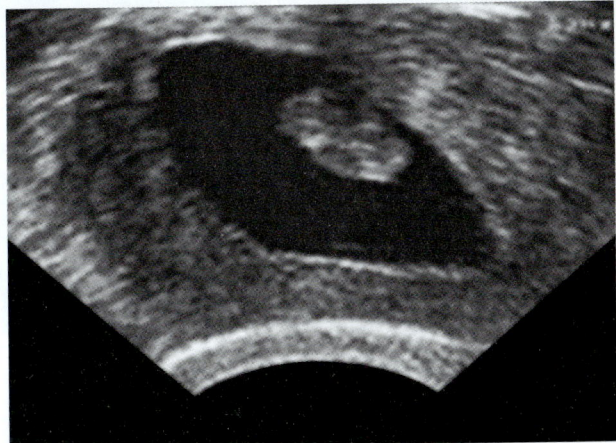

Fig. 1.7: Endometrial polyp.

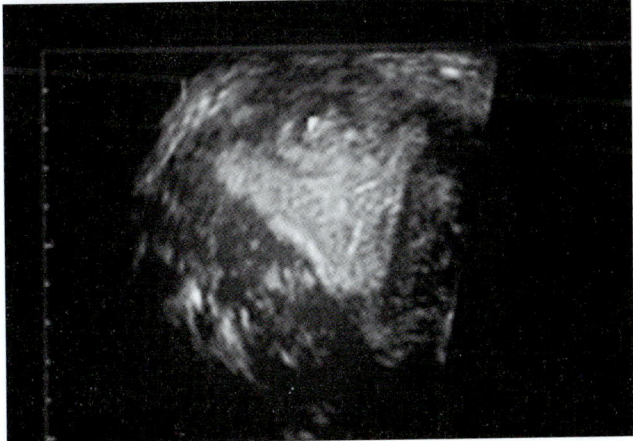

Fig. 1.8: Endometrial hyperplasia.

10 *Fibroids*

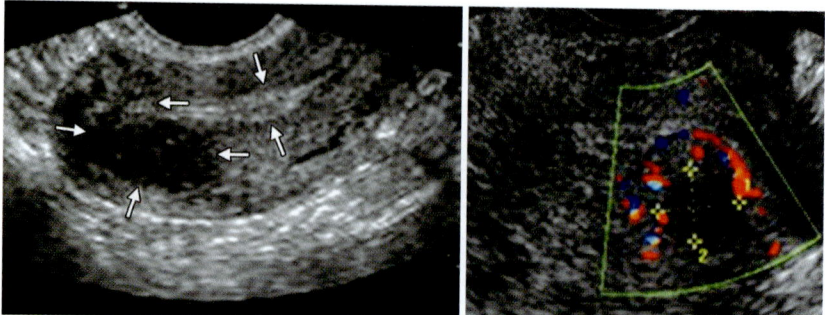

Fig. 1.9: Endometrial carcinoma.

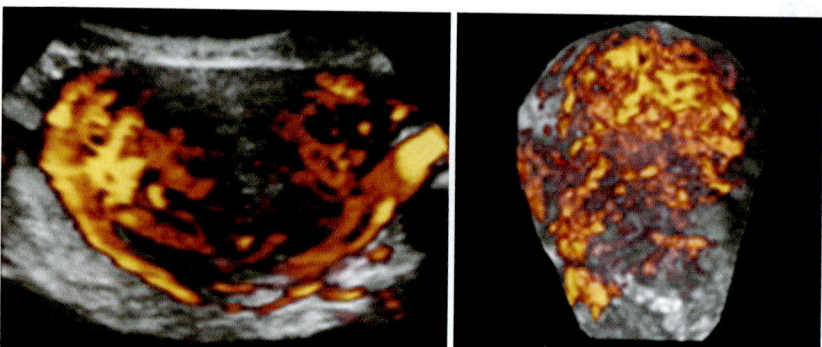

Fig. 1.10: Uterine sarcoma.

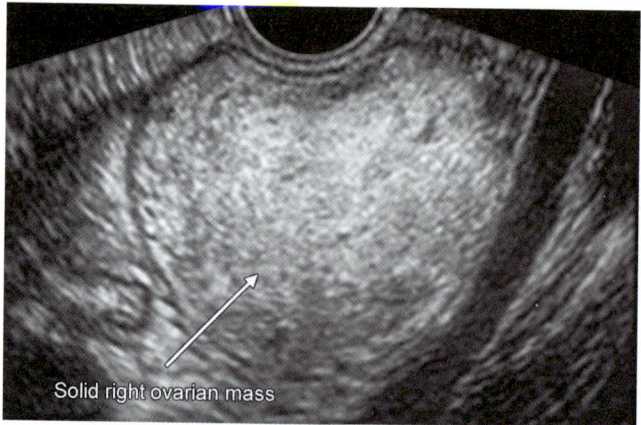

Fig. 1.11: Ovarian cancer.

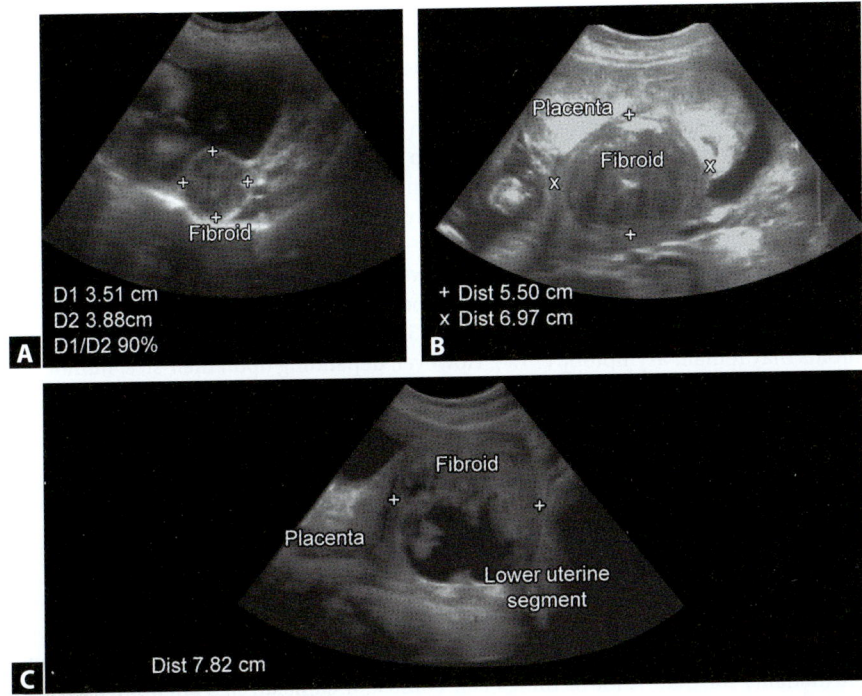

Figs. 1.12A to C: Pregnancy with fibroid disease.

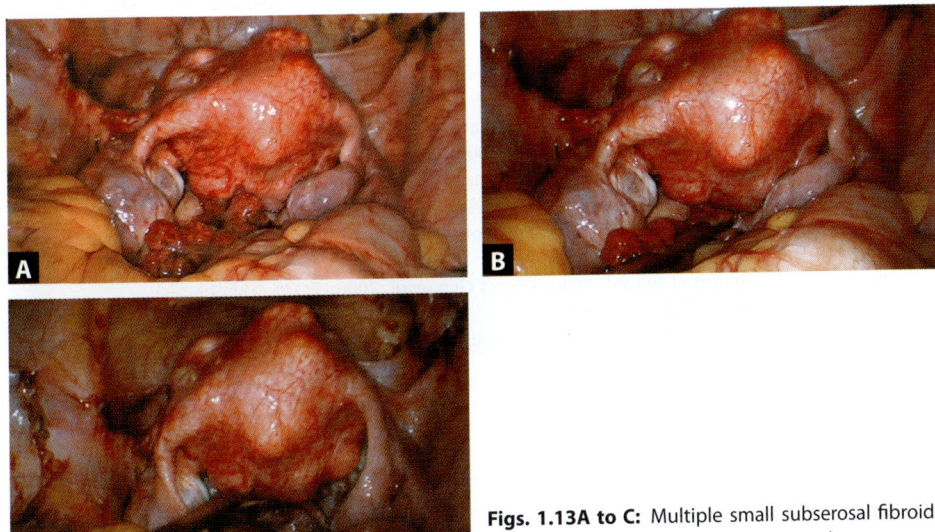

Figs. 1.13A to C: Multiple small subserosal fibroids with small fimbrial cyst as seen on endoscopy.

BIMANUAL EXAMINATION

- The uterus feels enlarged with regular or bossy margins depending upon the number and size of myomas.
- Cervical fibroid—normal uterus is perched on top of the tumor.
- Broad-ligament fibroid displaces the uterus to the opposite side.
- In a myomatous polyp—cervical os is open and its lower pole is felt.
- In submucous fibroids, the uterus is uniformly enlarged.
- Fibroid is the most common pelvic tumor.
- Incidence of symptomatic fibroids varies between 3% and 10%.
- Myomas are more common in nulliparous women.
- Prevalence is highest between 35 years and 45 years of age.
- Fibroids may remain asymptotic (75%). However, depending upon their size, number, and location, they may cause menstrual irregularities, pain, pressure symptoms, infertility, and complications during pregnancy.
- Hyaline degeneration is the most common secondary change.
- Sarcomatous change is extremely rare (<0.5%).
- Red degeneration occurs mainly in pregnancy and puerperium.

CONCLUSION

Fibroid tumors are very common and affect all age groups. They can grow at various sites and can clinically present in multiple ways. A clear diagnosis is required and ultrasound is the best modality for that. A lot of things can confuse a clinician like adenomyosis, polyps and solid ovarian tumors.

BIBLIOGRAPHY

1. Arulkumaran S. Acute complications of fibromyoma. Clin Obstet Gynaecol. 2009;5:23.
2. Dubuisson JB, Fauconnier A, Chapron C, et al. Reproductive outcome after laparoscopic myomectomy in infertile women. J Reprod Med. 2000;15(1):23-30.
3. Duncan J, Shulman LP. Yearbook of Obstetrics and Gynaecology. Elsevier: United States; 2010. p. 379.
4. Lichtinger M, Hallson L, Calvo P, et al. Laparoscopic uterine artery occlusion for symptomatic leiomyomas. J Am Assoc Gynecol Laparos. 2002;9(2):191-8.
5. Sarmini OR, Lefholz K, Froeschke HP. A comparison of laparoscopic supracervical hysterectomy and total abdominal hysterectomy outcomes. J Minim Invasive Gynecol. 2005;12(2):121-4.
6. Sengupta, Chattopadhyay, Varma. Textbook of Gynaecology for Postgraduates and Practitioners. Elsevier: US; 2007.
7. Studd J. Embolization of fibroid. Progr Obstet Gynaecol. 2006;17:333.
8. Studd J. Progr Obstet Gynaecol. 2005;16:277.
9. Sturdee. Yearbook of Obstetrics and Gynaecology. Elsevier: US; 2009. p. 9.

Diagnosis of Fibroids

Ankesh R Sahetya, Divya Sahetya

INTRODUCTION

Fibroid is the most common benign tumor of the uterus. It is more common among older nulliparous and obese women, particularly the ones with a family history of this disease. Based on the location of the tumor in the uterus, the various types of myoma are—subserous, intramural, and submucous fibroids as well as cervical and pseudocervical fibroids.

Women often consult their family physicians because of symptoms related to fibroid tumors or after the lesions have been diagnosed incidentally during physical or radiological examinations.

CLINICAL FINDINGS

History

Most leiomyomas are asymptomatic and are diagnosed incidentally.
- *Bleeding*:
    - Menorrhagia and menometrorrhagia
    - Continuous/irregular bleeding and blood-tinged discharge per vaginam may occur in cases of surface ulceration of submucosal fibroid polyp.
- *Pressure symptoms*:
    - Pelvic discomfort or feeling of heaviness in pelvis
    - Acute urinary retention
    - Urgency or frequency of micturition
    - Rarely dyspepsia or constipation.
- *Pain*:
    - Dysmenorrhea
    - *Lower abdominal and pelvic pain*: Not a common symptom, but may occur in cases of fibroid polyp, torsion of pedicle of subserous pedunculated fibroid, degeneration of fibroid, sarcomatous change in fibroid, and also dyspareunia.
- *Infertility*
- *Pregnancy-related complications*: Increase in size with red degeneration, abortions, preterm labor, and malpresentations
- *Labor complications*: Inertia, dystocia, postpartum hemorrhage.

General Physical Examination

Pallor may be present in cases of anemia due to menorrhagia.

Abdominal Examination (Fig. 2.1)

It may reveal a firm, nontender, rounded/lobulated mass with side-to-side mobility and which is dull to percuss (only in cases of huge fibroids).

Pelvic Examination

- *Pelvic (P/S) examination*: A submucosal fibroid polyp may be seen coming out of the cervix into the vagina with ulceration of the surface of the mass, seen as white discharge or bleeding, or blood stained discharge.
- P/V: Bimanual pelvic examination (Fig. 2.2) reveals an enlarged irregular firm uterus, but it may be symmetrically enlarged in cases of intramural and submucous fibroid.

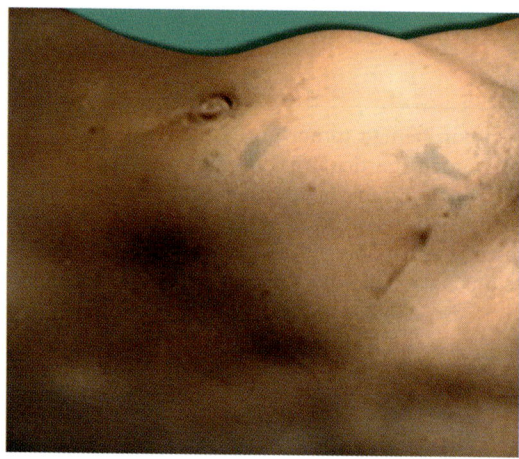

Fig. 2.1: Abdominal examination.

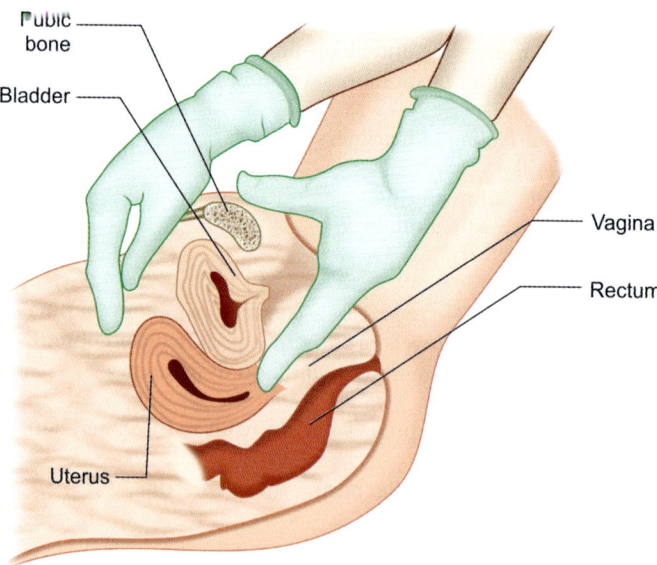

Fig. 2.2: Bimanual pelvic examination.

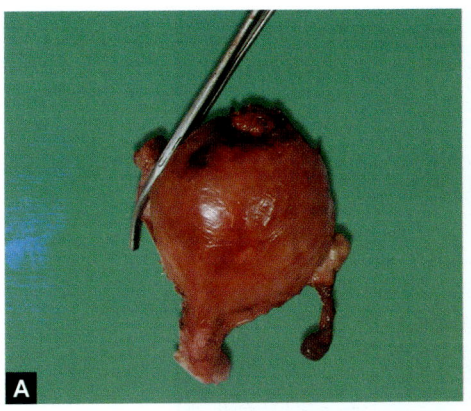 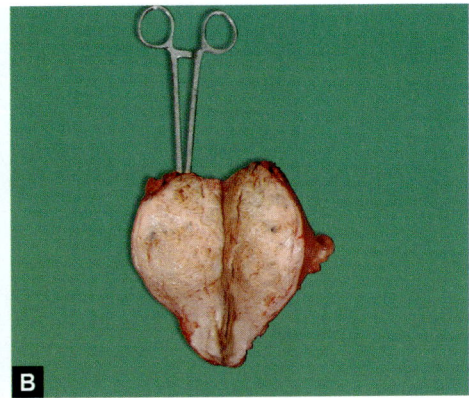

Figs. 2.3A and B: Bulky uterus with adenomyosis.

A subserous fibroid may be felt attached to the uterus or it may be felt as irregularity on one side or as an adnexal mass in case it is a pedunculated or broad-ligament fibroid. A submucosal fibroid polyp may be seen or felt coming out of the cervix into the vagina [differential diagnosis (D/D) with uterine inversion]. It should not be confused with uterine inversion. The swelling in uterine inversion is evidenced by the fact that uterus is not felt separately from the swelling and uterine fundus is not felt (Figs. 2.3A and B).

Routinely, ultrasound should be done to detect fibroids. However, submucous myomas often require saline-infusion sonography, hysteroscopy, or magnetic resonance imaging (MRI) for a definitive diagnosis. Fibroids must be differentiated from adenomyosis where uterus is bulky and globular in shape (Figs. 2.3A and B)

IMAGING

Precise uterine fibroid mapping (mapping is to know the location, measurement, characterization, and number of fibroids) is essential for research into clarifying the natural history of these tumors and for evaluating the therapeutic responses to investigational agents. The optimal selection of patients for medical therapy, noninvasive procedures, or surgery depends on an accurate assessment of the size, number, and position of myomas. Imaging techniques available for confirming the diagnosis of myomas include sonography, saline-infusion sonography, and MRI.

Ultrasonography and Color Doppler

Ultrasonography (USG) using the transabdominal and transvaginal routes (Fig. 2.4) has been employed most frequently, due to its accessibility and relatively low cost. While a cost-effective instrument, ultrasound has been criticized for its significant operator-dependence, resulting in inferior reproducibility when compared to MRI. Ideally, both transabdominal and transvaginal scans should be performed. Transvaginal scans are more sensitive for the diagnosis of small fibroids. However, when the uterus is bulky or retroverted, the uterine fundus may lie outside of the field of view. Transabdominal views are often of limited value, if the patient is obese. USG in skilled hands can detect fibroids as small as 5 mm on transvaginal ultrasounds. Typically, fibroids appear as well-defined, solid masses with a whorled appearance. These are usually of similar echogenicity to the myometrium, but sometimes may be hypoechoic. They cause the uterus to appear bulky or may cause an alteration of the normal uterine contour. Even noncalcified fibroids often show a degree of posterior acoustic

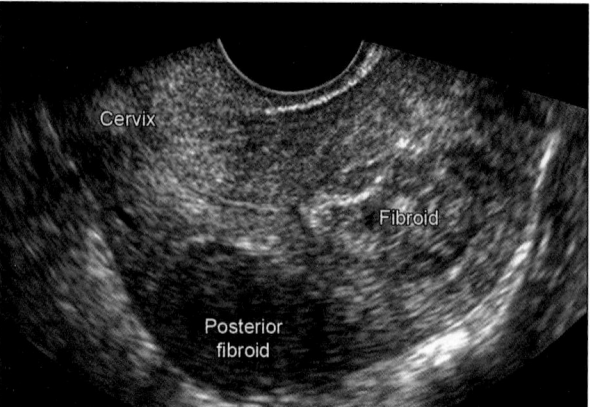

Fig. 2.4: Fibroids on transvaginal sonography.

shadowing, though this is of course more marked in calcified fibroids. Degenerated fibroids may have a complex appearance, with areas of cystic change.

Doppler ultrasound typically shows circumferential vascularity. However, fibroids, which are necrotic or have undergone torsion, will show absence of flow. Submucous fibroids are usually clearly visible separate from the endometrium under transvaginal ultrasound, but can be difficult to differentiate from polyps. Sonography may be inadequate for determining the precise number and position of myomas, although transvaginal sonography is reasonably reliable for uteri less than 375 mL in total volume or containing four myomas or fewer. Large fibroids can occasionally cause obstruction of the ureters, with secondary hydronephrosis. Therefore, ultrasound examination should include the urinary tract, whenever a large pelvic mass is identified. The diagnosis of fibroids on ultrasound is usually reasonably straightforward though focal adenomyosis can mimic a fibroid and a pedunculated uterine fibroid can sometimes be mistaken for an adnexal mass. Ultrasound cannot accurately determine the grade of a fibroid or whether its attachment point is simple (like a grape) or complex (broad based). When there is doubt about the origin of a pelvic mass at ultrasound, further evaluation with MRI should be performed.

In order to gain more complete information, other tests—saline infusion sonography (also called SIS or a sonohysterogram), hysteroscopy, ultrasound-guided hysteroscopy, or MRI may be required.

Saline Infusion Sonohysterography

Saline infusion sonography (Fig. 2.5) is a test that involves the use of ultrasound along with the injection of water into the uterus. The reason for the water injection is simple; water shows up as "jet black" on an ultrasound picture filled with various shades of "gray". The shades of gray can look confusing even to experienced physicians. The injection of water into the uterus let us know the exact location of the cavity and its relationship to the uterine fibroid.

During the test a catheter is inserted into the uterine cavity and water is injected through the cervix while an ultrasound examination is being performed. The water highlights the uterine cavity as well as any "masses" that occur within it—specifically fibroids and endometrial polyps. This turns out to be a very good method for measuring the fibroid or the polyp. In addition, SIS is able to clarify the type of fibroid—submucous or intramural—as well as its grade and the size of the attachment point.

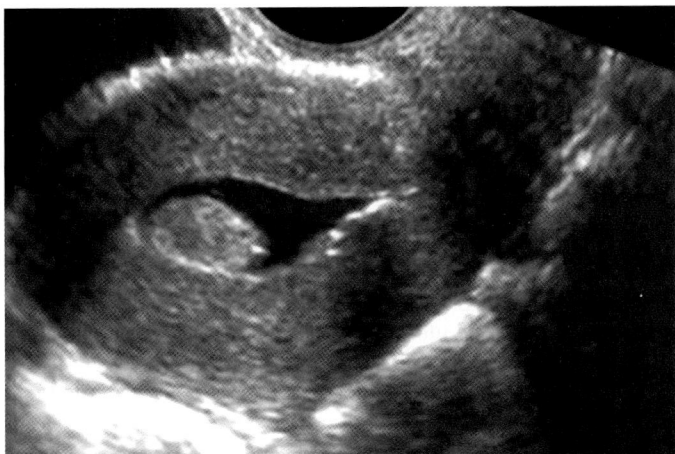

Fig. 2.5: Saline infusion sonography.

Saline infusion sonohysterography-based imaging is usually used as a supplementary or adjunct imaging modality for characterization of focal uterine masses diagnosed on B-mode ultrasound images. During transvaginal ultrasound, a uterine mass may appear as an area of increased echogenicity bulging into the endometrial cavity with echogenicity similar to that of the myometrium. In addition, it is difficult to distinguish a leiomyoma from a blood clot or a polyp, and leiomyomas also may obscure the endometrium on imaging or cause an overestimation of endometrial thickness. Transvaginal sonography may be used initially in the detection of endometrial polyps, which may appear as hyperechoic masses surrounded by a hypoechoic endometrium. However, it may be difficult to detect some polyps because they may appear as a diffusely thickened endometrium. Nevertheless, polyps may be better visualized during saline infusion sonohysterography, in which the saline pushes apart the uterine cavity, and the polyps appear as smoothly margined focal lesions that protrude into the endometrial cavity. Saline infusion sonohysterography is also effective in distinguishing diffuse endometrial changes and focal intracavitary protuberances. However, it is limited in its ability to differentiate between endometrial hyperplasia (premalignant polyps) and endometrial carcinoma.

The quality of the image obtained is dependent on the amount of deformation induced by the saline injection into the uterine cavity. If the amount of saline injected is too low, the deformation induced is too small to provide images with a reasonable signal-to-noise ratio. This situation has led to the generation of suboptimal strain images in some instances because of the minimal deformation of the tissue. The amount of deformation applied via saline injection is dependent on the ability of the patient to tolerate the discomfort induced due to saline injection into the uterus; in other cases, insufficient deformation is due to the presence of saline from a previous infusion and the inability to withdraw sufficient fluid before starting a new infusion.

Patient comfort is of paramount importance during the data acquisition because saline injection can be quite painful and distressing to the patient. Care should be taken to induce a sufficient deformation of the uterine wall that is tolerated by the patient to obtain high-quality strain images. The use of saline infusion sonohysterography-based strain imaging as a standalone imaging technique for the detection of uterine masses requires additional validation on a larger number of patients and at multiple clinical sites.

18 Fibroids

In conclusion, there seems to be limited diagnostic accuracy with saline infusion sonohysterography when better tolerated and more accurate imaging exists with USG and MRI imaging.

Magnetic Resonance Imaging

Magnetic resonance imaging (Fig. 2.6), while more costly, has been touted as the most sensitive modality for evaluating uterine myomas particularly for the detection of small fibroids. MRI is accurate in diagnosing a leiomyoma with a sensitivity of 88–93% and a specificity of 66–91%, and in differentiating leiomyoma from focal adenomyosis. Thus, MRI is more sensitive in identifying uterine fibroids than ultrasound, does not involve the use of ionizing radiation, and it can readily demonstrate the uterine zonal anatomy.

Submucosal, intramural, and subserosal fibroids are usually easily differentiated with MRI, and fibroids as small as 5 mm in diameter can be demonstrated. Fibroids in relatively unusual locations, such as within the cervix, can also be identified. MRI can be very helpful when investigating suspected acute fibroid complications when the patient presents to the emergency department and it is also a valuable tool that can be used to both predict and assess the response of fibroids to uterine artery embolization (UAE). Uterine fibroids are composed of a combination of smooth muscle cells and fibrous connective tissue. As these masses enlarge, they commonly outgrow their blood supply and undergo varying degrees of necrosis, which accounts for their variable signal intensities on MRI. Typically, leiomyomas are low in signal intensity relative to their surrounding myometrium on T2-weighted imaging and are isointense to myometrium on T1-weighted imaging. These signal characteristics are related to the most common form of degeneration (60%), which is hyalinization throughout the leiomyoma. Weinreb et al. defined diagnostic criteria for a leiomyoma to include a uterine mass that is predominantly hypointense compared to the myometrium on T2-weighted imaging and predominantly hypointense on T1-weighted imaging.

In some instances, it can be difficult to differentiate a large exophytic and subserosal leiomyoma from a solid adnexal mass such as an ovarian neoplasm. Differentiation is

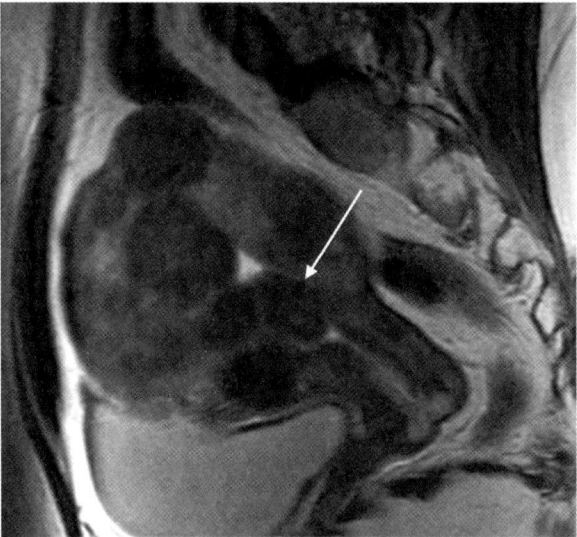

Fig. 2.6: Magnetic resonance imaging.

clinically very important because of differences in treatment and prognostic implications. MRI in combination with the patient's clinical findings can be invaluable in making this distinction and can avoid unnecessary laparoscopy and/or exploratory surgery. Location is an important distinguishing characteristic. If the mass can be definitively separated from the ovaries or is contiguous with the round ligament, then an ovarian etiology is unlikely. A well-described MRI feature that is helpful in the evaluation of large pelvic masses has been referred to as the "bridging vascular sign", which consists of vessels and/or signal voids that extend from the uterus to supply a pelvic mass. The identification of the bridging vascular sign increases the diagnostic confidence that a large pelvic mass is a uterine leiomyoma. The bridging vessels can be identified as enhancing tubular structures on contrast-enhanced T1-weighted imaging or as flow voids on a T2-weighted fast spin-echo sequence. In a study by Kim et al. the bridging vascular sign was present in 20 out of 26 exophytic leiomyomas and was absent in all other adnexal masses, resulting in a diagnostic accuracy of 80%.

Fibroids that have undergone acute degeneration show great diversity in their MRI appearances with cystic change and areas of nonenhancement. In cases of red degeneration, the patient often presents with an acute abdomen. The use of multiplanar views can enable localization of fibroids and can make it possible to distinguish fibroids from acute presentations of ovarian masses. MRI appearances show high-signal intensity centrally within the fibroid on T1-weighted images consistent with blood, with reduced signal at the periphery on T2-weighted images secondary to hemosiderin deposition. There may be heterogeneous signal intensity on T2, with no enhancement post-gadolinium administration (although gadolinium is not given to pregnant patients).

Fibroids that demonstrate high signal on T1-weighted images prior to embolization are likely to have a poor response to UAE, as they may already have outgrown their blood supply and undergone hemorrhagic necrosis. Conversely, high signal on T2-weighted images prior to embolization has been shown to be a predictor of good response. The vascularity of a fibroid is demonstrated by gadolinium enhancement and this is also a predictor of good response to UAE. Post-UAE fibroids typically show high signal on T1-weighted images due to hemorrhagic necrosis.

Magnetic resonance imaging is generally quite unhelpful in determining whether or not a fibroid can be removed hysteroscopically. Also to keep in mind is that MRI is quite expensive, and while it is very sensitive for detecting very small fibroids (less than 1 cm), these smaller fibroids are often of questionable clinical importance. The bottom line is that the best tools for evaluating the kind of fibroids that produce excessive menstrual bleeding are clearly a combination of ultrasound and hysteroscopy.

Magnetic resonance imaging may be the best tool, however, when evaluating a uterus containing numerous fibroids that require laparoscopic removal or procedures such as UAE and focused ultrasound destruction.

Hysteroscopy

Hysteroscopy (Fig. 2.7) is an excellent and relatively noninvasive tool in assessing the interior of the uterine cavity. This is extremely important for women who are experiencing menstrual issues as well as infertility. Hysteroscopy is one of the most important tests we require while trying out to figure out the location and the neighborhood of fibroids that are primarily responsible for heavy vaginal bleeding or infertility.

Hysteroscopy allows us to visualize the fibroid and determine how much of it lies within the uterine cavity. This simple test also allows us to determine the nature of the "attachment point". These assessments are very important in order to determine the best approach to remove a fibroid. Certain fibroids are best approached through the "hysteroscopic" approach, meaning through the natural openings of the vagina and the cervix, while other fibroids are

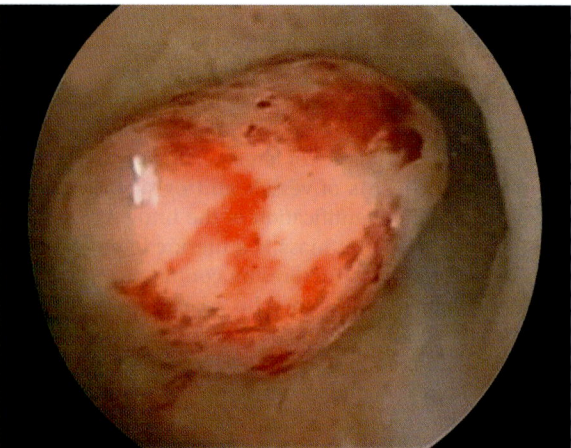

Fig. 2.7: Submucosal fibroid on hysteroscopy.

best approached laparoscopically. Importantly, hysteroscopy is also a tool, which helps in differentiating fibroids from polyps.

Finally, there is an important and often neglected advantage of hysteroscopy. Hysteroscopy simulates the environment for removing fibroids. Although tests such as magnetic resonance imaging can provide a great deal of information about fibroids, hysteroscopy allows a direct look and feel. Through hysteroscopy, we can see the blood vessels feeding the fibroid, watch the attachment site and also get an important idea about whether or not certain instrumentation can safely fit through the cervix in order to remove fibroids within the uterine cavity (submucous). No other test can provide this simulation.

Ultrasound-guided Hysteroscopy

If a woman has an abnormal ultrasound finding that needs to be further evaluated because of the suspicion of a fibroid or a polyp, she may undergo a hysteroscopy in a center where an ultrasound can be simultaneously available. Many, but not all women, with an abnormal ultrasound finding will require further evaluation with hysteroscopy and if this examination is done in a facility where ultrasound examinations are available at the time of her hysteroscopy then a great deal of information can be gained through this single test. This would include:
- The size, number, and grade of fibroids
- The size and number of endometrial polyps
- The type, size, and location of the attachment points
- The nature of the blood supply to the fibroid
- Information about the cervix, which is critical toward formulating a plan for removal of the fibroid or polyp
- Additional information that will be useful to the surgeon who is contemplating removal of the fibroid as well as which would be the better route of removal.

Laparoscopy

Laparoscopy (Fig. 2.8) is particularly helpful when the uterine size is less than 12 weeks and is associated with pelvic pain and infertility. Any associated pelvic endometriosis and tubal pathology can be revealed. It can also help in differentiating a pedunculated fibroid from an ovarian tumor, not revealed on clinical examination and ultrasound.

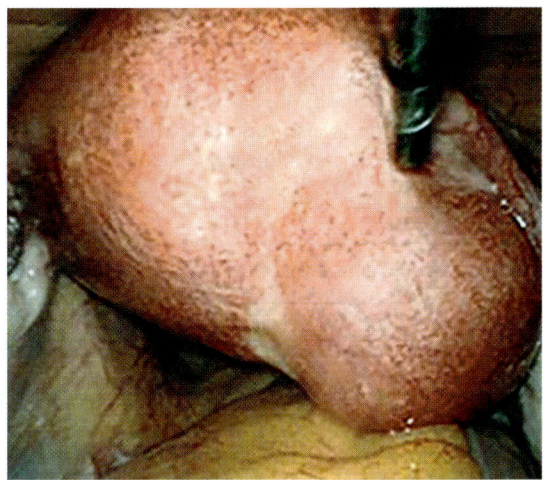

Fig. 2.8: Laparoscopy.

Endometrial Curettage

It is helpful in detecting any coexisting pathology in the presence of irregular bleeding and to study the endometrial pattern. It may help to diagnose a submucous fibroid by feeling a bump.

DIFFERENTIAL DIAGNOSIS

- Pregnancy
- Full bladder
- Adenomyosis
- Myohyperplasia
- Ovarian tumor
- Tubo-ovarian mass.

- *Pregnancy*: Many a times, enlarged uterus feels like fibroid especially if uterus is tense and history of irregular bleeding is there. USG and serum βhCG levels help in diagnosis.
- *Adenomyosis*: Many a times, adenomyosis is confused with fibroid on USG. For arriving at correct diagnosis, following points are critical: An adenomyotic uterus is generally bully or enlarged, maintaining its regular shape or becomes globular. But in fibroids, there is irregular contour of uterus.
  - There is disparity in size of anterior–posterior myometrium in adenomyosis.
  - Outer pseudocapsule not seen in case of adenomyoma but is there in fibroid.
  - Endometrial cavity may be distorted in fibroids, if they are multiple.
  - There is low velocity flow on Doppler in adenomyotic lesions.
  - Adenomyosis can be hyperechoic whereas fibroids are usually hypoechoic in nature.
- *Myohyperplasia*: It is again general enlarged uterus not focal lesion like fibroid.
- Solid ovarian lesions may be confused with subserosal fibroid and can be differentiated by pushing the probe in-between uterus and mass.
- *Tubo-ovarian mass*: Complex tubo-ovarian masses again may look like subserosal fibroid.
- *To conclude*: A careful Harding, examined and USG by good experienced operator can diagnose of fibroid. Rarely MRI is required.

CONCLUSION

Fibroids are tumors of uterine musculature which can grow to variable sizes. For diagnosis of and also for mapping of fibroids transabdominal as well as transvaginal scan should be done. However, a good clinical examination is also required. MRI is rarely indicated especially in obese females and also if there are uterine adhesions because of previous surgeries.

BIBLIOGRAPHY

1. ACOG Committee on Practice Bulletins-Gynecology. ACOG practice bulletin. Surgical alternatives to hysterectomy in the management of leiomyomas. Number 16, May 2000 (replaces educational bulletin number 192, May 1994). Int J Gynaecol Obstet. 2001;73(3):285-93.
2. Baird DD, Dunson DB. Why is parity protective for uterine fibroids? Epidemiology. 2003;14(2):247-50.
3. Barbieri RL, McShane PM, Ryan KJ. Constituents of cigarette smoke inhibit human granulosa cell aromatase. Fertil Steril. 1986;46(2):232-6.
4. Burbank F. Childbirth and myoma treatment by uterine artery occlusion: do they share a common biology? J Am Assoc Gynecol Laparosc. 2004;11(2):138-52.
5. Buttram VC Jr, Reiter RC. Uterine leiomyomata: etiology, symptomatology, and management. Fertil Steril. 1981;36(4):433-45.
6. Cantuaria GH, Angioli R, Frost L, et al. Comparison of bimanual examination with ultrasound examination before hysterectomy for uterine leiomyoma. Obstet Gynecol. 1998;92(1):109-12.
7. Cesen-Cummings K, Houston KD, Copland JA, et al. Uterine leiomyomas express myometrial contractile-associated proteins involved in pregnancy-related hormone signaling. J Soc Gynecol Investig. 2003;10(1):11-20.
8. Cramer SF, Patel A. The frequency of uterine leiomyomas. Am J Clin Pathol. 1990;94(4):435-8.
9. Daniel M, Martin AD, Drinkwater DT. Cigarette smoking, steroid hormones, and bone mineral density in young women. Calcif Tissue Int. 1992;50:300-5.
10. Day Baird D, Dunson DB, Hill MC, et al. High cumulative incidence of uterine leiomyoma in black and white women: ultrasound evidence. Am J Obstet Gynecol. 2003;188(1):100-7.
11. Farrer-Brown G, Beilby JO, Tarbit MH. Venous changes in the endometrium of myomatous uteri. Obstet Gynecol. 1971;38(5):743-51.
12. Ferenczy A, Richart RM, Okagaki T. A comparative ultrastructural study of leiomyosarcoma, cellular leiomyoma, and leiomyoma of the uterus. Cancer. 1971;28(4):1004-18.
13. Kawaguchi K, Fujii S, Konishi I, et al. Mitotic activity in uterine leiomyomas during the menstrual cycle. Am J Obstet Gynecol. 1989;160:637-41.
14. Lippman SA, Warner M, Samuels S, et al. Uterine fibroids and gynecologic pain symptoms in a population-based study. Fertil Steril. 2003;80(6):1488-94.
15. Lumbiganon P, Rugpao S, Phandhu-fung S, et al. Protective effect of depot- medroxyprogesterone acetate on surgically treated uterine leiomyomas: a multicentre case-control study. Br J Obstet Gynaecol. 1996;103(9):909-14.
16. Marino JL, Eskenazi B, Warner M, et al. Uterine leiomyoma and menstrual cycle characteristics in a population-based cohort study. Hum Reprod. 2004;19:2350-5.
17. Michnovicz JJ, Hershcopf RJ, Naganuma H, et al. Increased 2-hydroxylation of estradiol as a possible mechanism for the anti-estrogenic effect of cigarette smoking. N Engl J Med. 1986;315(21):1305-9.
18. Munro MG, Lukes AS. Abnormal uterine bleeding and underlying hemostatic disorders: report of a consensus process. Fertil Steril. 2005;84(5):1335-7.
19. Palomba S, Sammartino A, Di Carlo C, et al. Effects of raloxifene treatment on uterine leiomyomas in postmenopausal women. Fertil Steril. 2001;76:38-43.
20. Palomba S, Sena T, Morelli M, et al. Effect of different doses of progestin on uterine leiomyomas in postmenopausal women. Eur J Obstet Gynecol Reprod Biol. 2002;102(2):199-201.
21. Parazzini F, Negri E, La Vecchia C, et al. Oral contraceptive use and risk of uterine fibroids. Obstet Gynecol. 1992;79(3):430-3.
22. Parazzini F, Negri E, La Vecchia C, et al. Reproductive factors and risk of uterine fibroids. Epidemiology. 1996;7(4):440-2.

23. Ratner H. Risk factors for uterine fibroids: reduced risk associated with oral contraceptives. Br Med J (Clin Res Ed). 1986;293(6553):1027.
24. Reed SD, Cushing-Haugen KL, Daling JR, et al. Postmenopausal estrogen and progestogen therapy and the risk of uterine leiomyomas. Menopause. 2004;11(2):214-22.
25. Stewart EA, Nowak RA. New concepts in the treatment of uterine leiomyomas. Obstet Gynecol. 1998;92(4):624-7.
26. Wise LA, Palmer JR, Harlow BL, et al. Risk of uterine leiomyomata in relation to tobacco, alcohol and caffeine consumption in the Black Women's Health Study. Hum Reprod. 2004;19(8):1746-54.
27. Wegienka G, Baird DD, Hertz-Picciotto I, et al. Self-reported heavy bleeding associated with uterine leiomyomata. Obstet Gynecol. 2003;101(3):431-7.
28. Yang CH, Lee JN, Hsu SC, et al. Effect of hormone replacement therapy on uterine fibroids in postmenopausal women—a 3-year study. Maturitas. 2002;43(1):35-9.

Clinical Rainbow of Fibroids

Poonam Goyal

INTRODUCTION

Myomas are the most common tumors of female genital system. Commonly called fibroids, which is actually a misnomer as these are not tumors of fibrous tissue but are of muscle cell origin. These are abnormal growths, which develop in and on uterus. These are benign but burdensome tumors of uterus capable of wreaking havoc in woman's life. About 50-60% of the women are affected. The wide spectrum of clinical presentation is very intriguing; right from asymptomatic incidental finding to patient landing in hospital emergency in a state of shock. This chapter aims at discussing this clinical rainbow of fibroid disease.

EPIDEMIOLOGY

The literature of fibroid epidemiology treats fibroid as a single disease. Genetic predisposition is likely as is evident from association of fibroids with rare genetic syndromes. It is certainly possible that myometrium of some women is more prone to develop fibroids and once they develop they may grow more rapidly. Prevalence is different in different races and ethnic groups. Sex steroids can play important role in pathogenesis of fibroid disease along with growth factors, cytokines, and extracellular matrix.

Fibroids in accordance with their number, size, and location can lead to multiple and disabling symptoms. As already discussed, the range of presentation of fibroid disease is very widespread.

CLINICAL SPECTRUM OF FIBROID DISEASE (FLOWCHART 3.1)

- Asymptomatic incidental finding
- Gynecological symptoms
- Reproductive problems
- Obstetrical symptoms
- Generalized symptoms
- Rare fibroid syndromes
- Malignant change
- Pressure symptoms.

Asymptomatic

- Many a times when patient comes for routine checkup or gets an ultrasound scan done for another problem, an incidental diagnosis of fibroid is made. They are not affecting woman's quality of life and as there is no disruption of her wellbeing so she will not report to the doctor.

Flowchart 3.1: Presentation of fibroids.

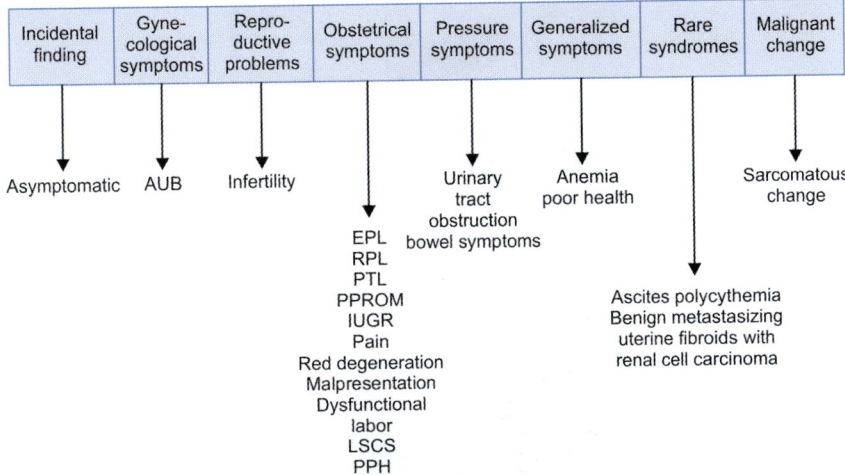

(AUB: Abnormal uterine bleeding; EPL: Early pregnancy loss; RPL: Recurrent pregnancy loss; PTL: Preterm labor; PPH: Postpartum hemorrhage; PPROM: Preterm premature rupture of membranes)

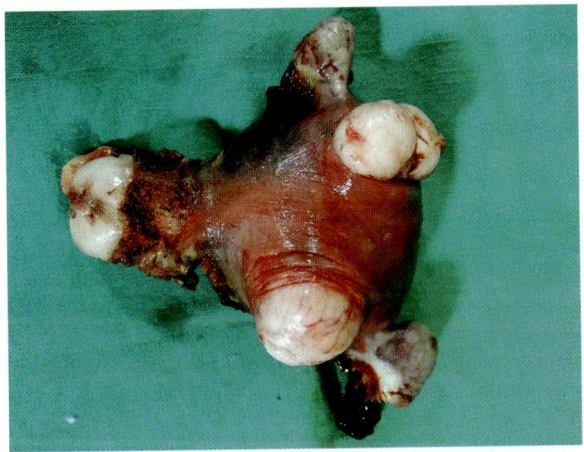

Fig. 3.1: Multiple subserosal fibroids in hysterectomy specimen.

- Clinical experience suggests that symptoms relate somewhat to the:
  - Size
  - Location of the existing fibroids:
  Smaller, less than 4 cm fibroids at intramural site or subserosal site will be asymptomatic whereas a fibroid of even 1 cm size in submucosal site will have lots of adverse symptoms like heavy bleeding and pregnancy loss.
    - Asymptomatic (Figs 3.1 and 3.2) fibroid disease most of the times does not require any treatment. A close follow-up is however advisable to keep watch on disease progress.

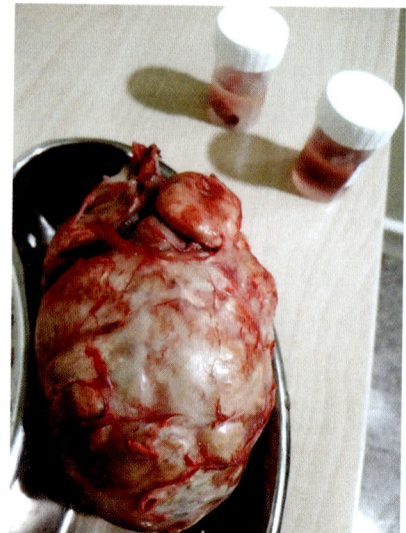

Fig. 3.2: Fibroid after myomectomy.

Gynecological Symptoms

- Abnormal uterine bleeding (AUB)—30%
  - Heavy menstrual bleeding (HMB)
  - Metrorrhagia
  - Short cycles
  - Dysmenorrhea.

The cause of excessive bleeding due to myomas has been associated with vascular alterations of the endometrium. The obstructive effect on uterine vasculature created by intramural myomas leads to endometrial venule ectasia, which results in myometrial and endometrial congestion leading to profuse menstrual bleed. Enlargement of cavity is another contributing factor. It increases surface area. It is also related to dysregulation of focal growth factors and abnormal angiogenesis.

Sometimes patient may present irregular profuse bleeding associated with foul smelling discharge due to necrosed fibroid polyp prolapsing through cervix.

Reproductive Problems

Infertility is the main Reproductive Problem
- *Few facts about infertility*: As the women are becoming carrier-oriented, late marriages and bearing first pregnancy at a much later age as compared to what was happening two decades earlier. Around 27% of infertile women will have associated fibroid disease. 50% of women with unexplained infertility will get pregnant after myomectomy. Around 10% of women with fibroids will have infertility. If all other causes of infertility are excluded, 2–3% cases are due to myoma.
- *Possible mechanism of action*:
  - Alteration of endometrial contour resulting in compromise in implantation.
  - Hampering endometrial and subendometrial vasculature resulting in implantation dysfunction.

- Distortion in uterine cavity may hamper sperm transport.
- Displaced cervix again has same effect.
- Prolonged bleeding intervals and presence of blood clots in cavity will hamper implantation.
- Poor myometrial contractility will alter gamete motility.
- Tubal ostia may get blocked due to mass effect.
- Large posterior myomas and multiple distorting fibroids will disturb the tubo-ovarian relationship.

Submucosal myomas, in particular, have proven bad effect. Endometrium covering the myoma will lead to atrophy of endometrium and the part at the periphery will have edema due to congestion. All this makes endometrium hostile for implantation.

In nutshell, it can be concluded that infertility patients with fibroids impinging on endometrium will have poor reproductive outcome. Such patients will have poor results on in vitro fertilization (IVF).

Factors Affecting Results of IVF in Patients where Uterine Cavity is not Distorted by Fibroids

- Intramural fibroid touching the endometrium can compromise the result.
- Intramural or subserosal fibroid if more than 4 cm in size will result in poor implantation rate.
- Fibroids if are affecting uterine blood flow, pregnancy rate will decline after ART treatment. Various studies are still being carried out to compare the pregnancy rates between women with and without fibroids. Till now, in IVF model, it seems that there is definite decrease in pregnancy rates in submucosal and fibroids indenting endometrium and results are negatively affected with large intramural and subserosal fibroids.

Obstetrical Symptoms

Being very common benign tumors, fibroids can co-exist with pregnancy. Reported incidence ranges up to 12.5%. Incidence is more in elderly primigravida. One important fact is that detection rate of fibroids during pregnancy drops to 42% and to 12.5% in fibroids smaller than 5 cm.

Antenatal Complications

Early pregnancy loss (EPL): Uterine myomas increase the risk of miscarriage during early pregnancy. In prospective studies, it has been revealed that spontaneous abortion were reduced from 41% to 19% after myomectomy. Uterine fibroids have been implicated in recurrent pregnancy loss. The proximity of fibroid to the placental site is more likely to cause miscarriage.

- Red degeneration of fibroid can occur resulting in acute pain abdomen. It is due to necrobiosis of fibroid.
- Increased risk of first trimester bleeding episodes.
- Impaction of fibroid rarely can occur causing pain.
- Preterm delivery: occurs in 15–20%.
- Premature rupture of membranes.
- Placental abruption.
- Breech presentation: malpresentation occurs in 20%.
- Fetal growth restriction (FGR) in 10%.

Intranatal Complications

Despite a reduction in fertility and antenatal complications, fibroid patients can conceive and deliver. There can be:
- Prolonged labor
- Dysfunctional labor or labor dystocia
- Increased chances of lower segment cesarean section (LSCS)
- Intrapartum hemorrhage due to poor myometrial contractility
- Placental anomalies like placenta accreta
- Retained placenta.

Postnatal Complications

- Postpartum hemorrhage can occur because of myometrial atonia
- Puerperal sepsis.

Effect of pregnancy on fibroid disease: There is controversy regarding the effect of pregnancy on fibroid whether it decreases or increases or remains same in size. Most of the increase in size takes place in the first trimester of pregnancy after which they remain same or decrease in size. Actually, they get stretched and become flat as the myometrial stretching occurs with advancement of pregnancy. At times, it becomes difficult to identify them in later stages of pregnancy.

Pressure Effects

Sometimes myomas become very large in size and can cause pelvic pressure. Uterine size increases as well as abdominal girth. Mass effect is more common than pain. As the tumor grows, pressure effect is on urinary tract, outflow obstruction leading to unilateral or bilateral hydronephrosis. There may be pressure on rectum and sigmoid colon leading to bowel problems. At times, there may only be heaviness in lower abdomen.

Generalized Symptoms

- There may be anemia due to regular episodes of HUB.
- There may be poor general health.
- Vaginitis foul smelling and blood-stained discharge due to prolapsing fibroid polyp.

Rare Fibroid Associations

- Ascites
- Polycythemia
- Hereditary leiomyomatosis and renal cell carcinoma
- Benign metastasizing uterine fibroids
- Leiomyomatosis peritonealis disseminata.

Malignancy

A malignant change in fibroid is very rare but can occur. Leiomyosarcoma can arise de novo also. Rapid growth of myoma is not related to malignant change. Incidence is less than 2% in postmenopausal and 0.23% in premenopausal women. Some fibroids are very vascular in nature (Fig. 3.3), but it is not associated with malignancy.

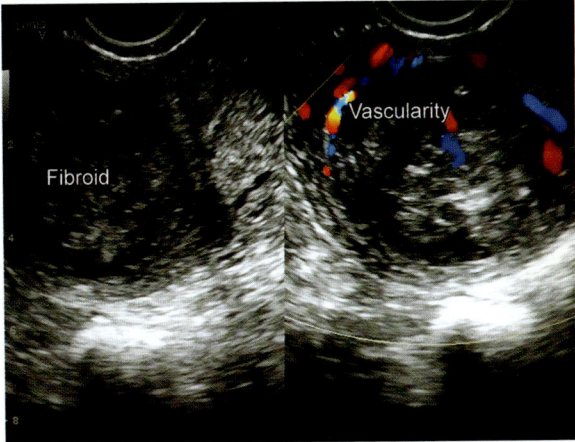

Fig. 3.3: Fibroid on USG with increased peripheral vascularity.

Pressure Symptoms

Large-sized fibroids produce pressure symptoms on urinary system leading to hydronephrosis and obstruction. When they press on gut loop, there is bloating sensation. Pressure on rectum may lead to painful defecation. There may be varicosity and pelvic congestion.

CONCLUSION

It has been rightly inferred that fibroids can surprise you even after decades of practicing gynecology. Fibroids are a very diverse disease with multiple presentations and infinite complexity. From a large asymptomatic fibroid to a fibroid of small size but with leiosarcomatous change anything can be there. All a doctor needs is experience and knowledge about them and art of counseling. If we understand the disease better, we can definitely manage it better.

BIBLIOGRAPHY

1. Abyoji A, Iljaiya M. Uterine fibroids: a ten-year clinical review in Ilorin Nigeria. Niger J Med. 2002;11:16-9.
2. Baird D, Dunson D, Hill M, et al. High cumulative incidence of uterine leiomyoma in black and white women: ultrasound evidence. Am J Obstet Gynecol. 2003;188:100-7.
3. Buttram Jr VC, Reiter RC. Uterine leiomyomata: etiology, symptomatology, and management. Fertil Steril. 1981;36:433-45.
4. Chen C, Buck G, Courey N, et al. Risk factors for uterine fibroids among women undergoing tubal sterilization. Am J Epidemiol. 2001;153:20-6.
5. Chiaffarino F, Parazzini F, Vecchia C, et al. Diet and uterine myomas. Obstet Gynecol. 1999;94:395-8.
6. Cramer SF, Patel A. The frequency of uterine leiomyomas. Am J Clin Pathol. 1990;94:435-8.
7. Day Baird D, Dunson DB, Hill MC, et al. High cumulative incidence of uterine leiomyoma in black and white women: ultrasound evidence. Am J Obstet Gynecol. 2003;188:100-7.
8. Deligdish L, Loewenthal M. Endometrial changes associated with myomata of the uterus. J Clin Pathol. 1970;23:676-80.
9. Dewaay D, Syrop C, Nygaard I, et al. Natural history of uterine polyps and leiomyomata. Obstet Gynecol. 2002;100:3-7.

10. Flake GP, Andersen J, Dixon D. Etiology and pathogenesis of uterine leiomyomas: a review. Environ Health Perspect. 2003;111:1037-54.
11. Hanafi M. Predictors of leiomyoma recurrence after myomectomy. Obstet Gynecol. 2005;105:877-81.
12. Kjerulff KH, Langenberg P, Seidman JD, et al. Uterine leiomyomas: racial differences in severity, symptoms and age at diagnosis. J Reprod Med. 1996;41:483-90.
13. Lumsden MA, Wallace EM. Clinical presentation of uterine fibroids. Baillieres Clin Obstet Gynaecol. 1998;12:177-95.
14. Marshall LM, Spiegelman D, Barbieri RL, et al. Variation in the incidence of uterine leiomyoma among premenopausal women by age and race. Obstet Gynecol. 1997;90:967-73.
15. Murta E, Oliveira G, Prado F, et al. Association of uterine leiomyomas. Obstet Gynecol. 1998;92:624-7.
16. Myers ER, Barber MD, Gustilo-Ashby T, et al. Management of uterine leiomyomata: what do we really know? Obtstet Gynecol. 2002;100:8-17.
17. Obstetrics and Gynecology Clinics of North America, Aydin Arici, MD.
18. Pretts EA. Fibroids and infertility: a systematic review of the evidence. Obstet Gynecol Surv. 2001;56:483-91.
19. Rice JP, Kay HH, Mahony BS. The clinical significance of uterine leiomyomas in pregnancy. Am J Obstet Gynecol. 1989;160(5pt 1):1212-6.
20. Ross R, Pike M, Vessey M, et al. Risk factors for uterine fibroids: reduced risk associated with oral contraceptives. BMJ. 1986;293:359-61.
21. Surrey ES, Lietz AK, Schoolcraft WB. Impact of intramural leiomyomata in patients with a normal endometrial cavity on in vitro fertilization-embryo transfer cycle outcome. Fertil Steril. 1998;70:687-91.
22. Velebil P, Wingo PA, Xia Z, et al. Rate of hospitalization for gynecologic disorders among reproductive age women in the United States. Obstet Gynecol. 1995;86:764-9.
23. Walker C, Stewart E. Uterine fibroids: the elephant in the room. Science. 2005;308:1589-92.
24. Wallach EE, Vlahos NF. Uterine myomas: an overview of development, clinical features, and management. Obstet Gynecol. 2004;104:393-406.
25. Wilcox LS, Koonin LM, Pokras R, et al. Hysterectomy in the United States, 1988-1990. Obstet Gynecol. 1994;83:549-55.
26. Yarali H, Bukulmez O. The effect of intramural and subserous uterine fibroids on implantation and clinical pregnancy rates in patients having intracytoplasmic sperm injection. Arch Gynecol Obstet. 2002;266:30-3.

4

Management of Fibroids in Adolescent Girl

Vimee Bindra, Shaik Meera Esha

INTRODUCTION

- Uterine myomas are the most common tumors of the female pelvis.
- Approximately one-third of women are diagnosed with fibroids.
- Myomas are rarely present in pediatric and adolescent age group but if suspected, on clinical history or examination, evaluation should be done properly to rule out adnexal pathologies in this age group.
- Biologic behavior of these tumors is unknown in this age group as well as there is a dilemma for appropriate management.
- Etiology of these tumors in this age group is not well-known; it has been suggested that there may be some intrinsic abnormalities in the myometrium due to elevated sex steroid levels or due to myometrial insult or injury during menstruation.

CLINICAL PRESENTATION

Symptomatic

- Most common complaints are irregular or heavy uterine bleeding
- Compression symptoms due to pelvic mass such as urgency and frequency of urine, and constipation
- Pelvic pain
- Symptoms in adolescent population usually are same as general population suffering from fibroids.

Incidental Findings

- Fifty percent of fibroids are asymptomatic which is not always correct because of under-reporting of cases.
- In adolescent population, approximately 87% of fibroids are symptomatic and rest is detected on routine ultrasound and examination.

DIAGNOSIS

Clinical Examination

Fibroids can be detected on clinical examination by determining the size and shape of uterus but in case of adolescent girls, bimanual examination is not possible so small fibroids may be missed. Clinically significant fibroids can be identified on abdominal examination in young girls. For big fibroids to differentiate from adnexal mass, we have to go for sonography or magnetic resonance imaging (MRI).

Ultrasound

Ultrasound uses the high frequency sound waves to create a picture of pelvic organs. Sonographic appearance of fibroids may widely vary but usually they appear as hypoechoic, well-defined heterogeneous masses. Sonography may not be accurate in determining the exact position and number of fibroids. Once the fibroids are diagnosed, it is also important to confirm the diagnosis in adolescent girls by doing MRI as it is very common to find an adnexal mass in this age group.

Magnetic Resonance Imaging

Magnetic resonance imaging by the use of magnetic field forms the images and once we diagnose the fibroids, it is important to know the exact location and number of fibroids which guides us in further management and decide the type of surgery as well. There are advantages of MRI that it is operator-independent and also low interobserver variations and does not use ionizing radiation. MRI has a sensitivity of 88–93% and a specificity of 66–91%. In some cases, it may be difficult to differentiate a large exophytic subserosal fibroid from an adnexal mass such as ovarian neoplasm which is a very common finding in adolescent age group. Differentiation is very imperative as it helps in deciding the treatment and also important for prognostic implications. MRI has a great advantage in making this distinction and it helps us in avoiding unnecessary laparoscopy or exploratory laparotomy. An important feature to identify uterine masses on MRI is "Bridging Vascular Sign" and in cases of exophytic fibroid away from the uterus, this sign helps in identifying it to be uterine in origin.

DIFFERENTIAL DIAGNOSIS

- Differential diagnosis of these tumors in adolescents is important. An increase in the abdominal volume due to pelvic mass should always alert the attending gynecologist to rule out the adnexal mass which is very common in this age group.
- Müllerian adenosarcomas are low-grade tumors which can affect teenagers and must be remembered.
- When leiomyoma protrudes through the cervical canal, it must be differentiated from sarcoma botryoides, a rare tumor originating from the vaginal mucosa which mainly affects adolescents.

MANAGEMENT (FLOWCHART 4.1)

There is no proved consensus on the type of treatment in adolescent population and treatment is usually extrapolated from general population suffering from fibroids.

Medical

Medical treatment is only used for short-term symptomatic relief because of risks associated with long-term treatment or the benefits with long-term treatment have not been proved till date. These are the following indications for medical treatment:
- For short-term symptomatic relief from pain or bleeding.
- As a preoperative adjunct to either reduce the size of fibroid before surgery or raise the hemoglobin level in case of concomitant anemia. Usually gonadotropin-releasing hormone (GnRH) analogs are currently used for this purpose.

Flowchart 4.1: Management.

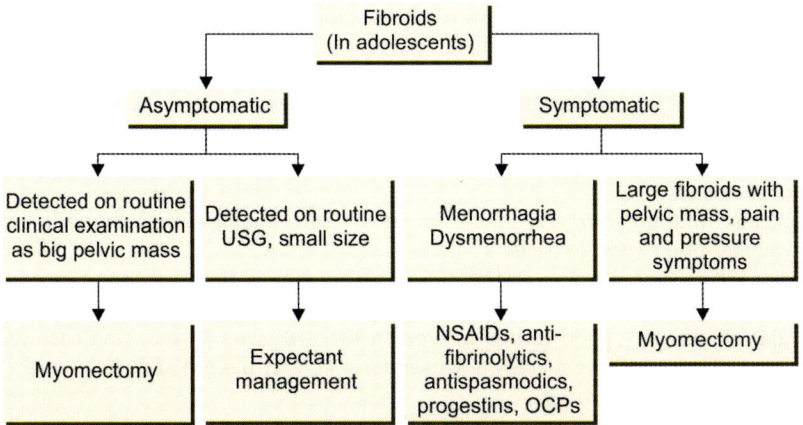

(USG: Ultrasonography; NSAIDs: Nonsteroidal anti-inflammatory drugs; OCPs: Oral contraceptive pills)

- As a part of research for newer drugs.
  - *Tranexamic acid (antifibrinolytic agents)*: It is used only during menstrual cycle to reduce the amount of blood loss. It has been shown to reduce bleeding by 60%.
  - *Progestins alone and medroxyprogesterone acetate can be given to reduce the bleeding.*
  - *Combined oral contraceptives* are widely used in cases of fibroids for reducing the amount of bleeding, but they also provide short-term relief.
  - *GnRH analogs* in adolescent girls for fibroids are only used as preoperative adjunct to reduce the size of fibroid and to raise the hemoglobin level in case of anemia. A Cochrane systematic review has shown that preoperative GnRH analog prior to myomectomy or hysterectomy has improved hemoglobin and hematocrit significantly. It also reduces the tumor volume, size, and pelvic symptoms significantly.
  - *Ormeloxifene*: It can be used if symptoms are of abnormal uterine bleeding. It does not have effect on size of fibroid. It is more patient- friendly drug.

Surgical

- Myomectomy is the best surgical treatment as it:
  - Preserves fertility
  - Most durable owing to low recurrence rate of fibroids
  - Does not interfere with the reproductive development of adolescent girl
  - Preferably if possible and surgical expertise is available, laparoscopic myomectomy should be preferred over abdominal myomectomy because of its well-known advantages of early recovery, less blood loss, less adhesions which will take care of her reproductive performance later in life.
  - Hysteroscopic myomectomy can be considered if the fibroid is completely submucous and she presents with bleeding problems and anemia. Proper counseling should be done prior to doing hysteroscopic myomectomy in an adolescent girl.
- Remote possibility of hysterectomy should always be discussed when planning myomectomy of adolescent patients.

Newer Conservative Methods

Newer conservative treatments are available, but still not sufficient evidence to determine their efficacy in adolescent population.
- Ulipristal acetate is a selective progesterone receptor modulator (SPRM); has been used in adult population and has given a success rate of reaching amenorrhea of 70–80% and also a faster onset of 4 median days to achieve it and also the adverse effects are much lesser as compared to GnRH analogs. But this drug has not been used in girls below 18 years of age.
- Aromatase inhibitors are very much similar to GnRH analogs, but have not been tested on younger population in trials.
- *Uterine artery embolization (UAE)*: It is a percutaneous image-guided procedure performed by highly trained interventional radiologist. No case series in young population but has shown very good results in women over 18 years of age. One case has been reported where UAE was successfully used for a 12-year-old girl and she was saved from life-threatening hemorrhage.
- High-intensity focused ultrasound (HIFU) or magnetic resonance-guided focused ultrasound surgery (MRgFUS) has also shown promising results in women more than 18 years of age but no studies in young women or adolescent girls. It is a new method of thermal ablation which uses high-intensity focused ultrasound through the anterior abdominal wall to a certain focused point to induce the coagulative necrosis of the fibroid. Use of MRI helps in targeting the right tissue and also helps in thermal control.

RISK OF MALIGNANCY

One must think of malignancy in older age group especially with a rapidly growing tumor. Chance of malignancy in adolescent age group is practically nil as uterine sarcomas are nonexistent in this age group. But in case of rapidly increasing tumor or sudden appearance of tumor, potential of malignancy or cellular leiomyoma must be kept in mind. There is a case report of cellular leiomyoma by Morad and El Said in 15-year-old girl.

IMPLICATIONS ON FUTURE FERTILITY

Fertility outcomes and pregnancy outcomes are similar across all types of surgical procedures, be it abdominal, laparoscopic or robotic myomectomy. As far as possible, minimally invasive approach is chosen over abdominal approach for better outcomes. Fibroids per se do not cause infertility; they are mostly associated with subfertility and rarely are a sole cause of infertility. If infertility is an issue in a patient with fibroids, she and her partner should be evaluated thoroughly to find out the associated causes of infertility as well.

COUNSELING

- Counseling, counseling, and counseling. It is very important whenever a decision to operate the patient is undertaken especially in adolescent age group. Appropriate preoperative counseling and discussion is very important also to decide the type of surgery and diagnosis as in most of these cases the diagnosis may be changed for adnexal mass in case of uterine fibroid and vice versa in case of adnexal mass and this should be properly informed to parents and they should be counseled in detail regarding the best course of action in either case.
- If uterine mass is suspected then preservation of fertility should be discussed in detail and also the need for hysterectomy if needed to save the patient.
- In case adnexal mass is suspected, counseling would center around the ovarian or tubal procedure and discussion about future fertility.

Flowchart 4.2: Follow-up.

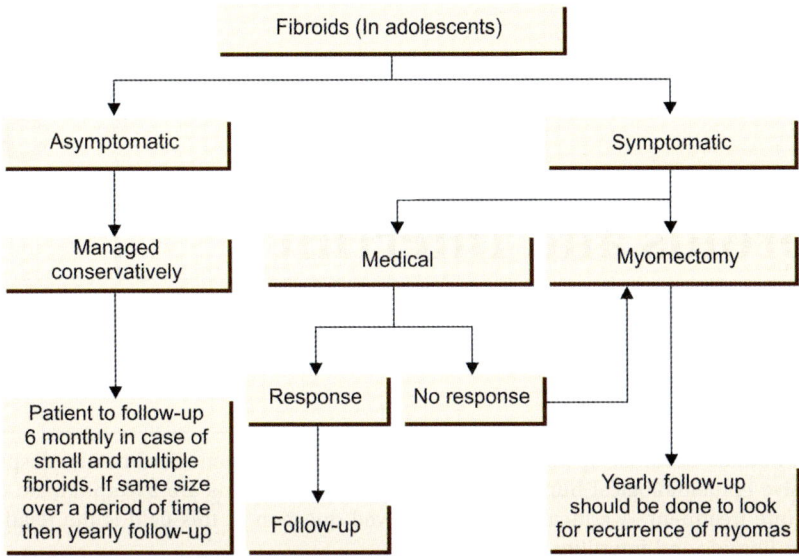

FOLLOW-UP (FLOWCHART 4.2)

- In young adolescent girl, if fibroids are detected incidentally and small in size, they should be called for 6 monthly follow-up to monitor the size and growth of fibroids and if it remains same over a period of time, they can be called for yearly follow-up.
- Multiple myomas and big myomas are a risk factor for recurrence and patient should be followed up after myomectomy regularly to look for its recurrence. Once a year follow-up is considered good to see for its recurrence.

CONCLUSION

- It is certain that the biologic behavior of fibroids in adolescents is different from other population.
- Ultrasound is usually sufficient for differentiating between the adnexal mass and myoma, but MRI is superior to ultrasound in case of doubt about the diagnosis.
- Best treatment is still not defined, but myomectomy for big fibroids is a preferable option to preserve their fertility.
- Myomas should always be kept in differential diagnosis in adolescents when dealing the pelvic masses.

BIBLIOGRAPHY

1. Bowkley C, Dubel G, Haas R, et al. Uterine artery embolisation for control of life threatening hemorrhage at menarche: brief report. J Vasc Interv Radiol. 2007;18:127-31.
2. Donnez J, Vazquez F, Tomaszewski J, et al. Long term treatment uterine fibroids with ulipristal acetate. Long term treatment of uterine fibroids with ulipristal acetate. Fertil Steril. 2014;101(6):1565-73.
3. Fields KR, Neinstein LS. Uterine myomas in adolescents: Case reports and review of literature. J Pediatr Adolesc Gynecol. 1996;9:195-8.
4. Lethaby A, Vollenhoven B, Sowter M. Preoperative GnRH analogue therapy before hysterectomy or myomectomy for uterine fibroids. Cochrane Database Syst Rev. 2000;(2):CD000547.
5. Livermore JA, Adusumilli S. MRI of benign uterine conditions. Appl Radiol. 2007;36(9):8-18.
6. Morad NA, El-Said MM. Cellular uterine myoma causing vaginal bleeding in a 15 year old girl. Aust NZ J Obstet Gynaecol. 1993:33;211-3.
7. Parker W. Etiology, symptomatology and diagnosis of uterine myomas. Fertil Steril. 2007;87:725-36.

5

Fibroids and Infertility

Bhavana Mittal

INTRODUCTION

Uterine fibroids occur in up to 30% of reproductive age women. Fortunately, despite this impressive epidemiological burden, the vast majority of fibroids are asymptomatic and do not require treatment. A critical and still unsolved question in this field is the relationship between fibroids and infertility.

This issue is assuming increasing relevance considering that, in the developed world, there is the tendency to start a family at an age when natural female fertility is in decline and the incidence of fibroids is increasing. It is essential to clarify whether these tumors affect fertility and, if so, which kind of lesions deserves treatment.

Although most women affected with fibroids are fertile, fibroids may interfere with fertility secondary to anatomical distortion and alterations to the uterine environment, with the effect being dictated largely by the location and size of the fibroid.

TYPES OF FIBROID

Submucous fibroids are those that distort the uterine cavity and are further divided into three subtypes—pedunculated (type 0), sessile with intramural extension of fibroid less than 50% (type I), and sessile with intramural extension more than or equal to 50% (type II). Intramural fibroids are those which do not distort the cavity and with less than 50% of the tumor protruding into the serosal surface of the uterus. Fibroids protruding more than or equal to 50% out of the serosal surface are considered subserosal. They are further divided into sessile or pedunculated.

FIBROIDS AND FERTILITY

Reviews focusing on the relationship between fibroids and infertility reported that these lesions may be responsible for only 2–3% of infertility cases.

Mechanisms by which fibroids may reduce fertility have been proposed. It is generally believed that fibroids may interfere with sperm migration, ovum transport, and embryo implantation. Detrimental effects on these phenomena may be mediated by alteration of the uterine cavity contour causing mechanical pressure or by the occurrence of abnormal uterine contractility. In addition, local inflammation associated with the presence of submucosal fibroids may result in a hostile endometrial environment that impairs sperm transport and embryo implantation. An inadequate blood supply to the endometrium has also been advocated to explain reduced embryo implantation. If fibroids are localized near the cervix or near the tubal ostia, the anatomical distortion may reduce access to the tubes by ejaculated sperm, whereas large corneal lesions might impair ovum retrieval by the tubes. A higher frequency of uterine peristalsis during the mid-luteal phase might be one of the causes of infertility associated with intramural-type fibroids.

A decreased risk of fibroids in parous women when compared with nulliparous women has been repeatedly reported. Parity may be a protective factor or, alternatively, fertility may be partly compromised in women with fibroids.

FIBROIDS AND IVF OUTCOME

With regards to in vitro fertilization (IVF) treatment, submucosal and intramural fibroids that protrude into the endometrial cavity have been associated with decreased pregnancy rates (PRs) and implantation rates (IRs). Studies have shown that IVF outcome is markedly improved in women with cavity-distorting submucosal fibroids following myomectomy. However, the effect of fibroids not distorting the uterine cavity on the outcome of IVF treatment remains poorly understood with studies yielding conflicting results.

Conclusions regarding intramural lesions have been conflicting. The two initial meta-analyses failed to document a harmful effect. On the contrary, results from the meta-analysis of Benecke et al. show a lower pregnancy rate in women with intramural fibroids.

Somigliana et al. published a meta-analysis of 17 studies investigating the influence of fibroids located at different sites in IVF cycles. Overall, their results showed that myomas negatively affect PRs. Although based on a small number of studies, submucous fibroids appeared to strongly interfere with the chance of pregnancy—odds ratio (OR) [95% confidence interval (CI)] for conception and delivery being 0.3 (0.1–0.7) and 0.3 (0.1–0.8), respectively. The impact of intramural fibroids was less dramatic although still statistically significant—OR (95% CI) for conception and delivery being 0.8 (0.6–0.9) and 0.7 (0.5–0.8), respectively. In general, these effects appeared to be more relevant when considering the delivery rate compared to the clinical PR. Conversely, subserosal fibroids did not seem to affect PRs.

Two limitations of studies focusing on IVF should be considered. First, they can do no more than evaluate the impact of fibroids on embryo implantation. Possible detrimental effects on tubal transport of oocytes and/or embryos are overcome by the technique. Second, recent findings suggest that the size of the fibroids is positively related to implantation failure, in particular when the diameter of the lesion exceeds 4 cm. The mean or median diameter of the fibroids included in studies on IVF and fibroids is rarely above 3 cm. Indeed, the policy of the units reporting on the influence of fibroids on IVF outcome is generally to recommend surgery for lesions exceeding 5 cm in diameter.

A recent updated systematic review evaluated the effects on fertility by location of fibroids. Their results were consistent in showing that women actively attempting to conceive and with submucous fibroids, compared to women without fibroids, demonstrated a significantly lower clinical PR [relative risk (RR): 0.36; 95% CI 0.17–0.73), implantation rate (RR: 0.28; 95% CI: 0.12–0.64), and ongoing pregnancy or live birth rate (RR: 0.31; 95% CI 0.11–0.85) and a significantly higher spontaneous abortion rate (RR: 1.67; 95% CI 1.37–2.05). Women with intramural fibroids also produced significantly lower implantation rate (RR: 0.79; 95% CI 0.69–0.90) and ongoing pregnancy or live birth rate (RR: 0.78; 95% CI 0.69–0.88) and a significantly higher spontaneous abortion rate (RR: 1.89; 95% CI 1.47–2.42). When women with subserous fibroids were compared with women without fibroids, no difference was observed for any outcome measure.

There is controversy on the impact of intramural fibroids that do not distort the uterine cavity on IVF treatment outcome. This was addressed in a recent systematic review, by Sunkara et al., that looked at 19 observational studies comprising a total of 6,087 IVF cycles. Meta-analysis of these studies showed a significant decrease in live birth rate by 21% and the clinical PR by 15% per IVF cycle in women with noncavity distorting intramural fibroids compared to those without fibroids, following IVF treatment. The relatively lower chance of achieving a live birth compared with clinical pregnancy probably reflects the adverse influence of intramural fibroids on the course of pregnancy.

The inverse relationship between IVF outcome and the presence of noncavity distorting intramural fibroid may be explained by altered uterine vascular perfusion, myometrial contractility, endometrial function, gamete migration or myometrial or endometrial gene expression.

Demonstration of reduction in IVF live births in women with non-cavity-distorting intramural fibroids does not necessarily mean that removal of such fibroids will restore the live birth rates to the levels expected in women without fibroids. Therefore, this evidence does not justify advocating routine myomectomy for these women, as a favorable risk—benefit analysis of this surgical intervention or any other interventions in this clinical context is currently lacking.

FERTILITY AFTER MYOMECTOMY

Several reviews of literature on PRs following myomectomy have been published. One of the early reviews focusing on studies published between 1933 and 1980 reported a 40% PR following abdominal myomectomy (480 out of 1,202 cases). This rate was 54% when patients with other causes of infertility were excluded. Another review by Vercellini et al. confirmed this rate of success following myomectomy. They reported a post-surgical PR of 57% across prospective studies. When including women with unexplained infertility, this rate was 61%. The advent of endoscopic surgery did not seem to modify this result. In a review by Donnez, the PR among women undergoing hysteroscopic and laparoscopic myomectomy was reported as 45% and 49%, respectively. These findings have further been confirmed by more recent and larger studies.

Despite a large number of series reporting on the PR after myomectomy, randomized studies are lacking. A recent Cochrane review on this issue failed to identify any randomized trial comparing surgery to expectant management.

IVF RESULTS AFTER MYOMECTOMY

Narayan and Goswamy investigated the effect of myomectomy on a small group of women with submucosal fibroids (n = 27). They found that the delivery rate was not significantly different in women who underwent myomectomy compared to women without fibroids (37% and 22%, respectively, P = 0.13). Surrey et al. reported a PR of 62% and 68%, respectively in women operated for submucous fibroids and controls without fibroids following IVF treatment. From these studies, we can infer that although the overall evidence is scarce, myomectomy for submucous fibroids did not seem to negatively affect the pregnancy rate following IVF treatment.

A comparative study by Bulletti et al. looked at the effectiveness of myomectomy prior to IVF treatment in women with intramural and/or subserosal fibroids with at least one lesion more than 5 cm. Women were allocated to myomectomy (n = 84) or no surgery (n = 84) based on their decision. They reported a live birth rate of 25% and 12%, respectively in women who did and did not undergo surgery prior to IVF treatment. It is worthy of note that this study involved small numbers and this evidence therefore does not justify advocating routine myomectomy for these women; as a favorable risk—benefit analysis of this surgical intervention or any other interventions, in this clinical context is currently lacking.

From this evidence, it can be concluded that fertility outcomes are decreased in women with submucosal fibroids, and removal seems to confer benefit. Subserosal fibroids do not affect fertility outcomes, and removal does not confer benefit. Intramural fibroids appear to decrease fertility, but the results of therapy are unclear.

FIBROIDS AND PREGNANCY OUTCOME

It has been claimed that the hormonal milieu of pregnancy can determine a rapid growth of fibroids and increased symptoms. In case-control studies, a history of miscarriage is more frequently reported by affected patients. Apart from placental abruption, placenta previa, intrauterine growth restriction (IUGR), and fetal malpresentation. Not surprisingly, a higher rate of cesarean section has also been repeatedly reported.

A role of fibroids in the determinism of pregnancy complications is also supported by the demonstration that the dimension and location of the lesions play a role in this regard. In particular, the location of the myomas in relation to the placental site has been reported to be a significant clue to the outcome of pregnancy.

MYOMECTOMY AND PREGNANCY OUTCOME

The rate of pregnancy wastage significantly decreases after surgery. One of the major concerns about myomectomy is the low, albeit clinically relevant, risk of uterine rupture during pregnancy or labor. But studies aimed at precisely quantifying this risk are scanty and controversial. Regardless of the surgical approach, fear about the risk of uterine rupture certainly leads to a high rate of cesarean section in pregnant patients who previously underwent myomectomy.

On the other hand, surgery is not without complications. Even if very rare, major intraoperative and postoperative complications may occur.

OTHER TREATMENTS FOR FIBROIDS

Several non-surgical approaches for the treatment of fibroid associated symptoms have emerged over the last several years with medical therapies (GnRH agonists, danazol, the antiprogestogen—mifepristone, the selective estrogen receptor modulator—raloxifene, and the aromatase inhibitor—fadrozole) as well as radiological interventions (fibroid embolization, laparoscopic myolysis, and MRI-guided focused ultrasound) being proposed. However, their use in the context of infertility treatment remains questionable.

CONCLUSION

Available evidence also suggests that submucosal, intramural, and subserosal fibroids interfere with fertility in decreasing order of importance. Although more limited, some data supports an impact of the number and dimension of the lesions. Drawing clear guidelines for the management of fibroids in infertile women is difficult due to the lack of large randomized trials aimed at elucidating which patients may benefit from surgery. At present, physicians should pursue a comprehensive and personalized approach clearly exposing the pros and cons of myomectomy to the patient, including the risks associated with fibroids during pregnancy on one hand, and those associated with surgery on the other hand.

At least four points have to be considered: (1) the age of the woman; (2) the location, dimension, and number of the fibroids; (3) the concomitant presence of fibroids-related symptoms such as menorrhagia or hypermenorrhea, and (4) the presence of other causes of infertility and whether or not there is an indication to IVF. The ultimate aim is to assume a shared decision with the patient.

BIBLIOGRAPHY

1. Bajekal N, Li TC. Fibroids, infertility and pregnancy wastage. Hum Reprod Update. 2000;6(6):614-20.
2. Benecke C, Kruger TF, Siebert TI, et al. Effect of fibroids on fertility in patients undergoing assisted reproduction. A structured literature review. Gynecol Obstet Invest. 2005;59(4):225-30.

3. Bernard G, Darai E, Poncelet C, et al. Fertility after hysteroscopic myomectomy: effect of intramural myomas associated. Eur J Obstet Gynecol Reprod Biol. 2000;88:85-90.
4. Bulletti C, DE Ziegler D, Levi Setti P, et al. Myomas, pregnancy outcome, and in vitro fertilization. Ann N Y Acad Sci. 2004;1034:84-92.
5. Buttram VC Jr, Reiter RC. Uterine leiomyomata: etiology, symptomatology, and management. Fertil Steril. 1981;36(4):433-45.
6. Donnez J, Jadoul P. What are the implications of myomas on fertility? A need for a debate? Hum Reprod. 2002;17(6):1424-30.
7. Griffiths A, D'Angelo A, Amso N. Surgical treatment of fibroids for subfertility. Cochrane Database Syst Rev. 2006;(3):CD003857.
8. Marchionni M, Fambrini M, Zambelli V, et al. Reproductive performance before and after abdominal myomectomy: a retrospective analysis. Fertil Steril. 2004;82(1):154-9.
9. Narayan R, Goswamy R. Subendometrial-myometrial contractility in conception and non-conception embryo transfer cycles. Ultrasound Obstet Gynecol. 1994;4(6):499-504.
10. Oliveira FG, Abdelmassih VG, Diamond MP, et al. Impact of subserosal and intramural uterine fibroids that do not distort the endometrial cavity on the outcome of in vitro fertilization-intracytoplasmic sperm injection. Fertil Steril. 2004;81(3):582-7.
11. Practice Committee of the ASRM, 2006.
12. Pritts EA, Parker WH, Olive DL. Fibroids and infertility: an updated systematic review of the evidence. Fertil Steril. 2009;91(4):1215-23.
13. Qidwai GI, Caughey AB, Jacoby AF. Obstetric outcomes in women with sonographically identified uterine leiomyomata. Obstet Gynecol. 2006;107(2 Pt 1):376-82.
14. Rackow BW, Arici A. Fibroids and in-vitro fertilisation: which comes first? Curr Opin Obstet Gynecol. 2005;17:225-31.
15. Seracchioli R, Manuzzi L, Vianello F, et al. Obstetric and delivery outcome of pregnancies achieved after laparoscopic myomectomy. Fertil Steril. 2006;86(1):159-65.
16. Sheiner E, Bashiri A, Levy A, et al. Obstetrics characteristics and perinatal outcome of pregnancies with uterine leiomyomas. J Reprod Med. 2004;49:182-6.
17. Somigliana E, Vercellini P, Daguati R, et al. Fibroids and female reproduction: a critical analysis of the evidence. Hum Reprod Update. 2007;13(5):465-76.
18. Sunkara SK, Khairy M, El-Toukhy T, et al. The effect of intramural fibroids without uterine cavity involvement on the outcome of IVF treatment: a systematic review and meta-analysis. Hum Reprod. 2010;25(2):418-29.
19. Surrey ES, Minjarez DA, Stevens JM, et al. Effect of myomectomy on the outcome of assisted reproductive technologies. Fertil Steril. 2005;83:1473-9.
20. Surrey ES, Minjarez D, Stevens J, et al. Effects of myomectomy on the outcome of assisted reproductive technologies. Fertil Steril. 2005;83:1473-9.
21. Ubaldi F, Tournaye H, Camus M, et al. Fertility after hysteroscopic myomectomy. Hum Reprod Update. 1995;1:81-90.
22. Vercellini P, Maddalena S, De Giorgi O, et al. Abdominal myomectomy for infertility: a comprehensive review. Hum Reprod. 1998;13(4):873-9.
23. Verkauf BS. Myomectomy for fertility enhancement and preservation. Fertil Steril. 1992;58:1-15.
24. Yoshino O, Hayashi T, Osuga Y, et al. Decreased pregnancy rate is linked to abnormal uterine peristalsis caused by intramural fibroids. Hum Reprod. 2010;25(10):2475-9.

6

Fibroids in Pregnancy

Dhaval A Baxi, Sonam D Baxi

INTRODUCTION

Fibroids or leiomyomata are benign tumors arising from the smooth muscle of the uterus. They are the most commonly encountered tumors in women with an incidence of 40–60% by age 35 and 70–80% by age 50 and incidence in pregnancy varies from 0.1% to 12.5%.

Fibroids are increasingly being diagnosed in pregnancy, which may be due to delay in childbearing, pregnancy following treatment for infertility or antiretroviral therapy (ART) and use of high-resolution ultrasound in pregnancy.

This chapter will cover aspects of dealing with fibroids during pregnancy and pregnancy after surgical or nonsurgical treatment of fibroids.

DIAGNOSIS

Diagnosis of fibroids during pregnancy can be tricky. Physical examination can detect only 42% of fibroids larger than 5 cm and 12.5% of fibroids less than 5 cm. Diagnosis by ultrasound can be tricky in pregnancy. The following points should be kept in mind for diagnosing a fibroid during pregnancy.

Clinical

- History of abnormal uterine bleeding preceding the pregnancy or poor obstetric history
- Size of uterus more than period of gestation
- Irregular or asymmetric uterine surface
- Presence of an eccentric mass in abdomen.

Ultrasound

- Spherical shape
- Distortion of myometrial contour
- Hypoechoic structure when compared to myometrium
- Speckled pattern of internal echoes
- Splaying of blood vessels around the mass when color Doppler is used.

EFFECT OF PREGNANCY ON FIBROIDS (FLOWCHART 6.1)

Growth

Fibroids are estrogen-dependent tumors. With the rapid increase in estrogen levels, leading to upscaling of progesterone receptors, fibroids are expected to increase in size during

Flowchart 6.1: Effects of pregnancy on fibroids.

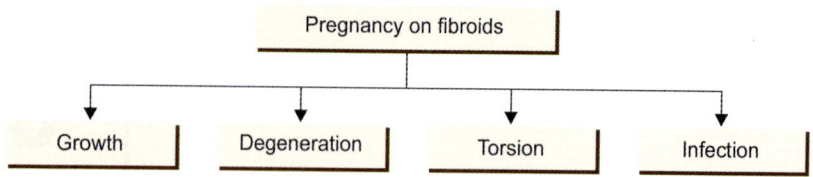

pregnancy. Stretching and hypertrophy of the myometrial fibers and an increase in blood supply are thought to contribute to increase in size of fibroids during pregnancy. However, there is a controversy regarding the growth patterns of fibroids during pregnancy. Contrary to overall belief, only 22–68% fibroids grow during pregnancy and some large fibroids more than 6 cm may also decrease in size. The fibroids that grew did so in the first trimester and shrinkage takes place in the third trimester. The increase in size may lead to pressure symptoms toward the end of the first trimester. Patients may have retention of urine and/or constipation, and other compressive symptoms depending upon the location and size of the fibroid, especially in the first trimester.

Degeneration

Degeneration of a fibroid may occur at any time of pregnancy. The mechanism is not clear but the most commonly accepted theories are rupture of arteries in the fibroid and peripheral venous obstruction. Degeneration may be cystic, hyaline, or red (carneous), which is the most common. It presents with severe lower abdominal pain usually around the 20th week accompanied with fever, leukocytosis, and raised erythrocyte sedimentation rate (ESR). Treatment is conservative with painkillers and rest. Tocolytic therapy may be required, if accompanied with uterine irritability and premature labor.

Torsion

Pedunculated large fibroids can undergo torsion during pregnancy and present as an acute abdomen. Management in such a situation involves myomectomy of the twisted fibroid only. The route of myomectomy is usually through laparotomy, but successful laparoscopic myomectomy during pregnancy has also been reported.

Infection

Infection of fibroids is common during the puerperium. With involution, the location of fibroids may change and become closer to the cavity. Infection of fibroids is usually polymicrobial. Treatment involves use of broad-spectrum antibiotics to control sepsis following which myomectomy may be required.

EFFECTS OF FIBROIDS ON PREGNANCY (FLOWCHART 6.2)

Antenatal

Early Pregnancy

Bleeding: The risk for bleeding in pregnancy is determined by the relationship between the fibroid and the placenta. There is a significant increase in risk for bleeding when the

Flowchart 6.2: Effects of fibroids on pregnancy.

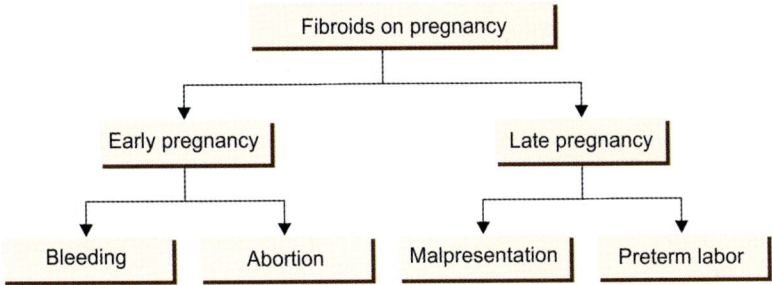

placenta implants close to the fibroid compared to when there is no contact between them (60% vs 9%).

Miscarriage: Presence of fibroids increases the risk of spontaneous miscarriage (14% vs 7.6%). The effect is influenced by the position and location of the fibroids. Fibroids more likely to cause miscarriage are usually submucous or large intramural fibroids. In patients with previous history of miscarriage with submucous or intramural fibroids, myomectomy decreases the chance of miscarriage from 57.1% to 13.8%. Overall, in patients with intramural and subserous fibroids the prognosis is favorable.

Difficulty in invasive prenatal testing: Failures of amniocentesis and chorionic villus sampling (CVS) increase in women with fibroids. This may be due to difficulty in approaching the target site due to distortion of anatomy.

Late Pregnancy

Preterm labor: Fibroids in pregnancy appear to increase the risk of preterm labor (16.1% vs 8.7%) compared to women without fibroids. Factors influencing the incidence include multiple fibroids, size of fibroids, and fibroids close to the placenta. Placental abruption diminished blood flow to the fibroid and surrounding tissues results in partial ischemia and decidual necrosis, which may increase. The incidence of placental abruption is seen to increase threefold in pregnancies complicated by fibroids. Risk factors for abruption include submucosal fibroids, retroplacental fibroids, and fibroid volume more than 200 mm^3.

Fetal growth restriction and malformations: Larger uterine fibroids may sometimes deform the uterine cavity leading to restriction in the available space for the fetus to grow. This restriction in space can lead to a growth restricted fetus or fetal malformations like limb deformities.

Labor and Puerperium

Malpresentation

Women with fibroids, particularly those which are large and present in the lower uterine segment are at increased risk of fetal malpresentations. This risk is almost 13% as compared to 4.5% in normal women. This increased risk of malpresentation further predisposes them to have a cesarean section, which is almost 3.7-folds higher.

Dystocia and Obstructed Labor

Fibroids can, at times, cause labor dystocia (two-fold) and obstructed labor, which may be due to the abnormal shape of the uterus causing difficulty in passage of fetal head. Cervical fibroids, even of very small size and fibroids present in the posterior wall below the sacral promontory are known to cause serious obstruction while those present in the anterior wall usually does not cause obstruction.

Postpartum Hemorrhage

Women with fibroids have an increased risk of postpartum hemorrhage (PPH) compared to pregnancies without fibroids (2.5% vs 1.4%). Fibroids may disturb the uterine anatomy, causing interference with myometrial contraction leading to atony and hemorrhage. This subjects patients to an increased risk of PPH and also of puerperal hysterectomy.

Adherent and Retained Placenta

Retained placenta is a significant cause of maternal morbidity and mortality. The cause has been suggested to be due to trapping of the placenta due to mechanical obstruction by fibroid, causing failure to be extracted manually after enucleation. Presence of fibroid in the uterus, though rarely, is associated with increased incidence of retained placenta in labor, especially if present in the lower segment. Other studies suggest the incidence to be high compared to the uterus without fibroids, irrespective of the location of fibroid (1.4% vs 0.6%). Management is by traditional methods but myomectomy may be required in some cases.

MANAGEMENT

Traditionally, fibroids are to be managed conservatively during pregnancy, which includes pain relief and fetal monitoring. In some situations, surgical management of fibroids may be required for maternal and fetal well-being, either during pregnancy or at the time of delivery. Contrary to popular belief, studies have reported favorable outcomes in women who underwent a second trimester myomectomy compared with conservative management. The main concern regarding surgical management is intraoperative hemorrhage, which may be life threatening. The pros and cons of the procedure need to be carefully evaluated before performing such procedures.

During Pregnancy

There are relatively few indications for performing a myomectomy during pregnancy. They include severe pain due to torsion of a pedunculated fibroid or pain refractory to symptomatic treatment following degeneration of a fibroid; and in cases of large fibroids leading to compressive symptoms. Around 2% of women with fibroids may require a myomectomy during pregnancy. Myomectomies have been performed via laparotomy and laparoscopy successfully followed by delivery at term in up to 92% cases undergoing trial of labor. Myomectomy for large intramural fibroids has also been reported with subsequent delivery via planned cesarean section. Myomectomies during the second and third trimester have been reported with favorable outcomes. First trimester myomectomy as an alternative to termination of pregnancy followed by myomectomy is an area that still needs to be explored. There are case reports of successful myomectomy in first trimester with term delivery of a healthy child. However, risks to the fetus need to be evaluated. Inadvertent opening of the endometrial cavity during myomectomy was reported in a woman who was later diagnosed to be pregnant and delivered a baby with a complex neurological malformation.

At the Time of Cesarean

Myomectomy during cesarean section may be a necessary procedure in the following situations:

- Anterior wall fibroid in the incision line
- Fibroid obstructing/interfering with delivery of the baby
- Fibroid interfering with repair of the uterine incision
- Pedunculated fibroids, which may undergo torsion during the puerperium
- While tackling PPH due to fibroids interfering with contraction of the uterus.

Performing a myomectomy during cesarean has always been discouraged as it is thought to have a high rate of complications, which include hemorrhage and hysterectomy. However, myomectomy during cesarean has the following advantages:
- Combination of two surgeries thus avoiding a second surgery and second anesthesia
- Reducing the incidence of subinvolution
- Preventing fibroid-associated symptoms in the long-term
- Reduces the incidence of pain and degeneration in subsequent pregnancies.

Points to consider while performing a myomectomy during pregnancy are:
- *Preoperative*:
  - Take consent for myomectomy and emergency hysterectomy
  - Cross-match or arrange adequate blood/blood products.
- *Intraoperative*:
  - Vasopressin infiltration, use of a tourniquet, and ligation of the uterine arteries can be used to create a relatively bloodless field/control hemorrhage
  - Remove only large fibroids
  - Avoid removing small fibroids and unnecessary prolongation of surgery
  - Use a cautery for incision
  - Take the help of a vessel sealer/bipolar forceps for enucleation
  - Repair in layers using absorbable suture
  - Calculation of blood loss.
- *Postoperative*:
  - Administration of uterotonic for 24–48 hours
  - Watch out for PPH
  - Monitor vitals to look for tachycardia and hypotension
  - Repeat blood counts after 24 hours and transfuse blood, if necessary.

A technique of an endometrial myomectomy during cesarean, which involves approaching the fibroid from the inside of the cavity has been reported to have a shorter operative time and decreased intraoperative bleeding when compared with the traditional approach. A study to evaluate the safety of cesarean myomectomy reported no significant differences in hemoglobin drop compared to controls.

Complications include intraoperative hemorrhage, which may require blood transfusion and hysterectomy, which has its own set of complications.

Every effort to avoid a myomectomy during cesarean must be taken. However, in fibroid endemic and low-resource settings with poor access to tertiary healthcare, a cesarean myomectomy appears to be an appealing surgical option. An experienced surgeon along with an adequately staffed and equipped center with blood banking facilities is a must for performing such procedures.

Special Situations

Pregnancy after Myomectomy

With delayed childbearing, fibroids are being frequently encountered in women wishing to conserve fertility, because of which myomectomies for fertility enhancement are being routinely performed via laparotomy, vaginally, and endoscopically.

In women conceiving after a myomectomy, the concerns are uterine rupture.

Adherent Placenta Cesarean Section

Uterine rupture in pregnancy after myomectomy has been reported to occur in 0.3–1%. Ruptures have been reported from as early as 10 weeks of gestation till labor.

The overall incidence of morbidly adherent placenta is 1.7 per 10,000 deliveries. Women with history of myomectomy have an increased risk of adherent placenta compared to women without any uterine surgery (OR 3.40, 95% CI 1.30–8.91). The incidence is highest in women who have undergone hysteroscopic resection for submucous fibroids.

The general consensus is to offer an elective cesarean section in women where the cavity was opened during surgery. However, the decision should also involve other factors including the size and number of incisions rather than just the breach of endometrium. 80.6% of women, who underwent a trial of labor following myomectomy delivered vaginally. Vaginal birth after myomectomy is possible and labor management should be similar to women with a previous cesarean section. Patients should be counseled in detail regarding the risks involved prior offering a trial of labor.

When techniques of myomectomy were compared, the time to conception and cesarean rate was found to be higher with abdominal myomectomy compared to the laparoscopic approach.

Pregnancy after Uterine Artery Embolization

Uterine artery embolization (UAE) is a safe and effective alternative treatment to surgery to relieve fibroid-related symptoms. However, the desire to maintain fertility is a relative contraindication to UAE. A recent review on pregnancy outcome after UAE, in their cumulative data, showed an increased risk of miscarriages, preterm delivery, malpresentation, intrauterine growth restriction (IUGR), PPH, and cesarean section. Studies have also the rate of live birth rate to be lesser as compared laparoscopic myomectomy. All these effects may be due to endometrial ischemia and atrophy following UAE, plus it only reduces the volume of uterine fibroid rather than eliminating it.

It is also important to note that apart from the effects on pregnancy, UAE can adversely affect the fertility potential by inducing transient or permanent amenorrhea accompanied by other symptoms of ovarian failure due to ovarian ischemia. Therefore, one should be cautious while considering UAE as a treatment option in women desiring future pregnancy.

Pregnancy after High-intensity Focused Ultrasound

High-intensity focused ultrasound (HIFU) is a noninvasive and thermoablative treatment for fibroids. It is offered as an alternative to surgery. It may potentially have a negative impact on fertility due to exposure to radiation, possible loss of ovarian function, adverse effect on Fallopian tubes, and disturbance in uterine function. Its effect on pregnancy has not been extensively studied. But available studies suggest that risk of miscarriage does not appear to increase significantly above the background risk. Moreover, there are no studies showing higher rates of obstetric, intrapartum, and postpartum complications in these patients.

However, current available studies are not large enough to provide sufficient evidence of its impact on fertility and obstetric outcome. Currently, HIFU treatment should be offered to women with symptomatic fibroids who reject surgery or have unacceptably high risk to surgery.

CONCLUSION

Fibroids are being increasingly encountered during pregnancy due to delayed childbearing. The effect of pregnancy on fibroids is yet not clear with regards to size. The effects of fibroids on pregnancy vary greatly depending on the size and location of the fibroids with data reporting an overall increase in the incidence of spontaneous miscarriage, preterm labor, placenta abruption, malpresentation, labor dystocia, cesarean delivery, and postpartum hemorrhage. Ultrasound is an invaluable tool for diagnosing fibroids in pregnancy. Pain is the most common symptom in pregnancy, which can be managed conservatively; however, surgical intervention may be required sometimes. Greater understanding, improved surgical technique, and growing experience are making cesarean myomectomy a popular and safe choice as a single-step surgical treatment. With good surveillance and management, a favorable outcome is routinely achieved.

BIBLIOGRAPHY

1. Agarwal K, Agarwal L, Agarwal A, et al. Caesarean myomectomy: prospective study. NJIRM. 2011; 2(3):11-4.
2. Aharoni A, Reiter A, Golan D, et al. Patterns of growth of uterine leiomyomas during pregnancy. A prospective longitudinal study. Br J Obstet Gynaecol. 1988;95(5):510-3.
3. Awoleke JO. Myomectomy during caesarean birth in fibroid-endemic, low-resource settings. Obstet Gynecol In. 2013;2013:520834.
4. Aziz SFA, Al-Sharkawy MK. Behavior of leiomyoma during pregnancy as evaluated by ultrasound. Sci J Al-Azhar Med Facul (Girls). 1996;17(2). [online] Available from: http://www.obgyn.net/fibroids/behavior-leiomyoma-during-pregnancy-evaluated-ultrasound. [Accessed June, 2018].
5. Benaglia L, Cardellicchio L, Filippi F, et al. The rapid growth of fibroids during early pregnancy. PLoS ONE. 2014;9(1):e85933.
6. Benson CB, Chow JS, Chang-Lee W, et al. Outcome of pregnancies in women with uterine leiomyomas identified by sonography in the first trimester. J Clin Ultrasound. 2001;29(5):261-4.
7. Campo S, Campo V, Gambadauro P. Reproductive outcome before and after laparoscopic or abdominal myomectomy for subserous or intramural myomas. Eur J Obstet Gynecol Reprod Biol. 2003;110(2):215-9.
8. Coronado GD, Marshall LM, Schwartz SM. Complications in pregnancy, labor, and delivery with uterine leiomyomas: a population-based study. Obstet Gynecol. 2000;95(5):764-9.
9. David M, Kröncke T. Uterine fibroid embolisation—potential impact on fertility and pregnancy outcome. Geburtsh Frauenheilk. 2013;73:247-55.
10. Day Baird D, Dunson DB, Hill MC, et al. High cumulative incidence of uterine leiomyoma in black and white women: ultrasound evidence. Am J Obstet Gynecol. 2003;188(1):100-7.
11. Donnez J, Pirard C, Smets M, et al. Unusual growth of a myoma during pregnancy. Fertil Steril. 2002;78(3):632-3.
12. Dubuisson JB, Fauconnier A, Deffarges JV, et al. Pregnancy outcome and deliveries following laparoscopic myomectomy. Hum Reprod. 2000;15(4):869-73.
13. Exacoustos C, Rosati P. Ultrasound diagnosis of uterine myomas and complications in pregnancy. Obstet Gynecol. 1993;82(1):97-101.
14. Fanfani F, Rossitto C, Fagotti A, et al. Laparoscopic myomectomy at 25 weeks of pregnancy: case report. J Minim Invasive Gynecol. 2010;17(1):91-3.
15. Faulkner RL. Red degeneration of uterine myomas. Am J Obstet Gynecol. 1947;53(3):474-82.
16. Fitzpatrick KE, Sellers S, Spark P, et al. Incidence and risk factors for placenta accreta/increta/percreta in the UK: a national case-control study. PLoS ONE. 2012;7(12):e52893.
17. Gambacorti-Passerini Z, Gimovsky AC, Locatelli A, et al. Trial of labor after myomectomy and uterine rupture: a systematic review. Acta Obstet Gynecol Scand. 2016;95(7):724-34.
18. Greenspoon JS, Ault M, James BA, et al. Pyomyoma associated with polymicrobial bacteremia and fatal septic shock: case report and review of the literature. Obstet Gynecol Surv. 1990;45(9):563-9.
19. Hatırnaz Ş, Güler O, Başaranoğlu S, et al. Endometrial myomectomy: a novel surgical method during cesarean section. J Matern Fetal Neonatal Med. 2017;23:1-15.
20. Homer H, Saridogan E. Pregnancy outcomes after uterine artery embolisation for fibroids. Obstet Gynaecol. 2009;11:265-70.
21. Hovsepian DM, Siskin GP, Bonn J, et al. Quality improvement guidelines for uterine artery embolization for symptomatic leiomyomata. Cardiovasc Intervent Radiol. 2004;27(4):307-13.

22. Kesseler A, Mitchell DG, Kulhman K. Myomas vs contraction in pregnancy: differentiation with colour Doppler imaging. J Clin Ultrasound. 1993;21(4):241-4.
23. Kim MS, Uhm YK, Kim JY, et al. Obstetric outcomes after uterine myomectomy: Laparoscopic versus laparotomic approach. Obstet Gynecol Sci. 2013;56(6):375-81.
24. Klatsky PC, Tran ND, Caughey AB, et al. Fibroids and reproductive outcomes: a systematic literature review from conception to delivery. Am J Obstet Gynecol. 2008;198(4):357-66.
25. Korczynski J. Uterine leiomyomas: a prenatal diagnosis group study. Ginekol Pol. 2002;73(4):276-9.
26. Kosmidis C, Pantos G, Efthimiadis C, et al. Laparoscopic excision of a pedunculated uterine leiomyoma in torsion as a cause of acute abdomen at 10 weeks of pregnancy. Am J Case Rep. 2015;16: 505-8.
27. Landon MB, Lynch CD. Optimal timing and mode of delivery after cesarean with previous classical incision or myomectomy: a review of the data. Semin Perinatol. 2011;35(5):257-61.
28. Leach K, Khatain L, Tocce K. First trimester myomectomy as an alternative to termination of pregnancy in a woman with a symptomatic uterine leiomyoma. J Med Case Rep. 2011;5:571.
29. Lev-Toaff AS, Coleman BG, Arger PH, et al. Leiomyomas in pregnancy: sonographic study. Radiology. 1987;164(2):375-80.
30. Lolis DE, Kalantaridou SN, Makrydimas G, et al. Successful myomectomy during pregnancy. Hum Reprod. 2003;18(8):1699-702.
31. Mann C, Karl K, Ertl-Wagner B, et al. Laparoscopic chromopertubation, myomectomy with opening of the uterine cavity and hysteroscopy during the early implantation phase of an undetected pregnancy: Delivery of a child with a complex brain malformation. Geburtshilfe Frauenheilkund. 2016;76(8):906-9.
32. Mara M, Maskova J, Fucikova Z, et al. Midterm clinical and first reproductive results of a randomized controlled trial comparing uterine fibroid embolization and myomectomy. Cardiovasc Intervent Radiol. 2008;31(1):73-85.
33. Mbamara S, Daniyan A, Osaro E, et al. Myomectomy for retained placenta due to incarcerated fibroid mass. Ann Med Health Sci Res. 2015;5(2):148-51.
34. Moir JC. Munro Kerr's Operative Obstetrics, 7th edition. Bailliere, Tindall and Cox: London; 1964. p. 417.
35. Mollica G, Pittini L, Minganti E, et al. Elective uterine myomectomy in pregnant women. Clin Exp Obstet Gynecol. 1996;23(3):168-72.
36. Muram D, Gillieson M, Walters JH. Myomas of the uterus in pregnancy: ultrasonographic follow-up. Am J Obstet Gynecol. 1980;138(1):16-9.
37. Okada Y, Hasegawa J, Mimura T, et al. Uterine rupture at 10 weeks of gestation after laparoscopic myomectomy. J Med Ultrason (2001). 2016;43(1):133-6.
38. Payne JF, Robboy SJ, Haney AF. Embolic microspheres within ovarian arterial vasculature after uterine artery embolization. Obstet Gynecol. 2002;100(5 Pt 1):883-6.
39. Rabinovici J, David M, Fukunishi H, et al. MRgFUS Study Group. Pregnancy outcome after magnetic resonance-guided focused ultrasound surgery (MRgFUS) for conservative treatment of uterine fibroids. Fertil Steril. 2010;93(1):199-209.
40. Rice JP, Kay HH, Mahony BS. The clinical significance of uterine leiomyomas in pregnancy. Am J Obstet Gynecol. 1989;160(5 Pt 1):1212-6.
41. Umezurike C, Feyi-Waboso P. Successful myomectomy during pregnancy: a case report. Reprod Health. 2005;2:6.
42. Vergani P, Locatelli A, Ghidini A, et al. Large uterine leiomyomata and risk of cesarean delivery. Obstet Gynecol. 2007;109(2 Pt 1):410-4.
43. Wang SW, He XY, Li MZ. High-intensity focused ultrasound compared with irradiation for ovarian castration in premenopausal females with hormone receptor-positive breast cancer after radical mastectomy. Oncol Lett. 2012;4(5):1087-91.
44. Winer-Muram HT, Muram D, Gillieson MS. Uterine myomas in pregnancy. J Can Assoc Radiol. 1984;35(2):168-70.
45. Yoshino O, Hayashi T, Osuga Y, et al. Decreased pregnancy rate is linked to abnormal uterine peristalsis caused by intramural fibroids. Hum Reprod. 2010;25(10):2475-9.

Management of AUB with Fibroids

7

Kundan Ingale, Ashish Kale

INTRODUCTION

Abnormal uterine bleeding (AUB) is one of the most common conditions for which women consult their gynecologists. Uterine leiomyomas, or fibroids, represent a large proportion of gynecological presentations in both general and specialist gynecology practice. They are estimated to affect 40-80% of women by age of 50 years.

- There is subset of patients with AUB who have fibroids. Fibroids are the benign tumors of corpus uteri with increased incidence in reproductive age. AUB and its subgroup, heavy menstrual bleeding (HMB), are common conditions affecting 14-25% of women of reproductive age. Chronic AUB was defined as "bleeding from the uterine corpus" that is abnormal in volume, regularity, and/or timing that has been present for the majority of the last 6 months.

Abnormal uterine bleeding with fibroids presents with both type may be acute or chronic AUB. The location of fibroids has an impact in bleeding pattern, usually submucous and intramural fibroids are the main causative factors in AUB with fibroids. Intramural fibroids over the time may merge with submucous fibroids then the AUB sets up.

CLINICAL PRESENTATION

Clinical presentation in AUB with fibroids depends on location of fibroids.
- Menorrhagia, polymenorrhea, and metrorrhagia
- Infertility and recurrent abortion
- Pelvic pain—spasmodic dysmenorrhea and backache
- Pressure symptoms—bladder, ureter, and rectum.
- Abdominal lump or mass protruding at introitus
- Vaginal discharge.

Almost, a third of women with leiomyomas will request treatment due to symptoms. Due to chronic AUB, patients may be anemic, which usually presents as easy fatigability, weakness, loss of concentration to daily work, if in severe case, may predispose to chronic illness. Their theories for the possible cause of menorrhagia included venous ectasia resulting from mechanical compression of veins by myomas, or altered function, expression, or storage of vasoactive growth factors produced by myomas.

EVALUATION OF PATIENT WITH BLEEDING

Evaluation of patients starts with detailed history of patients, and menstrual pattern with association of pain. Evaluation is incomplete without clinical examination as well as with diagnostic modalities.

Diagnosis

As asymptomatic fibroids are highly prevalent, so it is at most important to evaluate the uterus carefully to conclude that the fibroid is contributing to the clinical problem. It is not necessary that presence of both, i.e. fibroid and AUB have to be related as cause-effect fashion. The diagnosis can be achieved by on or the combination of hysteroscopy and radiological techniques such as transvaginal sonography (TVS), saline sonosalpingography, and magnetic resonance imaging (MRI).

Goals of Diagnosis

- To identify and characterize the lesions
- To distinguish fibroid from adenomyosis
- To find location of fibroid to decide whether close to submucosa or serosa (Flowchart 7.1).

Flowchart 7.1: Diagnosis of abnormal uterine bleeding.

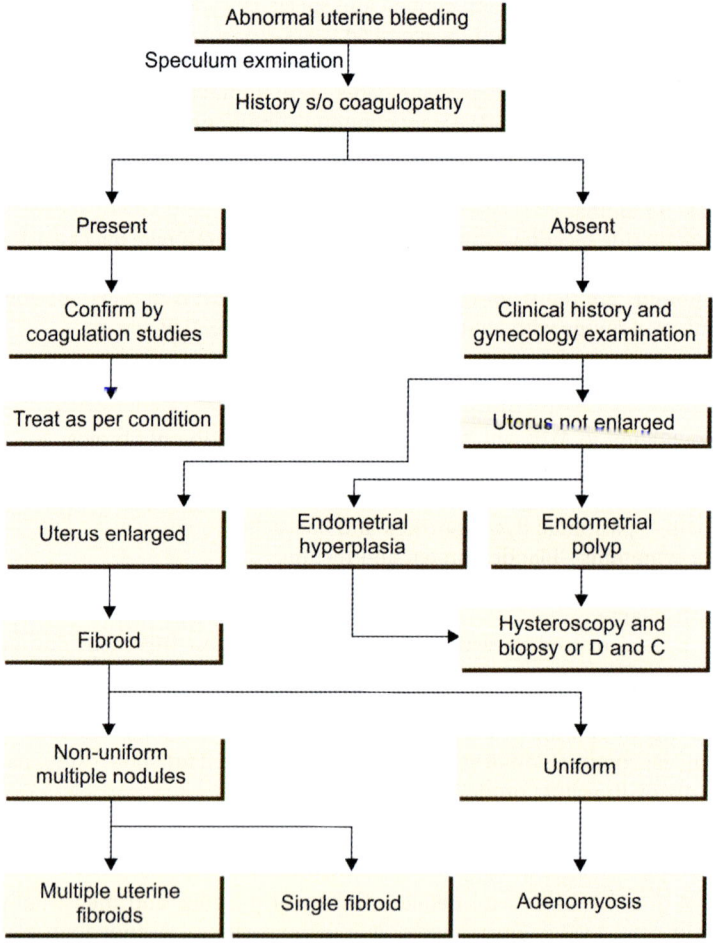

Lesions should be characterized by extent of myometrial penetration and the relationship to the uterine serosa. This will help us to decide whether fibroid lesion should be tackled transcervically or transabdominally.

Pelvic examination may reveal a palpable enlarged, firm, and irregular uterus.

Uterine size with fibroid is reported in the form of weeks of gravid uterus (size ore than 13 weeks may be palpated by abdominal examination).

On local examination, a fibroid polyp, which may be protruding outside the vagina, having ulcerations, can be seen.

Per speculum examination may reveal a fibroid polyp protruding through the cervical canal or a cervical fibroid at the external os.

Physical Examination

Transvaginal sonography: Ultrasonography is the imaging modality of choice in the detection and evaluation of uterine fibroids. Transvaginal ultrasound is a cost-effective, easily available, and most accurate modality for diagnosis of fibroids. It can accurately assess the myoma location, dimensions, and also any adnexal pathology.

The most frequent USG appearance is that of a concentric, solid, and hypoechoic mass (Figs. 7.1 and 7.2). Degree of echogenicity in appearance depends on extent of calcification or amount of fibrous tissue. In case of central necrosis, it can be seen as anechoic area in the center. If fibroid is close to uterine cavity then endometrial echo appears to be either displaced or indented by fibroid (Fig. 7.3). Ultrasound has a sensitivity of 60%, a specificity of 99%, and an accuracy of 87% in diagnosing fibroids.

There are four common locations of fibroid, accurately diagnosed by TVS—(1) intracavitary, (2) submucosal, (3) intramural, (4) subserosal (Fig. 7.4). TVS helps to classify submucosal fibroids to decide the surgical therapeutic options, including the surgical approach (Box 7.1).

Saline infusion sonography (sonosalpingography): This simple minimal invasive and effective sonographic procedure can be used to confirm the diagnosis of submucosal fibroid and to differentiate it from intracavitary fibroid. Compared with TVS, saline infusion sonography (SIS) typically permits superior detection of intracavitary masses and differentiation of lesions as being endometrial, submucous, or intramural. SIS has limitations. SIS is cycle dependent

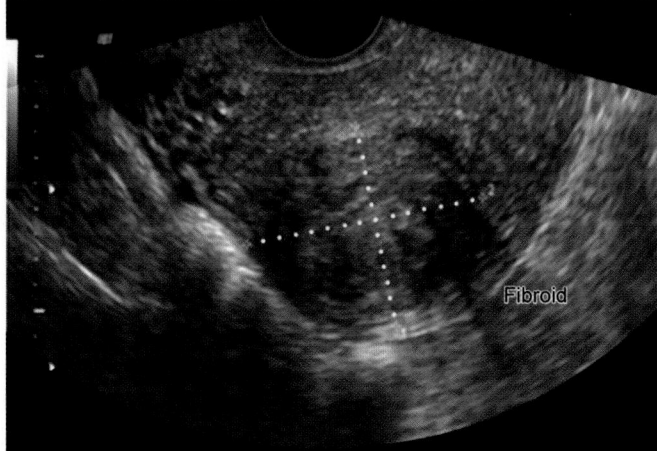

Fig. 7.1: Posterior wall fibroid on transvaginal USG.

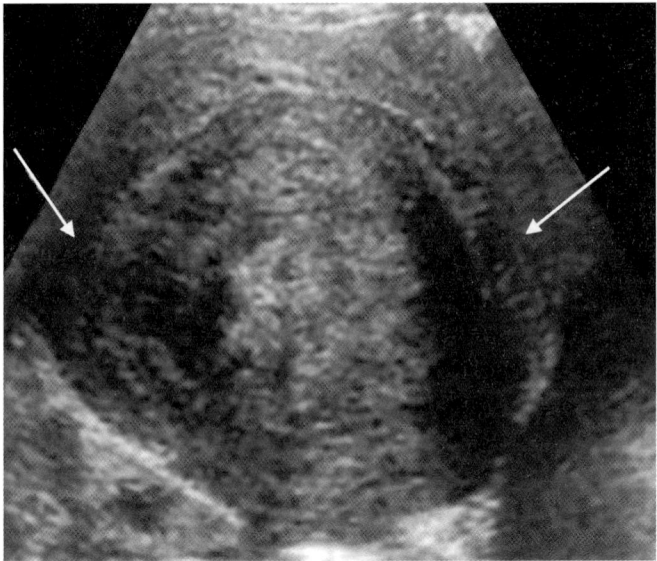

Fig. 7.2: Fibroid on transabdominal scan.

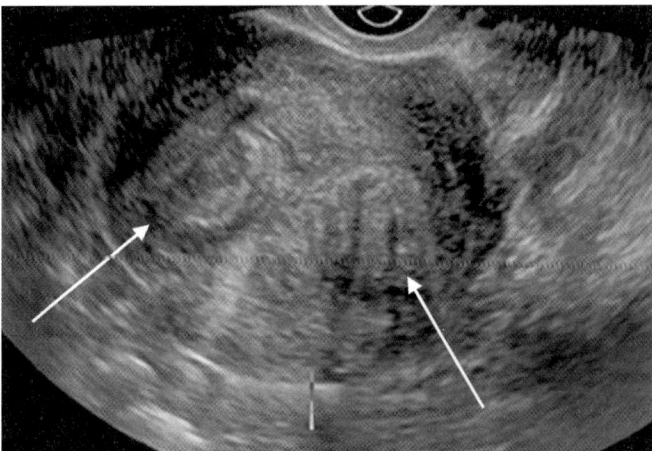

Fig. 7.3: Two intramural fibroids on TVS.

and should be performed in proliferative phase to minimize false-positive and false-negative results. SIS causes more discomfort to patient than TVS (Fig. 7.6).

Color Doppler: Color Doppler helps to distinguish uterine fibroids from other diffuse pathologies like adenomyosis. Uterine fibroid has typical circumferential peripheral vascularity, outlining the fibroid while in contrast to diffusely placed vascularity in adenomyotic lesions (Fig. 7.7).

Magnetic resonance imaging: Magnetic resonance imaging has an important role in defining the anatomy of the uterus and ovaries in patients in whom ultrasound findings are confusing or in cases of large fibroids. MRI is very valuable in diagnosing adenomyosis, deep endometriosis, and

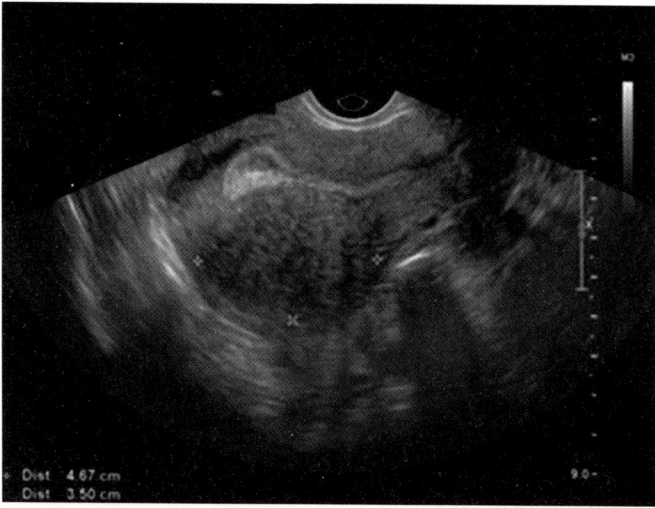

Fig. 7.4: Posterior wall intramural fibroid pushing endometrial cavity.

Box 7.1: The International Federation of Gynecology and Obstetrics (FIGO) system for classification of causes of abnormal uterine bleeding (AUB) in reproductive aged women uses the same system for categorization of submucosal fibroids but adds a number of other categories, including type 3 lesions that abut the endometrium without distorting the endometrial cavity (Fig. 7.5).

ESGE: Classification of submucous myomas

Type 0
 Entirely within endometrial cavity
 No myometrial extension (pedunculated)
Type I
 < 50% myometrial extension (sessile)
 < 90° angle of myoma surface to uterine wall
Type II
 ≥ 50% myometrial extension (sessile)
 ≥ 90° angle of myoma surface to uterine wall

Source: Modified from Wamsteker K, Emanual MH, dr Kruif JH. Transcervical hysteroscopic resection of submucosal fibroids for abnormal uterine bleeding: results regarding the degree of intramural extension. Obstet Gynecol. 1993;82(5):736-40.

pelvic masses. It helps in choosing between medical and surgical modalities of treatment. It has a sensitivity of 86–92%, specificity of 100%, and accuracy of 97% in evaluation of probable fibroids. MRI plays a role in selected patients with AUB and fibroids, also in the assessment of suitability for uterine artery embolization (UAE) (Fig. 7.8).

Hysteroscopy: Hysteroscopy is generally considered to be the gold standard of evaluation of the endometrial cavity for the presence of type 0 to 2 fibroids as well as characteristics such as diameter and location (Fig. 7.9). It also permits simultaneous removal of many lesions once identified (Fig. 7.10). There are certain studies, which suggest hysteroscopy as the primary tool

54 *Fibroids*

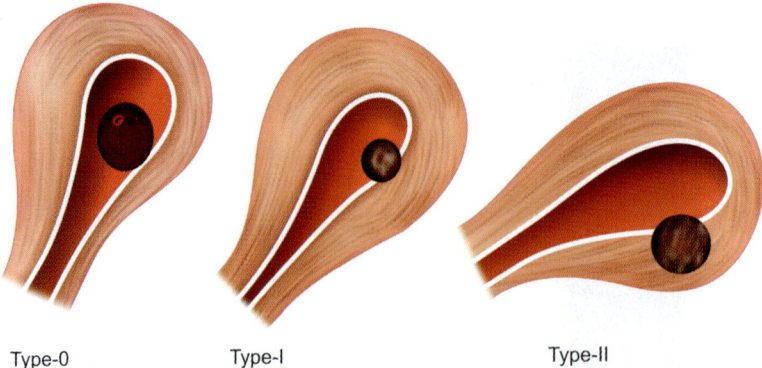

Type-0   Type-I   Type-II

Fig. 7.5: Classification of submucosal fibroid.

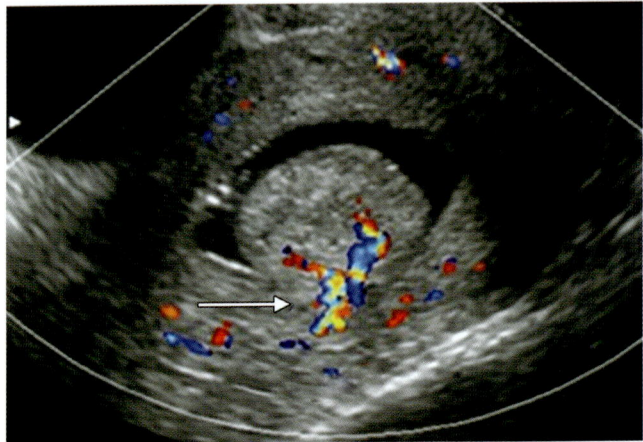

Fig. 7.6: Saline infusion sonography of fibroids.

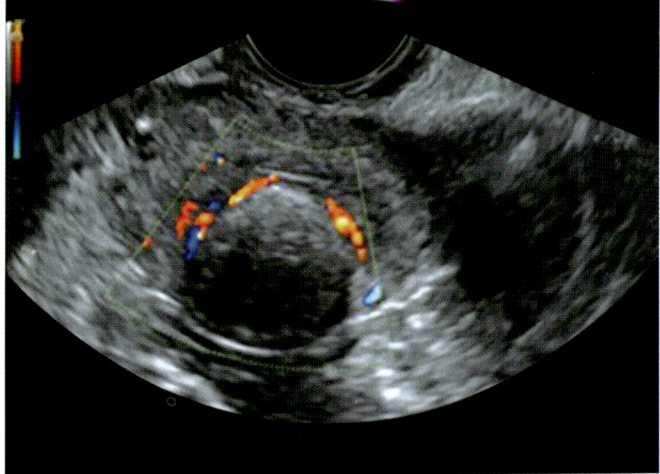

Fig. 7.7: Color Doppler of uterine fibroids.

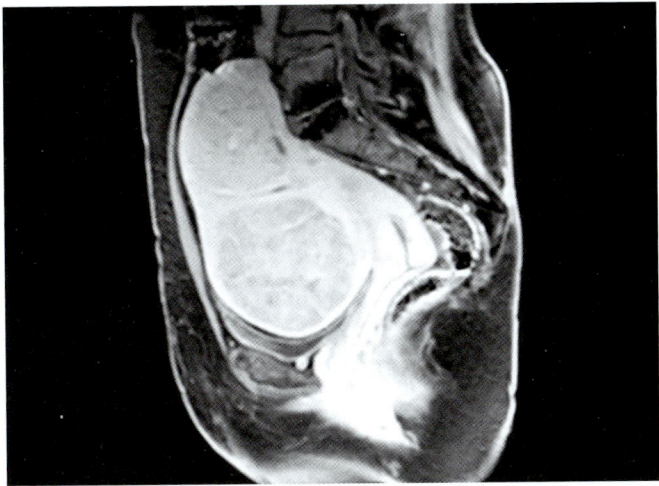

Fig. 7.8: Magnetic resonance imaging of fibroids.

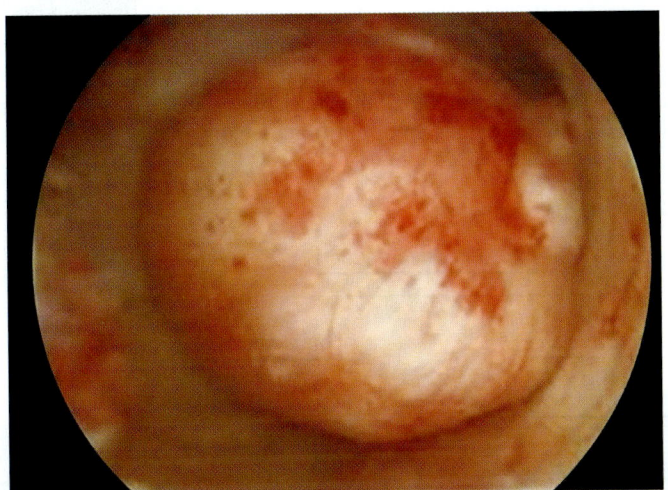

Fig. 7.9: Finding of diameter and location of fibroids using hysteroscopy.

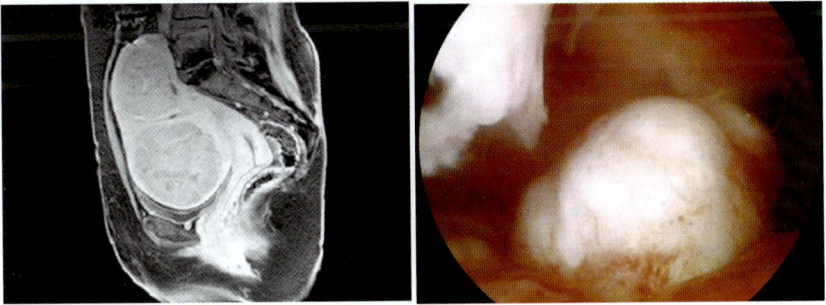

Fig. 7.10: Identification of lesions on hysteroscopy.

for AUB diagnosis. It is also expensive. The increasing use of saline infusion ultrasonography (SIS) and selected hysteroscopy will improve sensitivity and specificity for diagnosis of polyps and SM fibroids.

MANAGEMENT

Medical Management

Indications

- To preserve fertility in women with large fibroid prior to attempting conception
- Treatment of women near menopause in an effort to avoid surgery
- Women with medical contraindications to surgery
- Personal or medical indications for delaying surgery (Flowchart 7.2).

Gonadotropin-releasing Hormone Analogs

It acts by downregulating gonadotropin-releasing hormone (GnRH) receptors at the pituitary level resulting in significant reductions in follicle-stimulating hormone (FSH), luteinizing hormone (LH), and ovarian steroids thus, producing a hypoestrogenic state.

It can be given as a short-time course for preparation for surgery or built up her hemoglobin or as a long-term course to avoid surgical intervention. GnRha administration results in a reduction of both leiomyoma and total uterine volume by a mean of about 50% by 12 weeks. Short-term use (her circulating hemoglobin levels 2–3 months) of GnRha in conjunction with iron supplementation provides an opportunity for the women with AUB and associated

Flowchart 7.2: Management of fibroids.

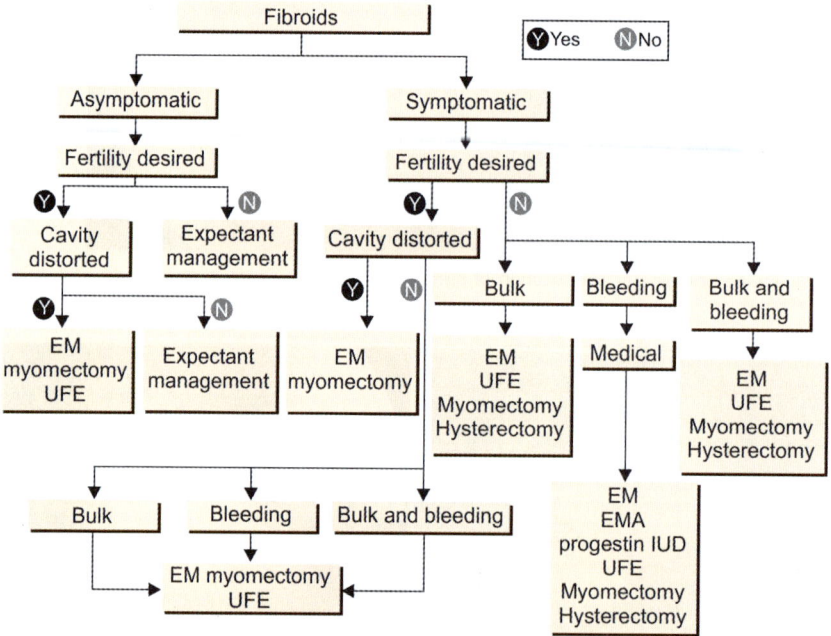

(EM: Expectant management; EMA: Endometrial ablation; UFE: Uterine fibroid embolization)

anemia to reconstitute her circulating hemoglobin levels without resorting to either blood transfusion or emergency surgery. Using GnRha preoperatively helps to reduce volume of fibroid, which makes surgery minimal invasive. It also helps to reduce intraoperative blood loss. Current recommendations do not warrant to use GnRha preoperatively prior to surgery due to absence of a difference in the incidence of blood transfusions in the literature.

Progestins

There is no currently available evidence regarding the use of systematic progestins for women with AUB in the presence of fibroid that do not distort the uterine cavity, but there is evidence that the levonorgestrel intrauterine system (LNG-IUS) may be effective in selected patients. The reduction in menstrual blood loss (MBL) at 3, 6, and 1 months postinsertion reached 90%, comparable with that of a group of women treated in the same center using a thermal balloon and expulsion rate were up to 5%. It would seem that LNG-IUS is a reasonable option for women with modestly enlarged uteri and at least selected type 2 leiomyomas.

Antiprogestins

The selective progesterone receptor modulator (SPRM) mifepristone has been shown to dramatically reduce or even eliminate the symptom of AUB while reducing the volume of fibroid by about 50% with few side effects. After 3 months of treatment, the mean volume of the largest leiomyoma was significantly reduced by mifepristone 10 mg or 25 mg. Most of the patients in all groups experienced amenorrhea after the treatment. There were also significant elevations in red blood cell count, hemoglobin, and hematocrit ($P < 0.0001$); and significant reductions in prevalence of dysmenorrhea, pelvic pressure, nonmenstrual abdominal pain ($P < 0.0001$) in each group. 10 mg is as effective as 25 mg mifepristone may provide an alternative for clinical application, especially for patient who are in perimenopause with uterine fibroids. Ulipristal acetate is a progesterone receptor modulator can inhibit ovulation and lead to amenorrhea, which will be of benefit to women who have HMB related to their fibroids. As progesterone promotes the growth of uterine fibroids, blocking its receptor may reduce their size. The common adverse effects of ulipristal include headache, nausea, and abdominal pain. The actions of ulipristal may cause some women to experience hot flushes. It can be a useful treatment in the emergency management of fibroid-related acute AUB. The effect of repeated courses on fertility is uncertain. For most women, menstruation resumes within a month of stopping ulipristal.

Surgical Management

Indications

- Anemia from AUB nonresponding to medical therapy
- Chronic pain, dysmenorrhea, dyspareunia, and lower abdominal pain
- Acute pain in case of prolapsing submucosal fibroid, and torsion of pedunculated fibroid
- Infertility due to fibroid
- Pressure symptoms due to big fibroid
- Rapidly enlarging fibroids in premenopausal patients or after menopause.

Uterine fibroid surgeries are:
- Hysteroscopic myomectomy
- Laparoscopic/open myomectomy
- Total laparoscopic or open hysterectomy with or without salpingo-oophorectomy.

Hysteroscopic Myomectomy

It is done for the management of symptomatic (AUB) intracavitary fibroids, with limitations related to the size, number, and locations of fibroids. The goals of the patients with respect to fertility are to excise fibroid completely with maximum preservation of endometrial and myometrial integrity. Lesions totally within endometrial cavity (Type 0 and Type 1) and that are less than or equal to 5 cm can be excised with relative ease.

Laparoscopic Myomectomy

Subserous and intramural fibroids and extrauterine fibroids are removed by laparoscopic myomectomy. AUB is associated with submucosal and intramural fibroids, less likely with subserous fibroid.

Uterine fibroid more than 24 weeks size should be better tackled by laparotomy than laparoscopy. After a ban on uterine morcellation by Food and Drug Administration (FDA), it is recommended to do fibroid morcellation in endobag. Currently available evidence suggests that patients selected for laparoscopic myomectomy and operated on by skilled surgeons will have similar pregnancy outcomes compared with those who have laparotomy and myomectomy.

Advantages of Laparoscopy over Laparotomy

- Lower analgesia requirement
- Shorter hospital stay
- Rapid recovery
- Greater patient satisfaction
- Lower rate of wound infection and hematoma formation.

Laparoscopic Hysterectomy

If women with AUB with fibroid do not desire to preserve fertility, laparoscopic total hysterectomy should be the first choice. Depending on her age at the time of surgery, decision should be take regarding salpingo-oophorectomy. Patients with large big fibroid or multiple fibroids are ideally subjected to laparoscopic hysterectomy, provided she does not desire fertility preservation.

Uterine Artery Embolization

Uterine artery embolization is the use of interventional radiographic technique to occlude both uterine arteries with polyvinyl alcohol microspheres positioned by a catheter passed through the right femoral artery. Complications are relatively infrequent but include postembolization syndrome (pain, fever, nausea, and vomiting), misembolization of tissues like ovary, ureter, etc. infection, and rarely death. In large study of 200 patients, mean MBL reduced in 87% of patients at 3 months and 90% at 12 months of follow up. By 5 years, 73% had continued symptoms control with 13.7% and 4.4% undergoing hysterectomy and myomectomy, respectively. Bilateral UAE seems to offer an option to women with AUB that may provide long-term resolution of symptoms without the need for traditional surgical interventions.

RISK OF MALIGNANCY

Malignant transformation of benign leiomyoma to leiomyosarcoma although a rare occurrence but can happen in certain patients with large myomas, postmenopausal women, rapid growing myomas, and in certain subset of leiomyoma. MRI and serum lactate dehydrogenase might be helpful in preoperative predetection of these changes. The hypothesis that uterine leiomyosarcoma arises from or as a result of the malignant transformation of benign leiomyomas have not been proved.

COUNSELING

Despite this high incidence, we know relatively little about their cause, growth, and development and contribution to the genesis of reproductive disorders. The prevalence of lesions puts women with associated but unrelated symptoms at risk for unnecessary and/or unsuccessful interventions, especially if they have not been carefully evaluated and counseled. If woman with fibroid and having desire for conception then she should be evaluated properly to counsel her best fertility-preserving strategy. Before any treatment, each patient of fibroid should be counseled for possibility of recurrence of fibroid at different location. Women should be counseled for long-term complications of myomectomy like uterine dehiscence or rupture.

CONCLUSION

Menstrual dysfunction in the form of heavy bleeding or intermenstrual bleeding with irregular cycles is the presenting symptom in majority of patients with fibroid and treatment should be aimed to alleviate symptoms keeping in mind the age of the patient. Estrogen has been implicated in the causation of uterine fibroids and, therefore, these patients may have associated endometrial hyperplasia contributing to HMB. Clinical diagnosis is important but for confirmation, ultrasound and newer imaging modalities may be of value. Medical management has got its own indications and should be offered, whenever it is indicated. GnRha are expensive and side effects of longer use have to be kept in mind. Hysteroscopic resection of fibroid is gold standard for the treatment of symptomatic submucous fibroids. Laparoscopic myomectomy is specifically for intramural and subserosal symptomatic fibroids in young patients with AUB. Laparoscopic hysterectomy should be considered for older patients with AUB. Uterine artery embolization is safe and effective method with significant fewer complications than hysterectomy. Patient's age and desire of future reproduction guide to plan the course of treatment to optimize the outcomes. The medical field has come a long way in developing alternative primary treatments top meet different needs and preferences.

BIBLIOGRAPHY

1. Benagiano G, Kivinen ST, Fadini R, et al. Zoladex (goserelin acetate) and the anemic patient: results of a multicenter fibroid study. Fertil Steril. 1996;66(2):223-9.
2. Donnez J, Vázquez F, Tomaszewski J, et al. PEARL III and PEARL III Extension Study Group. Long-term treatment of uterine fibroids with ulipristal acetate. Fertil Steril. 2014;101(6):1565-73.e1-18.
3. Farrer-Brown G, Beilby J, Tarbit M. Venous changes in the endometrium of myomatous uteri. Obstet Gynecol. 1971;38(5):743-51.
4. Fraser IS, Critchley HO, Broder M. The FIGO recommendations on terminologies and definitions for normal and abnormal uterine bleeding. Semin Reprod Med. 2011;29(5):383-90.
5. Fraser IS, Langham S, Uhl-Hochgraeber K. Health-related quality of life and economic burden of abnormal uterine bleeding. Expert Rev Obstet Gynecol. 2009;4:179-89.
6. Friedmann AJ, Rein MS, Harrison–Atlas D, et al. A randomized placebo-controlled, double blind study evaluating leuprolide acetate treatment before myomectomy. Fertil Steril. 1989;52(5):728-33.
7. Lethaby A, Vollenhoven B, Sowter M. Pre-operative GnRH analogue therapy before hysterectomy or myomectomy for uterine fibroids. Cochrane Database Syst Rev. 2001;2:CD000547.
8. Liu C, Lu Q, Qu H, et al. Different dosages of mifepristone versus enantone to treat uterine fibroids: A multicenter randomized controlled trial. Medicine (Baltimore). 2017;96(7):e6124.

9. Maiti S, Naidoo K. Patients' satisfaction survey at the outpatient hysteroscopy service at St Mary's Hospital, Manchester, UK. Menopause Int. 2008;14(1):5.
10. Munro MG, Chrichley HO, Broder MS, et al. The FIGO classification system for causes of abnormal uterine bleeding in non-gravid uterus in reproductive years, including guidelines for clinical investigations. Int J Gynecol Obstet. 2011;113:3-13.
11. Munro MG, Critchley HO, Fraser IS. The FIGO classification of causes of abnormal uterine bleeding. Int J Gynaecol Obstet. 2011;113(1):1-2.
12. Shapley M, Jordan K, Croft PR. An epidemiological survey of symptoms of menstrual loss in the community. Br J Gen Pract. 2004;54(502):359-63.
13. Stovali TG, Muneyyirci-Delale O, Summitt RL Jr, et al. GnRH agonist and iron versus placebo and iron in the anemic patient before surgery for leiomyomas: a randomized controlled trial. Leuprolide Acetate study group. Obstet Gynecol. 1995;85:65-71.
14. Valentin L. Imaging techniques in the management of abnormal vaginal bleeding in non-pregnant women before and after menopause. Best Pract Res Clin Obstet Gynaecol. 2014;28(5):637-54.
15. Wamsteker K, Emanual MH, dr Kruif JH. Transcervical hysteroscopic resection of submucosal fibroids for abnormal uterine bleeding: results regarding the degree of intramural extension. Obstet Gynecol. 1993;82(5):736-40.
16. Zagoria J, Brady M, Dyer B. Genitourinary Imaging: The Requisites. Elsevier Health Sciences: US; 2015. p. 448.

Management of Fibroids in Perimenopausal Women

8

Esha Sharma

INTRODUCTION

Leiomyoma also known as uterine fibroids are benign tumors of the smooth muscle of the uterus. These fibroids grow under the influence of the hormone estrogen and are most often seen after the menarche and tend to shrink after the menopause. Perimenopause refers to the time during which our body makes the natural transition to menopause, marking the end of the reproductive years. Around 50% of uterine fibroids remain asymptomatic, however, they cause significant morbidity affecting the quality of life in about 20–50% women. The prevalence of it ranges from 30% to 50% in reproductive age group, increasing the incidence to 70–80% by the age of 50.

CLINICAL PRESENTATION

Myomas may be asymptomatic and diagnosed incidentally on clinical examination or imaging. The symptoms associated with fibroids vary with their size, number, and location as well as with the concomitant degenerative changes. Most common symptoms of uterine leiomyoma are:
- *Abnormal uterine bleeding*: Premenopausal women with abnormal uterine bleeding constitute a large proportion of gynecologic consultations.
  - Heavy menstrual bleeding (30%) due to increased endometrial surface area, vascular dysregulation, and interference with endometrial hemostasis.
  - *Intermenstrual bleeding*: Submucosal fibroids may also present with intermenstrual.
- *Pain*: Spasmodic dysmenorrhea. Although rare pelvic pain in fibroids, usually signifies degeneration, torsion, or possibly-associated adenomyosis or endometriosis.
- *Pressure symptoms*:
  - Heaviness
  - Bloating
  - Constipation
  - Dyspareunia more likely with large fibroid
  - Urinary bladder (urinary retention)
  - Ureter (hydroureter and hydronephrosis)
  - Rectum (tenesmus)
  - Veins (mainly the left common iliac vein leading to varicosities), venous thromboembolism, and leg edema.
- *Infertility*
- *Others*: Anemia and infections.

DIAGNOSIS

- *Ultrasonography* (transabdominal and transvaginal) is the most widely used modality because of its availability, ease of use, and cost-effectiveness. In submucosal lesions, contrast infusion saline or gel sonography and 2D and 3D sonohysterography are very accurate diagnostic procedures with sensitivity and specificity of 98–100%.
- *Computed tomography (CT)* is of limited value in delineating the location of myomas relative to the endometrium or myometrium.
- *Magnetic resonance imaging (MRI)* is the most accurate modality in assessing the adnexae and the uterus because it provides information on the size, location, number, and perfusion of leiomyomas as well as the presence of other uterine pathology including adenomyosis and/or adenomyoma.

MANAGEMENT

Depending on the severity of symptoms, assessment of the size, number, and position of myomas, the needs and desires for preservation of fertility or the uterus, the availability of therapy, and the experience of the therapist, patient can be optimally selected for expectant management, medical therapy, noninvasive procedures, or surgery. Although most fibroids are asymptomatic, some women have significant symptoms that need interventions (Flowchart 8.1).

Flowchart 8.1: Management of fibroid in perimenopausal women.

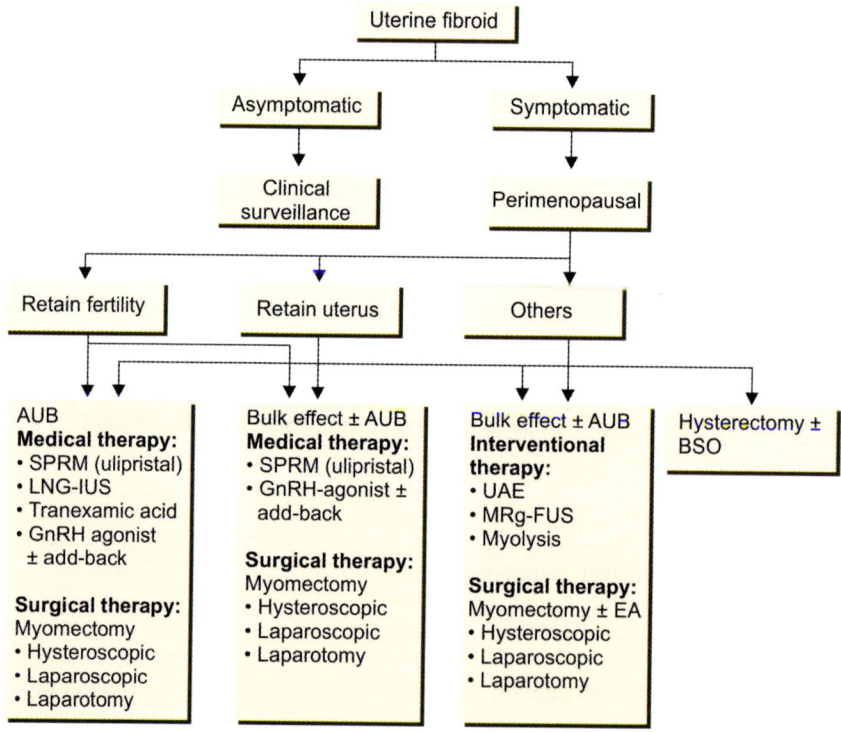

(AUB: Abnormal uterine bleeding; BSO: Bilateral salpingo-oophorectomy; GnRH: Gonadotropin releasing hormone; MRg-FUS: Magnetic resonance-guided focused ultrasound; LNG-IUS: Levonorgestrel intrauterine system; SPRM: Selective progesterone receptor modulator; UAE: Uterine artery embolization)

Management techniques:
- *Expectant*
- *Medical therapy*:
  - *Nonhormonal*: Nonsteroidal anti-inflammatory drugs (NSAIDs) and tranexamic acid.
  - *Hormonal*: Progestins, gonadotropin releasing hormone (GnRH) agonist selective estrogen receptor modulators (SERMs) (tamoxifen; raloxifene), selective progesterone receptor (PR) modulators (mifepristone, ulipristal acetate, asoprisnil, and telapristone acetate), and aromatase inhibitors (letrozole).
- *Minimally invasive technique*: Hysteroscopy, uterine artery embolization (UAE), MRI-guided focused ultrasound surgery.
- *Surgical*: Myomectomy and hysterectomy.

Expectant Management

In premenopausal women, prospective imaging studies indicate that 3–7% of untreated fibroids regress over 6 months to 3 years. Therefore, when women are approaching perimenopausal age, the general attitude is to avoid treatment and wait for menopause and a spontaneous resolution. Most women experience shrinkage of fibroids and relief of symptoms at menopause; therefore, depending on the severity of their symptoms, women who are approaching menopause may choose to wait for the onset of menopause before deciding on treatment.

Medical Therapy

Medical therapy may be beneficial in women who are in perimenopausal status with symptomatic uterine, although not considered a definitive treatment. Because of the significant risks with long-term therapy, or lack of evidence regarding the benefits—risks of long-term therapy with the newer medical agents, medical treatments are only used as short-term therapy.

Nonhormonal

- Nonsteroidal anti-inflammatory drugs are the first-line medical therapy in ovulatory menorrhagia. These drugs have been found to be better than placebo in reducing menstrual blood flow.
- *Tranexamic acid*: The mechanism of action in treating heavy menstrual bleeding is by prevention of fibrinolysis and the breakdown of clots via inhibiting endometrial plasminogen activator. In a study conducted by AS Lukes, women taking 3.9 g/day of tranexamic acid showed a significant reduction in menstrual blood loss and an increase in their quality of life compared with those taking placebo.

Hormonal

Progestin: The most frequently prescribed medicine for menorrhagia. Progestogen treatment is intended to reduce heavy menstrual bleeding by reducing the endometrial hyperplasia associated with fibroids. Although not a treatment for fibroids, they can be used to treat abnormal uterine bleeding associated with fibroids for a short or intermediate period.

Levonorgestrel intrauterine system—administered by the endouterine route has been recommended for treatment of the heavy bleeding associated with fibroid tumors. It reduces menstrual blood loss by as much as 97%. This is comparable to transcervical resection of the endometrium for reduction of menstrual bleeding.

Depo-medroxyprogesterone acetate (DMPA)—reduces menstrual bleeding, allows women to improve their hemoglobin prior to surgery. When used for a long time, DMPA also an anti-estrogen and can decrease bone density.

Gonadotropin releasing hormone agonist: GnRH agonists are useful preoperatively to shrink fibroids and to reduce anemia related to uterine bleeding. These are available as nasal spray, subcutaneous injections, and slow-release injections. In general, fibroids may be expected to shrink by up to 50% of their initial volume within 3 months of therapy. As it causes hypogonadal state, GnRH agonist treatment is restricted to a 3-6-month interval, following which regrowth of fibroids usually occurs within 12 weeks. To alleviate GnRH agonist-induced symptoms, add-back medications (estrogen/progestins) are initiated after 3 months, both together continued depending on the clinical situation and the patients adherence.

Newer Drugs

Selective estrogen receptor modulators: The SERMs (tamoxifen; raloxifene) are nonsteroidal drugs that bind to estrogen receptors and may act as agonists or antagonists to produce tissue-specific effects. Raloxifene, as it reduces cell proliferation and has no endometrial agonist activity, is the most studied SERM for treatment of leiomyomata.

Selective progesterone receptor modulators: Compared with the myometrium, fibroids overexpress estrogen (ER) and progesterone receptors, and there is "crosstalk" between ER and PR. Progesterone increases mitotic activity and cellularity in fibroids. SPRMs are PR ligands that have agonist, antagonist, partial, or mixed effects on progesterone target tissues. A number of clinical trials have investigated the efficacy and safety of selective PR modulators as a treatment for fibroids, showing that mifepristone ulipristal acetate, asoprisnil, and telapristone acetate are all effective in reducing fibroid and uterine volume. The selective PR modulators control tumor volume for a prolonged period of up to 6 months after treatment discontinuation, in contrast to GnRH agonist therapy but the possibility of endometrial hyperplasia requires prudence.

Aromatase inhibitors (letrozole): Myometrial-cultured cells overexpress aromatase P450 and synthesize sufficient estradiol to accelerate their own cell growth. Aromatase inhibitors may serve to block the aromatase activity and growth of leiomyomata. A clinical trial included in a recent Cochrane database review compared the aromatase inhibitor letrozole to the GnRH analog triptorelin. Letrozole reduced fibroid volumes by 46% (vs 32% in the GnRH analog group).

Surgical Management

As a definitive medical treatment is not available, surgical treatment remains the mainstream therapy for fibroids.

Indications for surgical intervention:
- Failure to respond to medical treatment
- Worsening vaginal bleeding
- Suspicion of malignancy.

Minimally Invasive Technique

Hysteroscopy: Hysteroscopic resection is the first-line treatment for perimenopausal women with symptomatic submucosal fibroids or who wish to retain their fertility. Risks of partial resection and of recurrence, as well as of the possibility of a second procedure, to be explained.

Uterine artery embolization: Premenopausal women with symptomatic fibroid aged 35–50 years who do not wish for fertility but want to retain the uterus are the most likely candidates for UAE. It acts by occluding or markedly reducing uterine blood flow at the arteriolar level to produce an irreversible ischemic injury to the fibroids, causing them to undergo necrosis and shrink, whereas the normal myometrium is able to recover. A Cochrane review has looked at the benefits and risks of UAE versus other medical or surgical interventions for symptomatic uterine fibroids.

MRI-guided focused ultrasound surgery: It is an emerging noninvasive and thermoablative technique for the management of symptomatic myomas. During the procedure, sonications or pulses of focused ultrasound energy are delivered to destroy target tissue as temperatures are raised in the treatment area to a range of 65–85°C. Administration approved MRI-guided focused ultrasound surgery as a safe, feasible, and effective alternative therapy for myomas.

Radiofrequency cryomyolysis: Cryomyolysis involves a probe with a cooling agent that is applied to the myoma, causing coagulation of the supporting blood vessels. Through this procedure, the blood flow is diminished, resulting in necrosis.

Myomectomy

Removal of fibroids should be considered in symptomatic fibroids, and in some cases, reproductive issues. Myomectomy is an alternative to hysterectomy for women who wish to retain their uterus, regardless of their fertility desire. The selection of the optimal approach like laparotomy, laparoscopy, minilaparotomy, and laparoscopically-assisted myomectomy depends on the patient's and the surgeon's preference.

Fibroids have a 15% recurrence rate and 10% of women undergoing a myomectomy will eventually require hysterectomy within 5–10 years. Risk of recurrence is associated with age, preoperative number of fibroids, uterine size, associated disease, and childbirth after myomectomy.

Hysterectomy

Hysterectomy is indicated as a permanent solution for symptomatic leiomyomas, in women who have completed childbearing. The only indication for hysterectomy in a woman with completely asymptomatic fibroids is enlarging fibroids after menopause without hormone replacement therapy (HRT), which raises concerns of leiomyosarcoma, even though it remains very rare.

Risk of Malignancy

Leiomyosarcoma

One of the most feared complications of fibroids by patients is if the fibroids can become cancerous. Case series have estimated the incidence of leiomyosarcoma at 0.22–0.49%, although in women in their 6th decade it may rise to 1% of hysterectomy specimens. Most recent reviews estimate that in women undergoing surgery for fibroids approximately 1 in 400 (0.25%) is at risk of having a leiomyosarcoma.

Hormone Replacement Therapy

Postmenopausal HRT is not contraindicated in the presence of fibroids as the estrogen content in HRT is too small to cause any change in size or the development of new fibroids.

Follow-up

Because the natural course of fibroids in perimenopausal women is unpredictable, the literature is devoid of evidence about the need for routine ultrasound monitoring of fibroids, but appearance of new symptoms, the aggravation of old ones, increase in size of persisting fibroid or their persistence after nonsurgical treatment require reassessment and justify exploration by supplementary imaging (CT, MRI, or Doppler ultrasound) and immediate hysterectomy in the event of suspicion of malignancy. The assumption that with the onset of the menopause fibroids will resolve is not always valid.

CONCLUSION

The management of uterine fibroids should not be overlooked in the perimenopausal period merely on the grounds that the pathology and symptoms are unlikely to persist after the menopause. The balance of the complications of the fibroids versus the risks of the treatment options is required. When it is decided that treatment is needed, the choice for peri- and postmenopausal women, surgical procedures have been the mainstay of definitive leiomyoma management over the last century. However, novel interventions and medical therapies with significant reductions in patient morbidity have been introduced with actual and promising results.

BIBLIOGRAPHY

1. Adusumilli S, Hussain HK, Caoili EM, et al. MRI of sonographically indeterminate adnexal masses. AJR Am J Roentgenol. 2006;187:732-40.
2. Andersson JK, Rybo G. Levonorgestrel-releasing intrauterine device in the treatment of menorrhagia. Br J Obstet Gynaecol. 1990;97(8):690-4.
3. Ang WC, Farrell E, Vollenhoven B. Effect of hormone replacement therapies and selective estrogen receptor modulators in postmenopausal women with uterine leiomyomas: a systematic review. Climacteric. 2001;4:284-92.
4. Baird DD, Dunson DB, Hill MC, et al. High cumulative incidence of uterine leiomyoma in black and white women: ultrasound evidence. Am J Obstet Gynecol. 2003;188:100-7.
5. Bouchard P, Chabbert-Buffet N, Fauser BC. Selective progesterone receptor modulators in reproductive medicine: pharmacology, clinical efficacy and safety. Fertil Steril. 2011;96:1175-89.
6. Bradley LD, Falcone T, Magen AB. Radiographic imaging techniques for the diagnosis of abnormal uterine bleeding. Obstet Gynecol Clin North Am. 2000;27:245-76.
7. Buttram VC, Reiter RC. Uterine leiomyomata: etiology, symptomatology and management. Fertil Steril. 1981;36:433-45.
8. Cardozo ER, Clark AD, Banks NK, et al. The estimated annual cost of uterine leiomyomata in the United States. Am J Obstet Gynecol. 2012;206:211.
9. Carranza-Mamane B, Havelock J, Hemmings R; Reproductive Endocrinology and Infertility Committee. The management of uterine fibroids in women with otherwise unexplained infertility. J Obstet Gynaecol Can. 2015;37:277-85.
10. Chegini N, Ma C, Tang XM, et al. Effects of GnRH analogues, 'add-back' steroid therapy, antiestrogen and antiprogestins on leiomyoma and myometrial smooth muscle cell growth and transforming growth factor-beta expression. Mol Hum Reprod. 2002;8:1071-8.
11. Chwalisz K, Larsen L, Mattia-Goldberg C, et al. A randomized, controlled trial of asoprisnil, a novel selective progesterone receptor modulator, in women with uterine leiomyomata. Fertil Steril. 2007;87:1399-412.
12. Chwalisz K, Perez MC, Demanno D, et al. Selective progesterone receptor modulator development and use in the treatment of leiomyomata and endometriosis. Endocr Rev. 2005;26:423-38.
13. Coulter A, Bradlow J, Agass M, et al. Outcomes of referrals to gynaecology outpatient clinics for menstrual problems: an audit of general practice records. Br J Obstet Gynaecol. 1991;98:789-896.
14. Deng L, Wu T, Chen XY, et al. Selective estrogen receptor modulators (SERMs) for uterine leiomyomas. Cochrane Database Syst Rev. 2012;10:CD005287.
15. DeWaay DJ, Syrop CH, Nygaard IE, et al. Natural history of uterine polyps and leiomyomata. Obstet Gynecol. 2002;100:3-7.
16. Donnez J, Tatarchuk TF, Bouchard P, et al.; PEARL I. Study Group. Ulipristal acetate versus placebo for fibroid treatment before surgery. N Engl J Med. 2012;366:409-20.

17. Donnez J, Tomaszewski J, Va´zquez F, et al.; PEARL II Study Group. Ulipristal acetate versus leuprolide acetate for uterine fibroids. N Engl J Med. 2012;366:421-32.
18. Farquhar C, Ekeroma A, Furness S, et al. A systematic review of transvaginal ultrasonography, sonohysterography and hysteroscopy for the investigation of abnormal uterine bleeding in premenopausal women. Acta Obstet Gynecol Scand. 2003;82:493-504.
19. Fletcher H, Wharfe G, Williams NP, et al. Venous thromboembolism as a complication of uterine fibroids: a retrospective descriptive study. J Obstet Gynaecol. 2009;29(8):732-6.
20. Friedman AJ, Hoffman DI, Comite F, et al. Treatment of leiomyomata uteri with leuprolide acetate depot: a double-blind, placebo-controlled, multicenter study. The Leuprolide Study Group. Obstet Gynecol. 1991;77:720-5.
21. Garcia CR. Management of the symptomatic fibroid in women older than 40 years of age: hysterectomy or myomectomy? Obstet Gynecol Clin North Am. 1993;20:337-48.
22. Gupta JK, Sinha A, Lumsden M, et al. Uterine artery embolization for symptomatic uterine fibroids. Cochrane Database Syst Rev. 2012;5:CD005073.
23. Johnson N, Fletcher H, Reid M. Depo medroxyprogesterone acetate (DMPA) therapy for uterine myomata prior to surgery. Int J Gynecol Obstet. 2004;85(2):174-6.
24. Knight J, Falcone T. Tissue extraction by morcellation: a clinical dilemma. J Min Invas Gynecol. 2014;21:319-20.
25. Leibsohn S, d'Ablaing G, Mishell DR Jr., et al. Leiomyosarcoma in a series of hysterectomies performed for presumed uterine leiomyomas. Am J Obstet Gynecol. 1990;162:968-74; discussion 974-6.
26. Lethaby A, Augood C, Duckitt K. Nonsteroidal anti-inflammatory drugs for heavy menstrual bleeding. Cochrane Database Syst Rev. 2002;(1):CD000400.
27. Lukes AS, Moore KA, Muse KN, et al. Tranexamic acid treatment for heavy menstrual bleeding: a randomized controlled trial. Obstet Gynecol. 2010;116(4):865-75.
28. Lumsden MA, Wallace EM. Clinical presentation of uterine fibroids. Baillieres Clin Obstet Gynaecol. 1998;12:177-95.
29. Makris N, Kalmantis K, Startados N, et al. Three dimensional hysterosonography versus hysteroscopy for the detection of intracavitary uterine abnormalities. Int J Gynecol Obstet. 2007;95:6-9.
30. Malek-Mellouli M, Ben Amara F, Youssef A, et al. Hysteroscopic myomectomy. Tunis Med. 2012; 90:458-62.
31. Marret H, Fritel X, Ouldamer L, et al.; CNGOF (French College of Gynecology and Obstetrics). Therapeutic management of uterine fibroid tumors: updated French guidelines. Eur J Obstet Gynecol Reprod Biol. 2012;165:156-64.
32. Maruo T, Ohara N, Wang J, et al. Sex steroidal regulation of uterine leiomyoma growth and apoptosis. Hum Reprod Update. 2004;10:207-20.
33. Murphy AA, Morales AJ, Kettel LM, et al. Regression of uterine leiomyomata to the antiprogesterone RU486: dose-response effect. Fertil Steril. 1995;64:187-90.
34. Nieman LK, Blocker W, Nansel T, et al. Efficacy and tolerability of CDB-2914 treatment for symptomatic uterine fibroids: a randomized, double-blind, placebo-controlled, phase IIb study. Fertil Steril. 2011;95:767-72.
35. Parker WH, Fu YS, Berek JS. Uterine sarcoma in patients operated on for presumed leiomyoma and rapidly growing leiomyoma. Obstet Gynecol. 1994;83:414-8.
36. Parker WH. Uterine myomas: management. Fertil Steril. 2007;88:255-71.
37. Parsanezhad ME, Azmoon M, Alborzi S, et al. A randomized, controlled clinical trial comparing the effects of aromatase inhibitor (letrozole) and gonadotropin releasing hormone agonist (triptorelin) on uterine leiomyoma volume and hormonal status. Fertil Steril. 2010;93:192-8.
38. Patel A, Malik M, Britten J, et al. Alternative therapies in management of leiomyomas. Fertil Steril. 2014;102:649-55. The study focuses on emerging less-invasive options.
39. Peddada SD, Laughlin SK, Miner K, et al. Growth of uterine leiomyomata among premenopausal black and white women. Proc Natl Acad Sci USA. 2008;105:19887-92.
40. Peng S, Hu L, Chen W, et al. Intraprocedure contrast enhanced ultrasound: the value in assessing the effect of ultrasound-guided high intensity focused ultrasound ablation for uterine fibroids. Ultrasonics. 2015;58:123-8.
41. Rahman M, Berenson AB. Predictors of higher bone mineral density loss and use of depot medroxyprogesterone acetate. Obstet Gynecol. 2010;115(1):35-40.
42. Rauramo I, Elo I, Istre O. Long-term treatment of menorrhagia with levonorgestrel intrauterine system versus endometrial resection. Obstet Gynecol. 2004;104(6):1314-21.

43. Sumitani H, Shozu M, Segawa T, et al. In situ estrogen synthesized by aromatase P450 in uterine leiomyoma cells promotes cell growth probably via an autocrine/intracrine mechanism. Endocrinology. 2000;141:3852-61.
44. Taylor DK, Holthouser K, Segars JH, et al. Recent scientific advances in leiomyoma (uterine fibroids) research facilitates better understanding and management. F1000Res. 2015;4:183.
45. Vercellini P, Crosignani PG, Mangioni C, et al. Treatment with a gonadotrophin releasing hormone agonist before hysterectomy for leiomyomas: results of a multicentre, randomized controlled trial. Br J Obstet Gynaecol. 1998;105:1148-54.
46. Wang PH, Chao HT, Lee WL. Rationale of myomectomy for perimenopausal women. Maturitas. 2007;58:406-7.
47. Weber AM, Mitchinson AR, Gidwani GP, et al. Uterine myomas and factors associated with hysterectomy in premenopausal women. Am J Obstet Gynecol. 1997;176:1213-7.
48. Yoo EH, Lee PI, Huh CY, et al. Predictors of leiomyoma recurrence after laparoscopic myomectomy. J Minim Invasive Gynecol. 2007;14:690-7.

Management of Fibroids in a Menopausal Woman

Selvapriya Saravanan

INTRODUCTION

In many instances, fibroids have been shown to shrink after menopause. This may not be the case always. Fibroids grow due to the amount of estrogen in a woman's body. So, technically, menopause can cause them to stop growing and even shrink. But it may not be enough to make the tumors go away completely.

It has to be kept in mind that postmenopausal woman on hormone replacement therapy (HRT) may experience two-fold increase in incidence of abnormal uterine bleeding (AUB).

CLINICAL PRESENTATION

- Asymptomatic
- Symptomatic
- Asymptomatic becoming symptomatic.

Asymptomatic

- Accidentally diagnosed during regular check-up or follow-up of pre-existing fibroids.
- The size of fibroid, location, HRT, and associated complications determine the management of asymptomatic fibroids.

Symptomatic

- Demands intervention irrespective of size, location, and HRT.
- Commonly associated with AUB, pelvic pain, pressure, and urinary urgency.

Asymptomatic becoming Symptomatic

- Possibility of malignancy should be ruled out first.
- HRT should be discontinued.
- Expectant management should be considered only if patient is not fit for surgery.

DIAGNOSIS

- Clinical history
- Clinical examination

Fibroids

- Investigations—ultrasonography (USG). Pelvis is gold standard.
  - Magnetic resonance imaging (MRI), if any associated pelvic pathology is suspected.

MANAGEMENT (FLOWCHART 9.1)

Expectant Management

Indications

- Asymptomatic fibroids
- Associated complications ruled out promptly
- Size less than 12 weeks
- Incidentally noticed:
  - Regular follow-up every 6 months
  - Routine pelvic examination
  - Baseline imaging to compare regression.

Medical Management

Indications

- Patient not fit for surgery
- Patient not willing for surgery
- When HRT in cause for the size of fibroid increase
- Temporary relief of symptoms for short period.

It has to be kept in mind that the effects are always short-term.
- Nonsteroidal anti-inflammatory drugs (NSAIDs) and tranexamic acid to control bleeding
- Gonadotropin-releasing hormone (GnRH) analogs for short-term in HRT patients
- Add back—tibolone, raloxifene, progesterone alone, estrogens alone, and combined estrogens and progesterones

Flowchart 9.1: Management of fibroid in a postmenopausal woman.

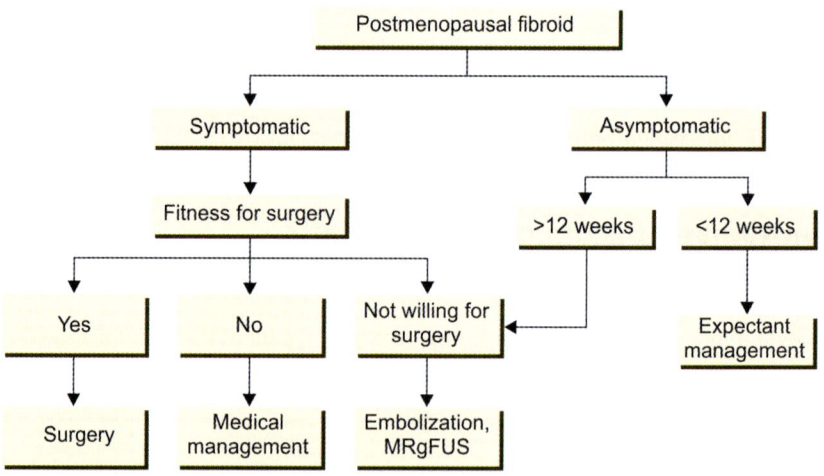

(MRgFUS: Magnetic resonance imaging-guided focused ultrasound)

- Selective estrogen receptor modulator (SERM) and aromatase inhibitors
- Antiprogesterones 5–10 mg/day for 1 year.

Surgical Management

- Myomectomy
- Hysterectomy
- Newer conservative methods
- Uterine fibroid embolization:
  - Minimally invasive procedure
  - Outpatient procedure or takes less than an hour
  - Recovery time is as short as 11 days.

Procedure

A small incision is made on the femoral artery and a catheter is inserted till it reaches artery to fibroid. Little spheres of embolic material are injected to the vessels supplying the tumor. Thus, blocking the supply and resulting in shrinkage.

MRI-guided Focused Ultrasound

- MRI-guided focused ultrasound (MRgFUS) is a noninvasive method of thermal ablation.
- MRI allows for 3D treatment planning and feedback of temperature deposition in the area to be treated.
- Suggested for safely-located symptomatic fibroids.
- Does not require anesthesia and hospital stay.
- Fibroid shrinkage can be seen in 6 months and sustains for 2 plus years.
- About 16–20% patients will require an additional treatment.

Counseling

- Need to concentrate on bone density should be emphasized.
- Patient not opting for surgeries should be given the follow-up chart.
- HRT should be stopped, if risks outweigh benefits.
- Patients must be encouraged to have a healthy and active lifestyle.
- After surgery:
  - HRT can be restarted 6 month after surgery after ensuring nonexistence of fibroid.

Risk of Malignancy

- Large fibroid, long standing are prone for degenerative changes.
- Long-standing degenerations rarely (0.5–1%) end up in sarcomatous change.
- Endometrial biopsy prior to surgical management is very safe.

Implications of HRT in Presence of Fibroid

- HRT should be stopped, if fibroid become symptomatic or increases in size.
- HRT can be continued, if fibroid size does not show any increase and no history of AUB persists.
- Following surgery HRT can be restarted after 6 months after ensuring normalcy.
- HRT is not advisable following embolization and MRgFUS.

Follow-up

- Biannual visits for 2 years after surgery
- If patient is asymptomatic:
  - Regular follow-up once in 6 months
  - Pelvic examination and USG to assess size of fibroid.

CONCLUSION

Hormone replacement therapy has major influence on postmenopausal fibroids. Symptomatic or asymptomatic, the size of fibroid and location determine the management of postmenopausal fibroids. The newer modalities like fibroid artery embolization and MRgFUS are showing good response and thus are gaining attention. Postmenopausal fibroids when symptomatic should be treated with additional alertness. Patients should be counseled regarding the follow-up and cautioned about the complications, which could be anticipated when HRT is discontinued, importance should be given for alternate methods of managing the postmenopausal flushes and bone mineral density by lifestyle modifications healthy diet and supplements. Regular follow-up of these patients will avoid further complications.

BIBLIOGRAPHY

1. Bourlev V, Pavlovitch S, Stygar D, et al. Different proliferative and apoptotic activity in peripheral versus central parts of human uterine leiomyomas. Gynecol Obstet Invest. 2003;55:199-204.
2. Bouwsma EV, Gorny KR, Hesley GK, et al. Magnetic resonance-guided focused ultrasound surgery for leiomyoma-associated infertility. Fertil Steril. 2011;96:e9-e12.
3. Bouwsma EV, Hesley GK, Woodrum DA, et al. Comparing focused ultrasound and uterine artery embolization for uterine fibroids—rationale and design of the Fibroid Interventions: Reducing symptoms Today and Tomorrow (FIRSTT) trial. Fertil Steril. 2011;96:704-10.
4. Chudnoff SG, Berman JM, Levine DJ, et al. Outpatient procedure for the treatment and relief of symptomatic uterine myomas. Obstet Gynecol. 2013;121:1075-82.
5. Donnez J, Tomaszewki J, Vazquez F, et al. Ulipristal acetate versus leuprolide acetate for uterine fibroids. N Engl J Med. 2012;366:421-32.
6. Friedman AJ. Combined oestrogen–progestin treatment of vaginal hemorrhage following gonadotropin-releasing hormone agonist therapy of uterine myomas. Hum Reprod. 1993;8:540-2.
7. Ghezzi F, Cromi A, Bergamini V, et al. Midterm outcome of radio frequency thermal ablation for symptomatic uterine myomas. Surg Endosc. 2007;21:2081-5.
8. Goldrath MH. Uterine tamponade for the control of acute uterine bleeding. Am J Obstet Gynecol. 1983;147:869-72.
9. Hamini Y, Ben-Shachar I, kailash Y, et al. Intrauterine balloon tamponade as a treatment for immune thrombocytopenic purpura-induced severe uterine bleeding. Fertil Steril. 2010;94:2769. e13-e5.
10. Lakhani KP, Marsh MS, Purcell W, et al. Uterine artery blood flow parameters in women with dysfunctional uterine bleeding and uterine fibroids: the effects of tranexamic acid. Ultrasound Obstet Gynecol. 1998;11:23-8.
11. Lindoff C, Rybo G, Astedt B. Treatment with tranexamic acid during pregnancy, and the risk of thromboembolic complications. Thromb Haemost. 1993;70:238-40.
12. Lukes AS, Moore KA, Mue KN, et al. Tranexamic acid treatment for heavy menstrual bleeding: a randomized controlled trial. Obstet Gynecol. 2010;116(4):865-75.
13. Munro MG; Southern California Permanente Medical Group's Abnormal Uterine Bleeding Working Group. Acute uterine bleeding unrelated to pregnancy: a Southern California Permanente Medical Group practice guideline. Perm J. 2013;17:43-56.
14. Naoulou B, Tsai MC. Efficacy of tranexamic acid in the treatment of idiopathic and nonfunctional heavy menstrual bleeding: a systematic review. Acta Obstet Gynecol Scand. 2012;91:529-37.
15. National Institute for Health and Clinical Excellence (NICE). (2011). IPG 413: Magnetic resonance image-guided transcutaneous focused ultra sound for uterine fibroids. [online] Available from

https://www.nice.org.uk/guidance/ipg413/resources/magnetic-resonance-imageguided-transcutaneous-focused-ultrasound-for-uterine-fibroids-pdf-1899869566932421. [Accessed September, 2018].
16. Pansky M, Cowan BD, Frank M, et al. Laparoscopically assisted uterine fibroid cryoablation. Am J Obstet Gynecol. 2009;201:571-7.
17. Sundstrom A, Seaman H, Kieler H, et al. The risk of venous thromboembolism associated with the use of tranexamic acid and other drugs used to treat Menorrhagia: a case–control study using the General Practice Research Database. BJOG. 2009;116:91-7.
18. Thomas MA, Gass ML, Scott MC, et al. Multiple therapies for vaginal bleeding secondary to large uterine myomas. Int J Gynaecol Obstet. 1991;36:239-41.
19. Thoro JM, Katz VL. Submucous myomas treated with gonadotropin-releasing hormone agonist and resulting in vaginal hemorrhage. A case report. J Reprod Med. 1991;36:625-6.
20. Zupi E, Sbracia M, Marcoin D, et al. Myolysis of uterine fibroids: Is there a role? Clin Obstet Gynecol. 2006;49:821-33.

Can We Leave Fibroids Alone?

Anuradha Khar

INTRODUCTION

Fibroids or leiomyomas are the most common gynecological tumors. Studies have shown that by the age of 50 years up to 70–80% of women may have fibroids when tested by ultrasonography for various indications. In the reproductive age group, various reports suggest the prevalence between 10% and 30%.

In India, the Ministry of Health data suggests that fibroids are found in 20% women in the reproductive age group. Uterine fibroids account for nearly 30% of all hysterectomies worldwide.

Treatment of uterine fibroids must be based on—*symptoms, size, and location* of the fibroids, age, comorbidities, and surgical risk for the patient, desire of the patient to preserve both fertility and uterus, and also the economic cost to the patient and community.

The question of conservative versus surgical treatment of uterine fibroids should address the following issues:
- Is there a role for conservative treatment in symptomatic women?
- Is there a need to treat asymptomatic women, either in the reproductive or in the postmenopausal age group?

SYMPTOMATIC FIBROIDS (BOX 10.1)

Abnormal Uterine Bleeding, Pain and Pressure Symptoms due to Fibroids

- Before planning surgical treatment for fibroids, it must be ascertained that the symptoms of abnormal uterine bleeding (AUB) or pelvic pain are due to the fibroid. Small, incidentally detected fibroids may be unrelated to the bleeding, pain or pressure symptoms.
- Submucous fibroids have been implicated in causation of AUB. Nearly 25% women with AUB were found to have submucous fibroids in a systematic review.
- Patients with symptomatic fibroids show excellent clinical response to both hysterectomy as well less invasive procedures such as myomectomy or newer modalities like uterine artery embolization (UAE) or MR-guided focused ultrasound surgery.
- *Conservative treatment for myomas and AUB*: Expectant management with levonorgestrel intrauterine system (LNG-IUS) or tranexamic acid may be effective in a proportion of patients with fibroids and AUB.
- Hysterectomy and myomectomy, both laparoscopic and hysteroscopic, have associated morbidity and risks. These procedures are to be advised only after conservative treatment is deemed inappropriate or failed.

Box 10.1: Clinical effects of fibroids.

Menstrual symptoms
   Menorrhagia
   Intermenstrual bleeding
   Anemia
Pressure effects
   Urinary symptoms: Frequency or retention; hydroureters or hydronephrosis; constipation; venous edema; venous thrombosis
Pain
   Spasmodic dysmenorrhea
   Pain due to degeneration or infarction
Fibroid degeneration
Infection
Infertility
Complications during pregnancy:
Red degeneration, placenta previa, intrauterine growth restriction (IUGR), fetal malpresentation, obstructed labor, postpartum hemorrhage, and puerperal infection
Malignant transformation

- Similarly, techniques such as UAE have been compared with conservative treatment for uterine fibroids and it was shown that there was no significant difference in satisfaction rates between the two groups in spite of a higher rate of post-procedural complications and further re-interventions in the UAE arm.

Infertility Associated with Fibroids

The association of fibroids and infertility is a matter of debate.
- About 5–10% of women with infertility have fibroids in various numbers. But only 1–2% women with no other cause of infertility are found to have myomas.
- Women with submucous myomas compared with infertile women without such myomas showed significantly lower clinical pregnancy rates, implantation rates, and live birth rates. The same study also showed that higher spontaneous abortion rates are seen in women with submucous myomas.
- Pregnancy rates are higher after hysteroscopic myomectomy for submucous myomas than no or "placebo" procedures.
- There is no evidence to suggest that subserosal and intramural myomas impact clinical pregnancy rates or live birth rates. Therefore, there is no indication for surgical management of these fibroids in women with otherwise unexplained infertility.

Fibroids and Pregnancy

- The estimated incidence of fibroids in pregnancy depends on the trimester of examination and size threshold for diagnosis. In one study of 72,373 women undergoing routine second-trimester examination, 3.2% were found to have myomas.
- Contrary to popular view, during pregnancy, fibroid sizes remain relatively stable in nearly 60% of cases, increase in about a quarter of the patients, and actually shrink in up to 20% patients.
- An increased risk of malpresentation, cesarean delivery, and preterm birth is seen in pregnancies associated with fibroids.
- Also, a higher incidence of placenta previa, abruption, premature rupture of membranes, and intrauterine fetal death were reported from an analysis of 72,000 pregnancies, but the frequency of complications was considered low.

- For a large majority of pregnant women with fibroids, expectant management with adequate analgesia is all that is warranted.
- Prior to pregnancy, myomectomy can be considered in patients with recurrent unexplained pregnancy loss.
- Myomectomy during the first and second trimester have been reported to be safe, in case of:
  - Intractable pain from a degenerating fibroid
  - Painful subserosal or pedunculated fibroid
  - Large or rapidly growing fibroid
  - Large fibroid in the lower segment.
- Therefore, most patients with fibroids diagnosed during pregnancy can be treated conservatively, although the ones with large fibroids may need close monitoring during antenatal period.

ASYMPTOMATIC WOMEN (FLOWCHART 10.1)

- Nearly 50% of all women with fibroids are asymptomatic. In fact, a large number of women may not get noticed clinically.
- There is no evidence to suggest that incidentally detected asymptomatic fibroids require treatment. In a study comparing conservative treatment versus surgery for fibroids presenting with AUB or chronic pelvic pain, it was seen that in women with fibroids with minimal or no symptoms had no worsening in quality of life or symptom status when managed conservatively.
- Patients who come to know that they have fibroids may suffer from anxiety related to general health, fertility, pregnancy course as well as malignant transformation. Such patients need adequate counseling.
- Patient's desire to get treated, comorbid medical conditions, and cost should be important consideration in patients with mild to moderate symptoms. This is especially important for women with symptoms who have small fibroids but are close to menopause.

Flowchart 10.1: Managing uterine fibroids.

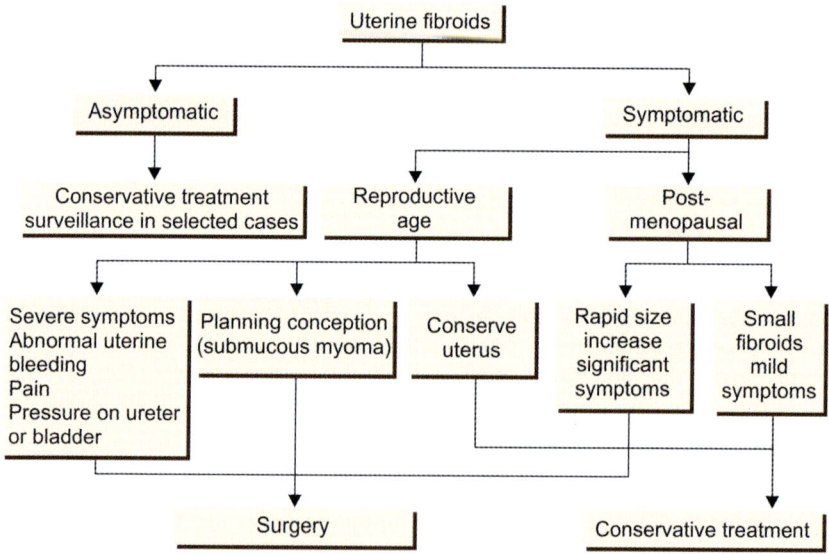

- *Shrinkage of myomas*: Small fibroids and fibroids in older women tend to regress. Therefore, it is recommended that in women in late reproductive years who have minimal symptoms, waiting for menopause and possible regression of the tumor is perhaps more desirable than surgery.

IMPACT ON QUALITY OF LIFE

- In addition to direct symptoms, women diagnosed with fibroids report concerns about fibroids affecting overall physical and emotional health. In one study, 20–40% of women with symptomatic fibroids reported feeling depressed and worn out.
- Women who are incidentally detected to have fibroids also exhibit signs of anxiety including that of *malignant transformation*.
- In a large review of patients undergoing myomectomy, only 18 out of 6,815 patients (0.26%) had leiomyosarcomas. This rate was similar even in those patients in whom the myomas had grown rapidly, suggesting that rapid growth of a fibroid alone does not seem to be a predictor of leiomyosarcoma. Therefore, patients incidentally found to myomas who are otherwise asymptomatic need not be treated for suspected or prevention of malignancy.

CONCLUSION

- The true incidence of uterine myomas may be underestimated. Up to 30% women in reproductive age and nearly 70% women by the age of 50 years may have fibroids.
- About half of all patients with fibroids are asymptomatic.
- Asymptomatic women with myomas should be treated conservatively. The only exception is perhaps rapidly growing myomas, especially in the post-menopausal.
- Mild to moderate symptoms of abnormal uterine bleeding, pain and pressure symptoms should be managed conservatively with analgesics, hematinics, and even expectant management.
- Levonorgestrel-releasing intrauterine contraceptive devices and tranexamic acid is useful in treatment of less severe AUB associated with leiomyomas.
- Hysterectomy, myomectomy or other nonsurgical procedures such as UAE and MR-guided focused ultrasound treatment are all effective. However, nonconservative treatment should depend on symptoms, nature of the fibroids, age, and comorbidities of the patient that determine surgical and patients' expectation in terms of fertility and uterine preservation in addition to cost.
- Fibroids cause infertility in a small number of patients, especially when submucous in location. In such cases, surgical treatment is recommended. However, in case of subserosal and intramural myomas, there is no evidence that surgical management is superior to conservative treatment to improve chances of conception.
- Most fibroids associated with pregnancy are to be treated conservatively. In select cases, large fibroids especially in the lower segment, those causing intractable pain or fibroids growing rapidly may be subjected to first or second trimester myomectomy.
- Fibroids cause an impact on psychological quality of life. Anxiety regarding malignant transformation is seen in patients incidentally detected to have fibroids. Prophylactic surgery to prevent complications of pregnancy or malignancy is of no proven benefit. Such patients should be actively counseled.

Thus, asymptomic fibroids of up to 5 cm intramural fibroid and up to 7 cm subserosal can be left as such with active proper counseling and proper follow-up with scan after 6 months to see changes in fibroid. Submucosal are most of the time symptomatic and treatment is required. Specially in perimenopausal and postmenopausal women asymptomatic fibroids can be ignored provided proper counseling and follow-up schedule has been given to the patient.

BIBLIOGRAPHY

1. Baird DD, Dunson DB, Hill MC, et al. High cumulative incidence of uterine leiomyoma in black and white women: ultrasound evidence. Am J Obstet Gynecol. 2003;188:100-7.
2. Carlson KJ, Miller BA, Fowler FJ. The Maine women's Health study: II. Outcomes of non-surgical management of leiomyomas, abnormal bleeding and chronic pelvic pain. Obstet Gynecol. 1994;83:566-72.
3. Cook H, Ezzati M, Segars JH, et al. The impact of uterine leiomyomas on reproductive outcomes. Minerva Gynecol. 2010;62:225-36.
4. De Carolis S, Fatigante G, Ferrazzani S, et al. Uterine myomectomy in pregnant women. Fetal Diagn Ther. 2001;16:116-9.
5. DeWaay DJ, Syrop CH, Nygaard IE, et al. Natural history of uterine polyps and leiomyomata. Obstet Gynecol. 2002;100:3-7.
6. Donnez J, Jadoul P. What are the implications of myomas on fertility? A need for a debate? Hum Reprod. 2002;17:1424-30.
7. Gupta JK, Sinha A, Lumsden M, et al. Uterine artery embolization for symptomatic uterine fibroids. Cochrane Database Syst Rev. 2012;5:CD005073.
8. Klatsky PC, Tran ND, Caughey AB, et al. Fibroids and reproductive outcomes: a systematic literature review from conception to delivery. Am J Obstet Gynecol. 2008;198:357-66.
9. Lethaby A, Vollenhoven B, Sowter M. Efficacy of pre-operative gonadotrophin releasing hormone analogues for women with uterine fibroids undergoing hysterectomy or myomectomy: a systematic review. BJOG. 2002;109:1097-108.
10. Marshall LM, Spiegelman D, Barbieri RL, et al. Variation in the incidence of uterine leiomyoma among premenopausal women by age and race. Obstet Gynecol. 1997;90:967-73.
11. Neiger R, Sonek JD, Croom CS, et al. Pregnancy-related changes in the size of uterine leiomyomas. J Reprod Med, 2006;51:671-4.
12. Parker WH, Fu YS, Berek JS. Uterine sarcoma in patients operated on for presumed leiomyoma and rapidly growing leiomyoma. Obstet Gynecol. 1994;83:414-8.
13. Pritts EA, Parker WH, Olive DL. Fibroids and infertility: an updated systematic review of the evidence Fertil Steril. 2009;91:1215-23.
14. Sawin SW, Pilevsky ND, Berlin JA, et al. Comparability of perioperative morbidity between abdominal myomectomy and hysterectomy for women with uterine leiomyomas. Am J Obstet Gynecol. 2000;183(6):1448-55.
15. Shokeir T, El-Shafei M, Yousef H, et al. Submucous myomas and their implication sin the pregnancy rates of patients with otherwise unexplained primary infertility undergoing hysteroscopic myomectomy: A randomized matched control study. Fertil Steril. 2010;94:724-9.
16. Soysal S, Soysal ME. The efficacy of levonorgestrel-releasing intrauterine device in selected cases of myoma-related menorrhagia: a prospective controlled trial. Gynecol Obstet Invest. 2005;59:29-35.
17. Stewart EA, Nicholson WK, Bradley L, et al. The burden of uterine fibroids for African-American women: results of a national survey. J Women's Health. 2013;22:807-16.
18. Stewart EA, Rabinovici J, Tempany CM, et al. Clinical outcomes of focused ultrasound surgery for the treatment of uterine fibroids. Fertil Steril. 2006;85:22-9.
19. Stout MJ, Odibo AO, Graseck AS, et al. Leiomyomas at routine second-trimester ultrasound examination and adverse obstetric outcomes. Obstet Gynecol. 2010;116:1056.
20. van Dongen H, de Kroon CD, Jacobi CE, et al. Diagnostic hysteroscopy in abnormal uterine bleeding: a systematic review and meta-analysis. BJOG. 2007;114:664-75.
21. Walker WJ, Pelage JP. Uterine artery embolization for symptomatic fibroids: Clinical results in 400 women with imaging follow-up. Br J Obstet Gynecol. 2002;109:1263-72.

Surgical Management of Fibroids

Rajalaxmi Walavalkar, Garima Sharma, Vimee Bindra

INTRODUCTION

The terms fibroid, myoma, and leiomyoma are synonymous. They are the most common gynecological tumors. The prevalence increases with age and reaches at peak in women in their 40s.

Myomas are usually asymptomatic and are found incidentally on either clinical examination or pelvic imaging. However, myomas can lead to significant morbidity by causing menstrual irregularities (heavy, irregular, and prolonged bleeding), fertility issues, pelvic pressure or pain, obstructive symptoms, and iron-deficiency anemia.

BASIS OF SELECTING PATIENT FOR SURGERY

- Abnormal uterine bleeding (AUB) not responsive to medical management
- Pressure symptoms
- Infertility
- Associated pathology such as ovarian mass, endometriosis, or adenomyosis
- Rapid growth of the tumor
- Persistent growth even after menopause.

PLANNING OF SURGERY

The factors to be considered during planning of surgery:
- Appropriate indication
- Fertility concerns
- Accurate mapping of the location, size, and number of fibroids with preoperative imaging
- Surgeon's training, experience, and comfort
- Building of hemoglobin
- Counseling the patient about implications of surgery, types and route of surgery, complications (immediate and long-term), and recurrence rate.

Counseling

A detailed patient counseling should be done and should include following points:
- Various management options should be explained with their respective advantages and disadvantages.
- Possibility of recurrence of symptoms and fibroid regrowth with conservative, medical, and uterus-preserving surgeries.

- Possibility of conversion to hysterectomy, while performing myomectomy should be explained and an informed consent should be taken before performing the procedure.
- Intraoperative blood loss and, hence, need for blood transfusion to be explained.

Types of Surgery and Routes (Tables 11.1 and 11.2)

- Myomectomy can be performed through following routes:
  - Laparoscopy
  - Hysteroscopy
  - Robotic
  - Laparotomy.
- Hysterectomy can be performed through following routes:
  - Laparoscopy
  - Abdominal

Table 11.1: Comparison of various routes of surgery.

Features	Laparoscopic	Hysteroscopic	Open
Duration of surgery	Short	Short	Long
Hospital stay	1–2 days	1–2 days	3–5 days
Resumption of activities	Early	Early	Late
Postoperative pain	Less	Less	More
Complications	Injury to adjacent organs	Fluid imbalance Perforation Bleeding Intrauterine adhesion formation in case of removal of type 2 fibroids	Injury to adjacent organs Bleeding Intra-abdominal adhesions

Table 11.2: Comparison of various surgeries for fibroid.

Features	Hysterectomy	Myomectomy	Endometrial ablation
Advantages	Definitive surgery and hence no recurrence	Preserves uterus	Only requires vaginal insertion Preserves uterus
Disadvantages	Surgical risks of infection, bleeding, and anesthesia complications	Surgical risks of infection, bleeding, and anesthesia complications Recurrence	Contraindicated, if woman is attempting for pregnancy Treats only symptoms and not fibroid Regrowth of fibroid
Duration of procedure	1.5–3 hours	1–3 hours	45 minutes
Surgery	Yes	Yes	No
Duration of hospital stay	1–5 days	1–3 days	Day care procedure
Efficacy	100%	80%	NA
Fertility preserved	No	Yes	Contraindicated

- Vaginal
- Robotic.
- Endometrial ablation.

Choice of Surgery

Following factors should be considered before deciding the type and route of surgery:
- Patient desire for fertility and/or to preserve uterus.
- Surgeon's skill, experience, and comfort
- Fibroid mapping by imaging to determine number, location, and size of fibroids.
- Any other associated pelvic pathology.
- Suspected malignancy.

According to the Society of Obstetricians and Gynaecologists (SOGC) Clinical Practice Guideline 2015: The Management of Uterine Leiomyomas

- Treatment of women with uterine leiomyomas must be individualized based on symptomatology, size and location of fibroids, age, need, and desire of the patient to preserve fertility or the uterus, the availability of therapy, and the experience of the therapist. (Level of Evidence III-B)
- Concern about possible complications related to fibroids in pregnancy is not an indication for myomectomy except in women who have had a previous pregnancy with complications related to these fibroids. (III)
- Hysterectomy is the most effective treatment for symptomatic uterine fibroids. (III)
- In women who do not wish to preserve fertility and/or their uterus and who have been counseled regarding the alternatives and risks, hysterectomy by the least invasive approach possible may be offered as the definitive treatment for symptomatic uterine fibroids and is associated with a high level of satisfaction. (II-2A)
- Myomectomy is an option for women who wish to preserve their uterus or enhance fertility, but carries the risk of requiring further intervention. (II-2)
- Hysteroscopic myomectomy should be considered first-line conservative surgical therapy for the management of symptomatic intracavitary fibroids. (II-3A)

MYOMECTOMY

Principles

- Removal of as many fibroids as is feasible through least number of uterine incisions.
- Main incision to be placed over the largest fibroid and other fibroids should be approached through tunneling incisions in the uterine bed.
- The incisions should be placed carefully in order to avoid impinging on the cornua and involvement or kinking of Fallopian tubes.
- Vertical incisions are preferred for anterior and posterior wall fibroids. Transverse incisions are preferred for fundal fibroids to avoid kinking of tubes.
- Adequate hemostasis.

Hemostasis during Myomectomy

Various methods to reduce intraoperative blood loss and ensure hemostasis:
- Vasoconstrictive agents such as synthetic vasopressin (Pitressin 20 units diluted in 20 mL of saline).

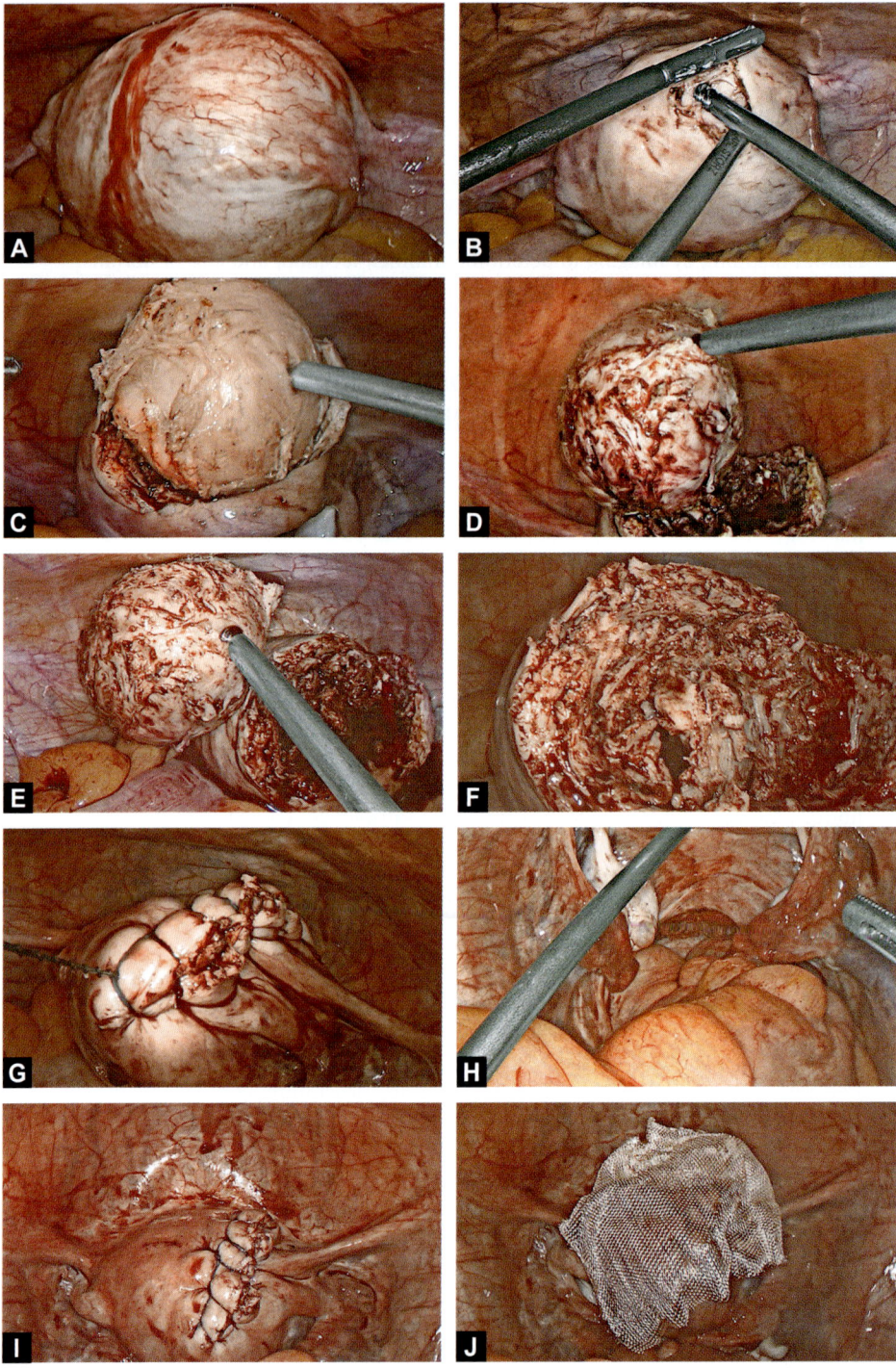

Figs. 11.1A to J: (A) Fundal right cornual fibroid after vasopressin injection; (B) Incision on fibroid surface; (C to E) Stepwise slow enucleation of fibroid; (F) After comlete enucleation; (G) Stitching with barbed suture; (H) Inspecting pod for collection; (I) Inspecting anterior surface for confirming hemostasis; (J) Putting interceed to prevent adhesions.

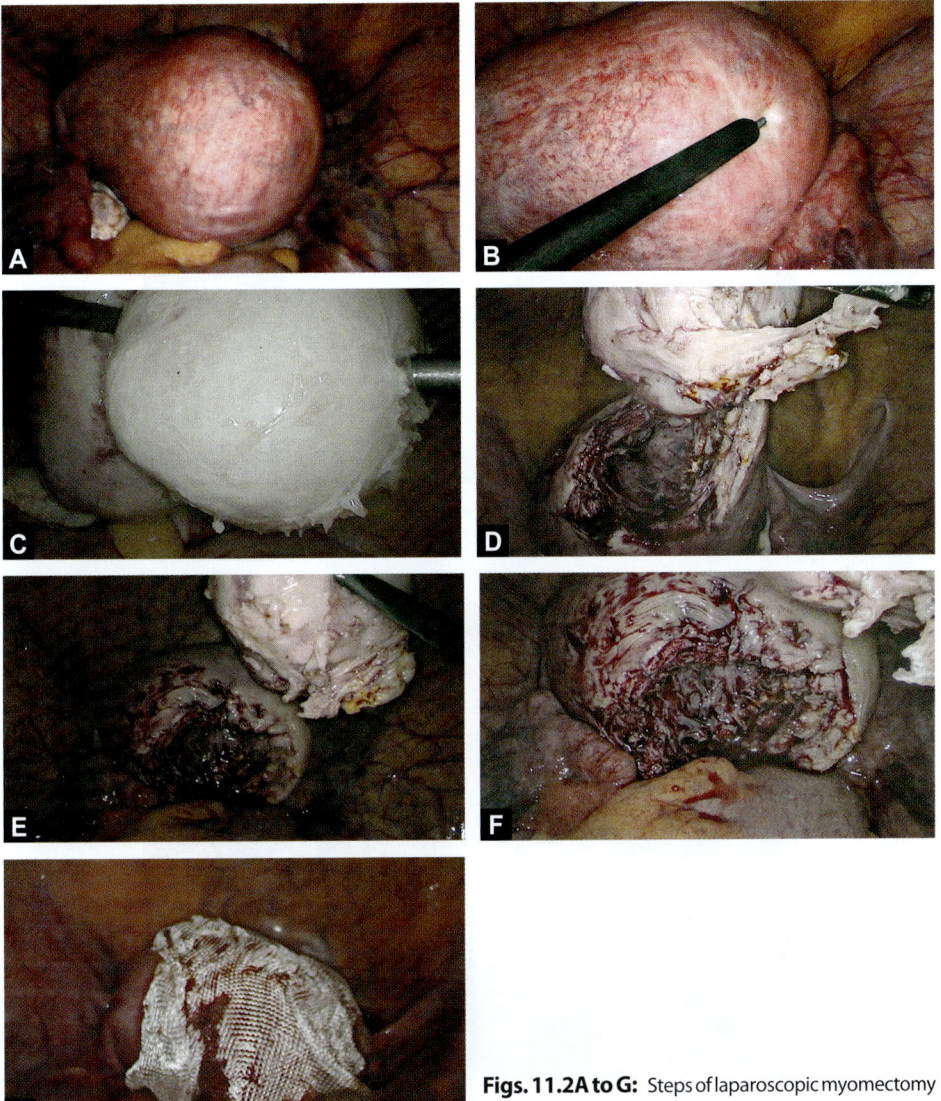

Figs. 11.2A to G: Steps of laparoscopic myomectomy in an intramural fibroid.

- 1:300,000 adrenaline, another vasoconstrictive agent can also be used. However, its use is contraindicated in women with hypertension, cardiac arrhythmias, and vascular insufficiency.
- *Bonney's myomectomy clamp*: It compresses the uterine vessels between lateral uterine walls and round ligaments. Simultaneously, ovarian vessels are compressed by placing the sponge holding forceps on the infundibulopelvic ligaments. This technique effectively reduces pulse pressure in the uterine and ovarian vessels.
- Use of tourniquets encircling the cervix along with rubber-shod clamps placed over infundibulopelvic ligaments.
- Use of lasers or harmonics.

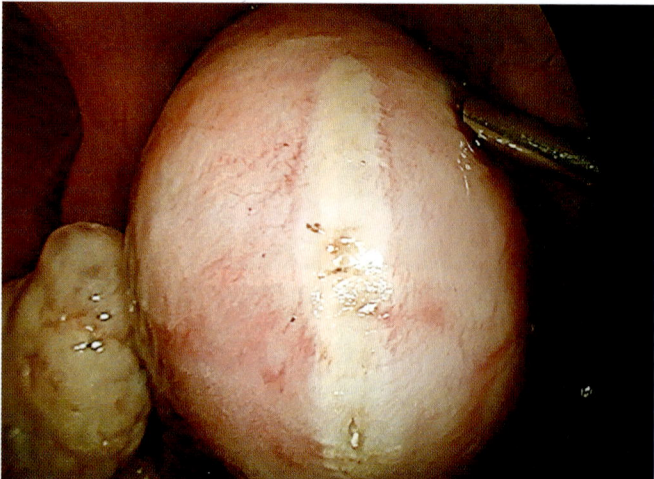

Fig. 11.3: Blenching the fibroid after giving vasopressin before giving incision.

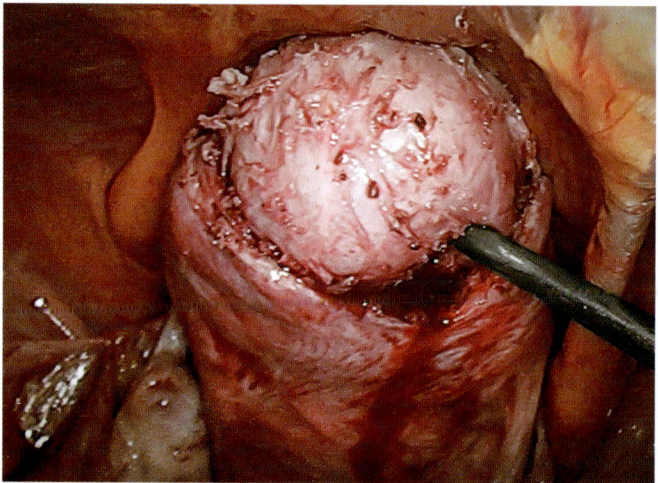

Fig. 11.4: Slow enucleation.

- Reduction of mean blood pressure by use of regional anesthesia, ganglion blockers such as phentolamine, vasodilators, and the Trendelenburg position.

According to Cochrane review 2014, 18 randomized controlled trials (RCTs) with 1,250 participants were studied. The authors concluded:
- At present, there is moderate-quality evidence that misoprostol or vasopressin may reduce bleeding during myomectomy.
- Low-quality evidence that bupivacaine plus epinephrine, tranexamic acid, gelatin–thrombin matrix, ascorbic acid, dinoprostone, loop ligation, a fibrin sealant patch, a pericervical tourniquet or a tourniquet tied round both cervix, and infundibulopelvic ligament may reduce bleeding during myomectomy.

- There is no evidence that oxytocin, morcellation, and temporary clipping of the uterine artery reduce blood loss.
- Further well-designed studies are required to establish the effectiveness, safety, and costs of different interventions for reducing blood loss during myomectomy.

HYSTEROSCOPIC MYOMECTOMY

European Society of Gastrointestinal Endoscopy (ESGE) classification of submucous myomas:
- *Type 0*: Entirely within endometrial cavity and no myometrial extension (pedunculated)
- *Type I*: Less than 50% myometrial extension (sessile), less than 90° angle of myoma surface to uterine wall.
- *Type II*: More than or equal to 50% myometrial extension (sessile), more than or equal to 90° angle of myoma surface to uterine wall.

The first and most common hysteroscopic technique for myomectomy is transcervical resectoscopic myomectomy (TCRM) with a modified urological resectoscope. This was first reported in 1976.

However, now various hysteroscopic techniques are available for dissection, vaporization, or morcellation and excision of submucous myomas. Submucous myomas (types 0, 1, and 2) up to 4–5 cm diameter can be effectively removed by hysteroscopic route in the hands of an experienced surgeon. Larger and multiple myomas (more than 3) are best removed abdominally. Multistaged procedure is usually required for type 2 myomas.

One of the greatest concerns to the hysteroscopic surgeon is the risk of perforation. An abdominal approach is appropriate when the submucous myoma is a type 1-5 or 2-5, i.e. traversing the myometrium and reaching the uterine serosa. In such circumstances, resectoscopic myomectomy may be neither feasible nor safe.

American Association of Gynecologic Laparoscopists (AAGL) Practice Report: Practice Guidelines for the Diagnosis and Management of Submucous Leiomyomas 2012

- For women desiring future fertility, or who are currently infertile, an abdominal approach to submucous myomectomy should be considered when there are three or more submucous myomas or in other circumstances where hysteroscopic myomectomy might be anticipated to damage a large portion of the endometrial surface.
- Hysteroscopic myomectomy with the removal of the entire myoma is effective for the relief of heavy menstrual bleeding.
- If hysteroscopic myomectomy is performed for AUB, and future fertility is not an issue, concomitant endometrial ablation may reduce the risk of subsequent uterine surgery.
- Postoperative bleeding can be managed either with intracervical prostaglandin F2α (carboprost) or with tamponade by use of an inflated balloon catheter.
- Distention media complications can be minimized with strict monitoring of fluid deficit, preferably with weighted monitoring systems and the adherence to institutionally predetermined fluid loss guidelines.
- The risk of monopolar current diversion resulting in lower genital tract burns may be reduced by maintaining contact of the external sheath with the cervix, avoiding activation of the electrosurgical unit when the electrode is not in contact with tissue, ensuring the sustained integrity of the electrode insulation, and minimizing the use of high-voltage ("coagulation") current when performing hysteroscopic submucous myomectomy.

86 *Fibroids*

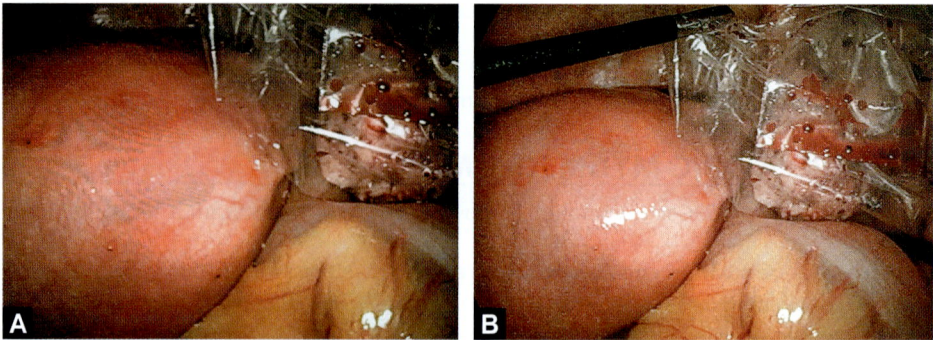

Figs. 11.5A and B: Putting the encleated myoma in the plastic endo bag.

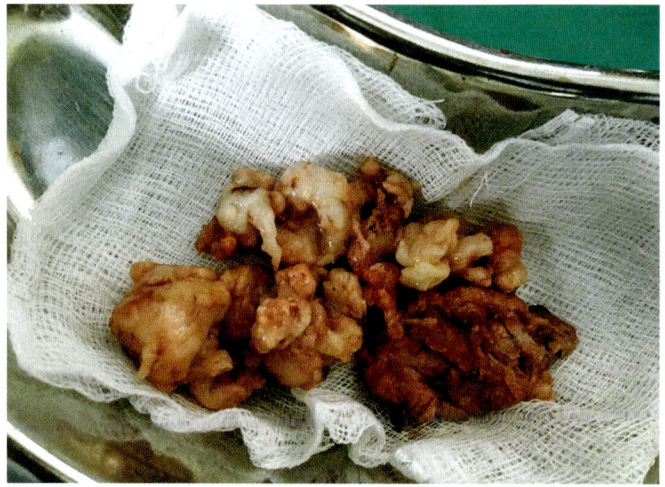

Fig. 11.6: Piecemeal removal from endo bag.

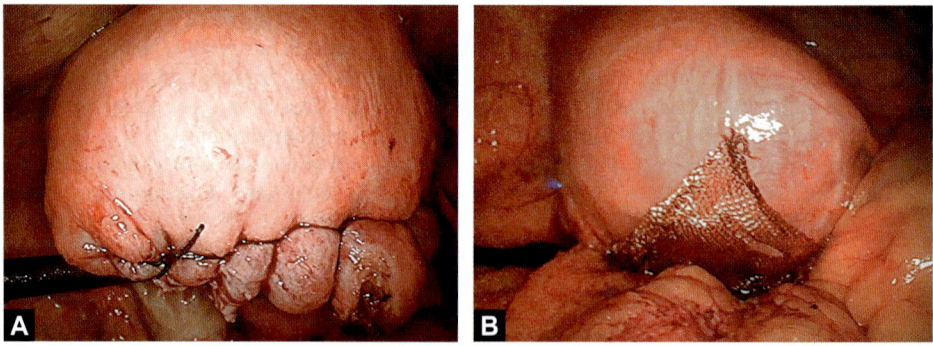

Figs. 11.7A and B: Covering the scar with interceed.

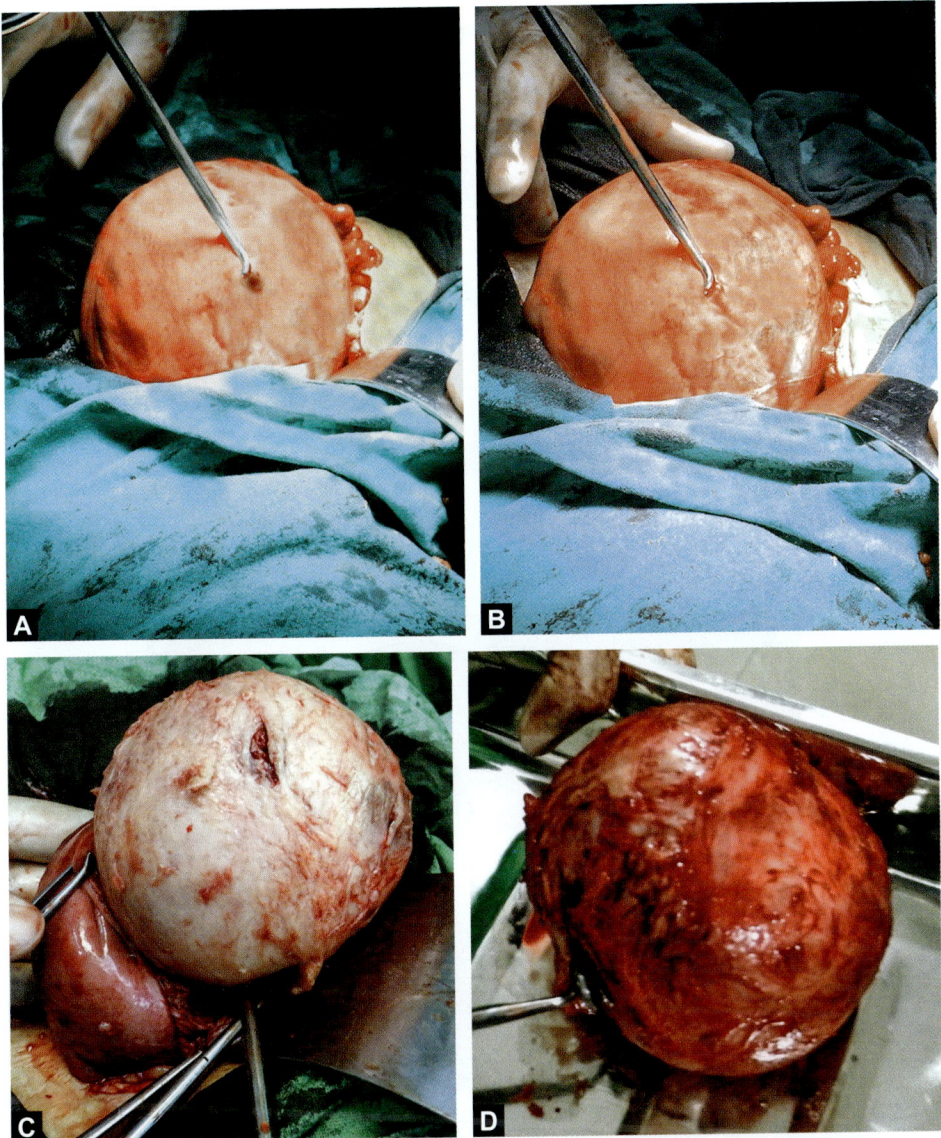

Figs. 11.8A to D: Steps of open myomectomy.

- Postmyomectomy intrauterine synechiae are more common after multiple submucous myomectomies. In such circumstances, and when fertility is an issue, second look hysteroscopy and appropriate adhesiolysis should be considered.

Advantages of Hysteroscopic Resection
- Decreased hospitalization
- Less pain
- Less operative morbidity

88 *Fibroids*

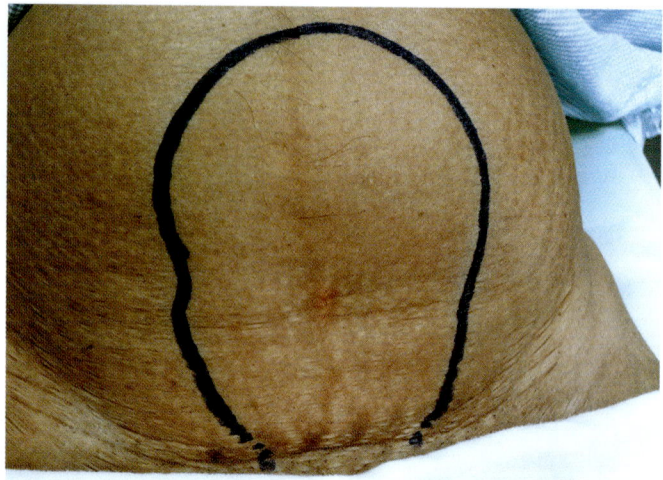

Fig. 11.9: Large myoma evident on P/A in perimenopausal lady marking done.

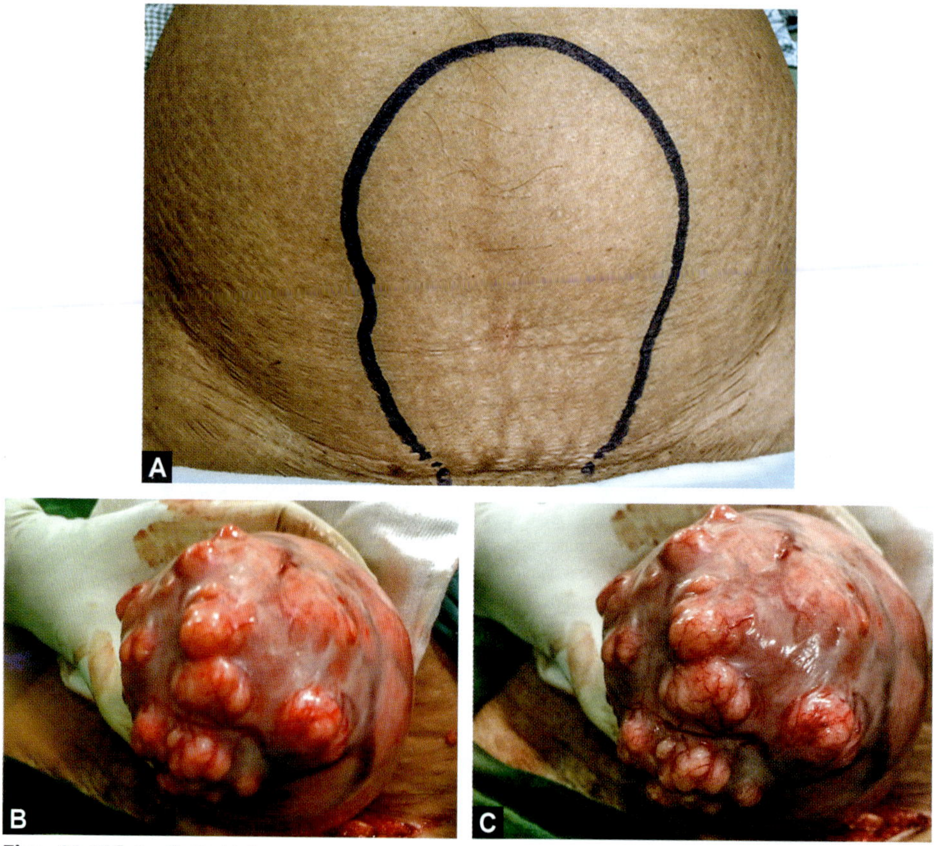

Figs. 11.10A to C: Multiple myomas on open myomectomy.

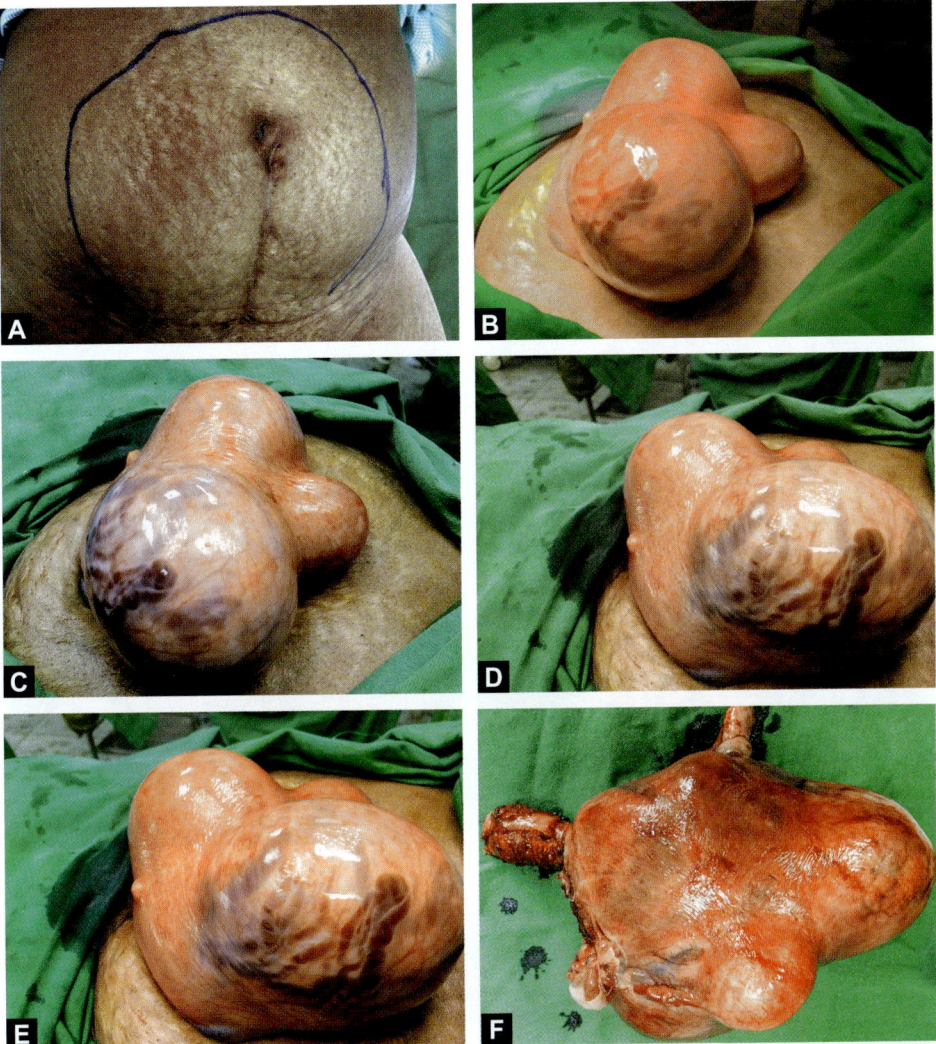

Figs. 11.11A to F: Another case of multiple large myomas on open myomectomy.

- Early mobilization
- Vaginal route of delivery can be offered.

Complications

Intraoperative

- Perforation in 1–2% of cases.
- Excessive fluid absorption:
  - Excess absorption of noncrystalloid distension media (1.5% glycine, 3% sorbitol, and 5% mannitol solutions) can cause serious fluid and electrolyte imbalance, pulmonary and cerebral edema, cardiac failure, and death.
  - Excess absorption of saline can lead to volume overload and pulmonary edema.

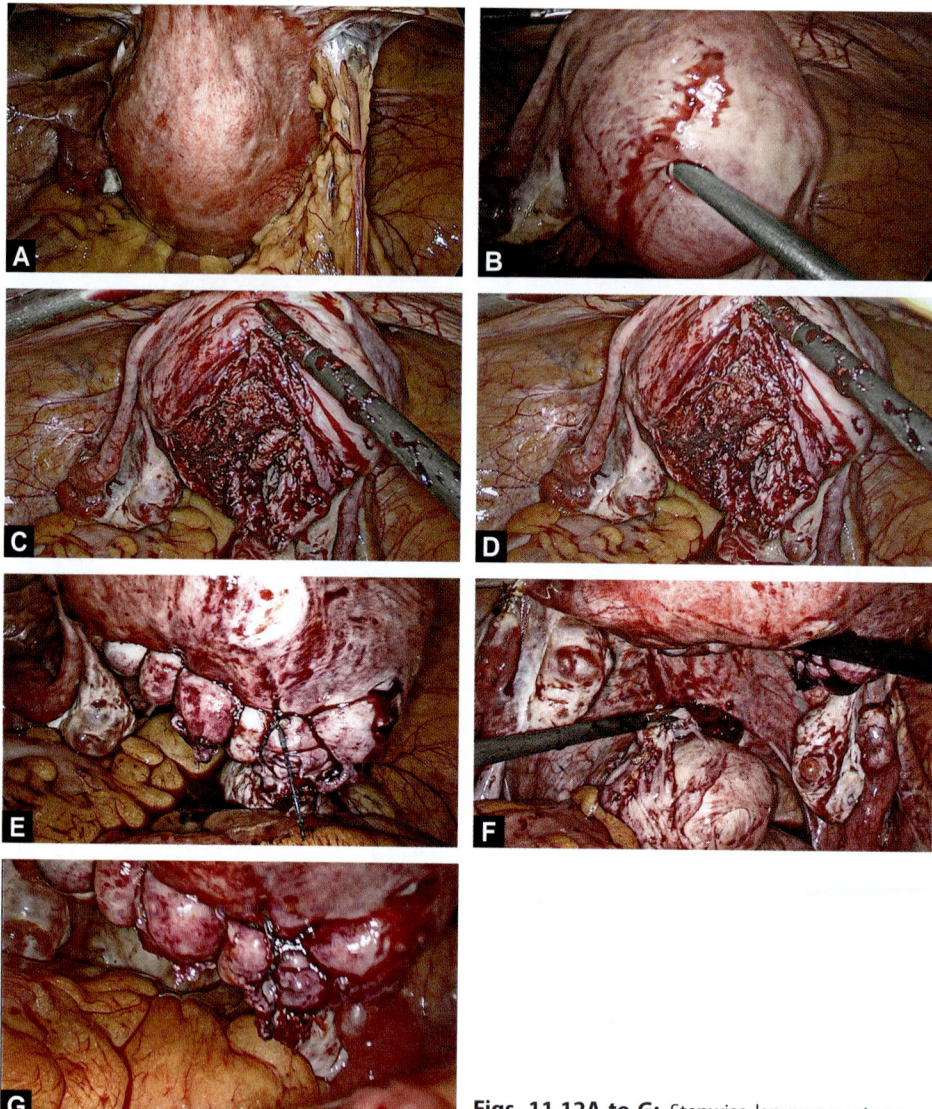

Figs. 11.12A to G: Stepwise lap myomectomy.

- Hemorrhage.
- Air embolism is rare.
- Anesthesia complications.

Postoperative

- Intrauterine adhesions especially with removal of type-2 fibroids
- Endomyometritis
- Recurrence
- Dissemination of tumor cells with endometrial cancer is controversial.

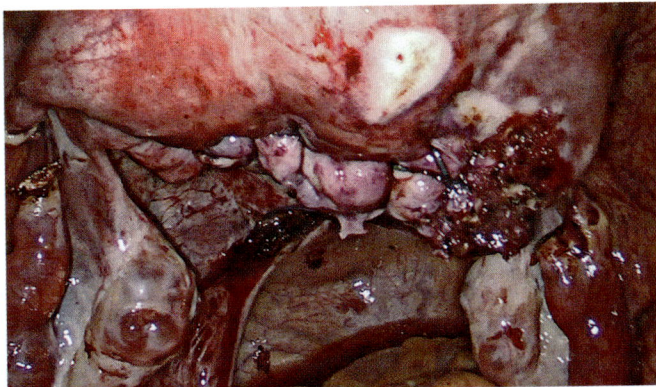

Fig. 11.13: Inspecting abdomen for hemostasis before closing.

LAPAROSCOPIC MYOMECTOMY

Advantages

- Shorter hospitalization
- Faster postoperative recovery
- Reduced postoperative pain
- Fewer adhesions
- Less blood loss
- Comparable pregnancy rates with abdominal myomectomy.

Hemostatic Options at Laparoscopy

- Vasopressin (0.05–0.3 U/mL, i.e. 20 units in 60–400 mL saline)
- Vaginal misoprostol
- Uterine artery ligation
- Vicryl tourniquet.

Tips and Tricks for Laparoscopic Closure of Uterine Muscle

- Do not push when using laparoscopic needle drivers. Set the needle perpendicular and rotate the wrist, letting the needle glide through the tissue.
- Use a multilayer closure.
- Intracorporeal knots can be used to secure the suture.
- Barb suture self-anchors every 1 mm to maintain constant tension and do not require knots.
- Avoid excessive use of electrocautery.

Specimen Morcellation

Morcellator use can lead to seeding of peritoneal cavity with fibroid cells leading to parasitic leiomyomas or dissemination of incidental leiomyosarcoma. The patient should be informed about possible risks and complications, including the fact that in rare cases fibroid(s) may contain unexpected malignancy and that laparoscopic power morcellation may spread the cancer, and potentially worsening their prognosis.

Summary of Recommendations regarding Uterine Morcellation

American Association of Gynecologic Laparoscopists (April, 2014):
- Most women with uterine cancer can be diagnosed prior to surgical intervention.
- Between 1 in 400 and 1 in 1,000 women who undergo hysterectomy for presumed benign uterine myomas will be diagnosed with uterine leiomyosarcoma.
- The prognosis of patients with uterine leiomyosarcoma is universally poor and may be worsened in the setting of power morcellation.

US Food and Drug Administration (April, 2014):
- 1 in 350 women undergoing hysterectomy or myomectomy for the treatment of fibroids is found to have an unsuspected uterine cancer.
- Laparoscopic power morcellation poses a risk of spreading unsuspected cancerous tissue, notably uterine sarcomas, beyond the uterus.
- The Food and Drug Administration (FDA) discourages the use of laparoscopic power morcellation during hysterectomy or myomectomy for uterine fibroids.

Complications

Early
- Persistent bleeding
- Intraoperative damage to bowel or bladder.

Late
- Recurrence
- Incisional hernia
- Rupture uterus at delivery. Usually linked to absence of multilayer closure or excessive use of electrosurgical energy.

Robotic-assisted Laparoscopy

The AAGL states that in current times, robotic surgery offers no significant advantage in benign gynecological surgery over laparoscopy and is more costly than conventional laparoscopic surgery.

HYSTERECTOMY

It is the definitive treatment for fibroids. It can be attempted through following routes:
- Abdominal
- Vaginal
- Laparoscopy
- Robotic.

Abdominal Hysterectomy

Common guidelines for abdominal approach include:
- Uterine size greater than 12 weeks (relative indication)
- Narrow vaginal caliber

- Lack of uterine descent and mobility
- Adnexal disease
- Previous pelvic surgery [myomectomy and lower section cesarean section (LSCS)]
- Malignancy.

Intraoperative and Immediate Postoperative Complications

- Hemorrhage
- Injury to adjacent organs
- Postsurgical infections
- Deep-venous thrombosis
- Pulmonary embolus.

Long-term Complications

- Apical vaginal prolapse
- Urinary incontinence
- Fistula formation
- Postprocedure regret.

Vaginal Hysterectomy

Prerequisites

- Uterine size usually below 12–14 weeks
- Mobile uterus with accessible paracervical tissue and uterine vessels
- Accessible lateral pelvic space and absence of pathology (endometriosis and broad-ligament fibroid)
- Experienced and competent vaginal surgeon.

Complications

- Bleeding
- Vaginal cuff dehiscence
- Pelvic abscess.

Complications of Laparoscopic Hysterectomy

Intraoperative:
- Bladder injury
- Ureteric injury
- Bowel injury
- Hemorrhage.

Late onset:
- Hematoma
- Ileus
- Thromboembolism.

INTRAOPERATIVE ADJUNCTS

Misoprostol

It reduces uterine blood flow and increases myometrial contractions thereby reducing the blood loss. It also plays a role in cervical ripening before operative hysteroscopy. Placebo-controlled randomized studies have shown statistically significant reduction in operative time, blood loss, postoperative hemoglobin drop, and need for transfusion following the use of 400 μg of tablet misoprostol either vaginally or by rectal route.

Vasopressin

The use of synthetic vasopressin, i.e. Pitressin prevents bleeding during uterine surgery by causing vascular spasm and myometrial contractions. However, its use is contraindicated in women with hypertension, cardiac issues, and vascular insufficiency. Several reports of sudden cardiovascular collapse have been seen with intramyometrial instillation of this drug. Thus, it should be administered in properly diluted form and after communication with anesthetist.

In a systematic review, two trials comparing vasopressin to placebo showed a pooled mean difference of 298.7 mL in blood loss. No statistical difference was seen in duration of surgery, blood transfusion requirement, duration of hospital stay, and pregnancy rates after 1 year of myomectomy.

Antiadhesion Barriers

Adhesion formation can be reduced but not completely prevented. Measures to reduce abdominal adhesion formation include:
- Gentle tissue handling
- Meticulous hemostasis
- Excision of necrotic tissue
- Use of fine and nonreactive sutures
- Adhesion barriers like oxidized regenerated cellulose.

SUMMARY

- Uterine fibroids are common and appearing in 70% of women by age of 50 years.
- The presence of uterine fibroids can significantly affect the quality of life.
- Concern about possible complications related to fibroids in pregnancy is not an indication for myomectomy. However, myomectomy can be considered in women who have had a previous pregnancy with complications related to these fibroids.
- Hysterectomy is the most effective and definitive treatment for symptomatic uterine fibroids.
- Myomectomy is an option for women who wish to preserve their uterus or enhance fertility, but carries the potential for further intervention.
- Use of vasopressin, bupivacaine and epinephrine, misoprostol, pericervical tourniquet, or gelatin-thrombin matrix reduces blood loss at myomectomy.

CONCLUSION

Fibroids are the most common benign gynecological tumors, which may cause significant morbidity and affect the quality of life. Treatment of women with uterine leiomyomas must be individualized based on symptomatology, size and location of fibroids, age, need, and desire of the patient to preserve fertility or the uterus, the availability of therapy, and the experience of the surgeon.

BIBLIOGRAPHY

1. AAGL Advancing Minimally Invasive Gynecology Worldwide. AAGL position statement: robotic-assisted laparoscopic surgery in benign gynecology. J Minim Invasive Gynecol. 2013;20(1):2-9.
2. AAGL Advancing Minimally Invasive Gynecology Worldwide. AGL practice report: Morcellation during uterine tissue extraction. J Minim Invasive Gynecol. 2014;21(4):517-30.
3. American Association of Gynecologic Laparoscopists (AAGL): Advancing Minimally Invasive Gynecology Worldwide. AAGL Practice Report: Practice Guidelines for the Diagnosis and Management of Submucous Leiomyomas. J Minim Invasive Gynecol. 2012;19(2):152-71.
4. Baird DD, Dunson DB, Hill MC, et al. High cumulative incidence of uterine leiomyoma in black and white women: ultrasound evidence. Am J Obstet Gynecol. 2003;188(1):100-7.
5. Celik H, Sapmaz E. Use of a single preoperative dose of misoprostol is efficacious for patients who undergo abdominal myomectomy. Fertil Steril. 2003;79(5):1207-10.
6. Fletcher H, Frederick J, Hardie M, et al. A randomized comparison of vasopressin and tourniquet as hemostatic agents during myomectomy. Obstet Gynecol. 1996;87(6):1014-8.
7. Food and Drug Administration. (2014). Quantitative assessment of the prevalence of unsuspected uterine sarcoma in women undergoing treatment of uterine fibroids: summary and key findings. [online] Available from: http://www.fda.gov/downloads/MedicalDevices/Safety/AlertsandNotices/UCM393589.pdf. [Accessed June, 2014].
8. Frederick S, Frederick J, Fletcher H, et al. A trial comparing the use of rectal misoprostol plus perivascular vasopressin with perivascular vasopressin alone to decrease myometrial bleeding at the time of abdominal myomectomy. Fertil Steril. 2013;100(4):1044-9.
9. Ginsburg ES, Benson CB, Garfield JM, et al. The effect of operative technique and uterine size on blood loss during myomectomy: a prospective randomized study. Fertil Steril. 1993;60(6):956-62.
10. Istre O, Bjoennes J, Naess R, et al. Postoperative cerebral oedema after transcervical endometrial resection and uterine irrigation with 1.5% glycine. Lancet. 1994;344(8931):1187-9.
11. Kongnyuy EJ, Wiysonge CS. Interventions to reduce haemorrhage during myomectomy for fibroids. Cochrane Database Syst Rev. 2014;(8):CD005355.
12. Lasmar RB, Barrozo PR, Dias R, et al. Submucous myomas: a new presurgical classification to evaluate the viability of hysteroscopic surgical treatment–preliminary report. J Minim Invasive Gynecol. 2005;12(4):308-11.
13. Neuwirth RS, Amin HK. Excision of submucus fibroids with hysteroscopic control. Am J Obstet Gynecol. 1976;126(1):95-9.
14. Pritts EA, Parker WH, Olive DL. Fibroids and infertility: an updated systematic review of the evidence. Fertil Steril. 2009;91(4):1215-23.
15. SOGC Clinical Practice Guideline. (2015). The Management of Uterine Leiomyomas. [online] Available from: https://sogc.org/wp-content/uploads/ 2015/02/gui318CPG1502ErevB1.pdf. [Accessed June, 2018].
16. Wamsteker K, Emanuel MH, de Kruif JH. Transcervical hysteroscopic resection of submucous fibroids for abnormal uterine bleeding: results regarding the degree of intramural extension. Obstet Gynecol. 1993;82(5):736-40.

Controversies Regarding Fibroid Morcellation

Prakash Trivedi, Soumil Trivedi, Sandeep Patil

INTRODUCTION

Most gynecologists are well aware of the recent developments surrounding laparoscopic morcellation. Things have unfolded rapidly since the December 18th, 2013 coverage by *The Wall Street Journal*.

The article was sparked by the case of a physician who underwent a routine laparoscopic hysterectomy for presumed symptomatic uterine fibroids. A preoperative workup did not indicate a suspicion for malignancy, and laparoscopic morcellation was performed for tissue extraction. Unfortunately, pathological examination revealed an occult leiomyosarcoma.

Significant media coverage followed *The Wall Street Journal* article and there was a strong call for a change in morcellation practices. Later, it was decided to significantly limit the use of laparoscopic morcellation for patients undergoing surgery for uterine fibroids, encouraging morcellation inside of a containment bag, based on pioneering work by Dr Anthony Shibley, who first introduced this concept 2 years ago.

On April 17th, the Food and Drug Administration (FDA) issued an advisory discouraging the use of power morcellation during hysterectomy or myomectomy for uterine fibroids. The FDA did not issue a moratorium on the use of power morcellation, but encouraged physicians to seek alternatives.

It did not take long for industry to respond. On April 28th, a major company announced that it would discontinue supplying its morcellator until further notice. At that time, its morcellator had approximately 80% market share, so the impact of this decision will have widespread implications.

BACKGROUND SITUATION

Electromechanical morcellation was first introduced to the market almost 20 years ago and has since enabled surgeons to offer patients a minimally invasive approach to hysterectomies and myomectomies.

The benefits of minimally invasive surgery are well known and include faster recovery, less pain, less blood loss, and lower risk of overall morbidity and mortality. However, laparoscopic morcellation has important drawbacks that include the risk of severe trauma, tissue disruption that makes pathological diagnosis more difficult, and dispersion of the morcellated tissue throughout the abdominal cavity. Less-serious consequences of tissue dispersion include cases of endometriosis and adenomyosis as well as leiomyomatosis, which are estimated to occur in 0.9% of patients having laparoscopic morcellation.

A more serious consequence is dissemination of occult malignancy. The estimated incidence of occult leiomyosarcoma in patients having surgery for presumed leiomyomata is between 1:200 and 1:1,100, with the FDA quoting a risk of 1 in 350 based on its comprehensive review of the literature. Many have challenged these numbers, especially because most of the publications come from large referral centers, which could inflate the prevalence estimates.

Tissue retrieval is a unique challenge since long time. Originally, it was for dermoid cyst, doubtful ovarian masses removed in lap sac or endobag reducing the risk of spillage, though if the spillage was from a nonmalignant mass, the consequences were not dangerous. However, laparoscopic power morcellation, if performed in women with unsuspected uterine sarcoma, there is a risk that the procedure will spread the cancerous tissue within the abdomen and pelvis, significantly worsening the patient's likelihood of long-term survival. Evaluation by sonography, Doppler, or markers is also not completely reliable to diagnose a case of sarcoma. In a recent meta-analysis, the estimated rate of leiomyosarcoma was 0.51 per 1,000 procedures or approximately 1 in 2,000; restricting the meta-analysis to the 64 prospective studies resulted in a substantially lower estimate of 0.12 leiomyosarcomas per 1,000 procedures or approximately 1 leiomyosarcoma per 8,300 surgeries. By withdrawing morcellation and not giving the benefits of laparoscopic surgery, especially in young infertile women with fibroids or laparoscopic hysterectomy in patients with low risk for uterine leiomyosarcoma (ULMS) is debatable.

Thus, any kind of tissue disruption at the time of surgery may significantly worsen the prognosis for patients with an occult sarcoma or other pathology.

What should the gynecologist do?
Given the risk of occult malignancy, does it make sense to abandon all minimally invasive approaches for patients who are having surgery for symptomatic uterine fibroids?

Because a myomectomy ultimately involves some tissue disruption, should myomectomy be abandoned as a surgical procedure? What about noninvasive treatment options that leave the presumed fibroid inside the body, such as uterine artery embolization, magnetic resonance imaging (MRI)-guided focused ultrasound, and radiofrequency ablation?

It would be a step in the wrong direction to counsel all patients with symptomatic uterine fibroids to undergo total abdominal hysterectomy. That would result in increased patient morbidity and remove the option of future fertility for women who would rather retain their uterus.

In our opinion, patients with symptomatic fibroids who desire future fertility should still be offered this treatment option. However, they need to be adequately counseled that removing fibroids from the uterus involves some tissue disruption and that this must be balanced against their desire for future fertility.

One can predict that the extent of the tissue disruption and dispersion may be limited, if open morcellation is avoided in these cases. In addition, it is likely that providers may counsel patients more toward a total laparoscopic hysterectomy versus a supracervical hysterectomy because the former may not involve morcellation, provided that the specimen is small enough to fit through the vagina intact.

On May 9th, American College of Obstetricians and Gynecologist (ACOG) released a special report titled "Power Morcellation and Occult Malignancy in Gynecologic Surgery". It advises practitioners to quote patients a rate of 1/500 for undiagnosed sarcoma and also recommend extensive patient counseling as well as offering alternatives to laparoscopic power morcellation.

American Association of Gynecologic Laparoscopists (AAGL) issued a statement as a reply to FDA stating that it is possible that different risk profiles exist among the various methods of morcellation, but specific data are lacking with respect to these differences

(Level C). Hysteroscopic removal of symptomatic submucosal uterine myoma in premenopausal women need not be exchanged for definitive treatment (i.e. hysterectomy) simply to avoid morcellation (Level A). Women with asymptomatic uterine myoma can be managed expectantly (Level A). Laparoscopy has well-documented advantages over laparotomy regarding surgical complications and patient outcomes (Level A). Sarcomas have been diagnosed after alternative uterine-preserving treatments such as uterine artery ligation. The same challenges in preoperative diagnosis of uterine sarcoma apply to these surgical alternatives (Level C). The use of morcellation within specimen retrieval pouches for containment of benign or malignant uterine tissue requires significant skill and experience, and the use of specimen retrieval pouches should be investigated further for safety and outcomes in a controlled setting (Level C).

It would be ideal to be able to predict preoperatively whether a presumed fibroid is actually a malignancy. Unfortunately, we do not have reliable ways to determine this. Demographic factors such as age or rapid tumor growth are not helpful, especially because occult malignancy may be present in women in their 20s and 30s.

Preoperative imaging shows promise, but its clinical utility is yet to be determined. Two preliminary studies using MRI with lactate dehydrogenase isoenzyme-3 measurements or with diffusion-weighted imaging demonstrate promising results, but more research is needed before recommending routine MRIs before all surgeries for presumed leiomyomas.

The cost of such a measure would be significant and the chance of false-positive results is high and given the rarity of these conditions.

What technique should we adopt?
Laparoscopic myomectomy is an art of three in one technique:
1. Removal of fibroid from the uterus
2. Reconstructing the uterus with very efficient methods of laparoscopic suturing
3. Removing the separated fibroid from the abdominal cavity either vaginally or by morcellation.

Total healthcare technique of doing in-bag morcellation of fibroids and uterus: The steps of laparoscopic myomectomy and laparoscopic hysterectomy remain the same as done in a standardized fashion leaving the fibroid or uterus separated in the peritoneal cavity. The left lower port is widened to pass a 10-mm port and further with a finger mechanically stretched to make easy passage of the soft plastic sleeve carrying the bag.

As shown in Figure 12.1 there is a medium size strong plastic bag in the shape like stomach but with a wider opening. The wide opening of the bag is folded and introduced in a one side openable plastic cannula, which is designed to carry the bag inside the abdomen replacing the left lower 10 mm port (Fig. 12.2). Once the bag is seen inside the sleeve in the abdomen through the laparoscope, the assistant holds only the bag with a 5 mm atraumatic grasper allowing the removal of introducing plastic sleeve. The remaining part of the mouth of the bag is pulled systematically with atraumatic graspers held in sequence by the surgeon and assistant (Fig. 12.3). Once full bag is inside the abdomen, the 10 mm port is reintroduced with a reducer to carry a 5 mm instrument. The wide ring of the opening of the bag is identified and held by the assistant and surgeon, with a single tooth grasper surgeon holds the specimen and transfers it inside the bag (Fig. 12.4). The opening of the bag is systematically closed bringing one end close to the left lower 10 mm port carrying a 5 mm grasper. The two parts of the opening of the bag are held together and pulled out withdrawing the 10 mm trocar. And then holding the two margins of the mouth, the bag is mechanically pulled by two hands of the surgeon bringing the entire mouth of the bag outside the left lower port. The camera keeps a constant watch to see that the specimen is always inside the bag. Now from the right lower port with a 5 mm grasper, the duodenum-shaped part of the bag, which we call as the ear with a hole, is held at the tip and rail-roaded inside the

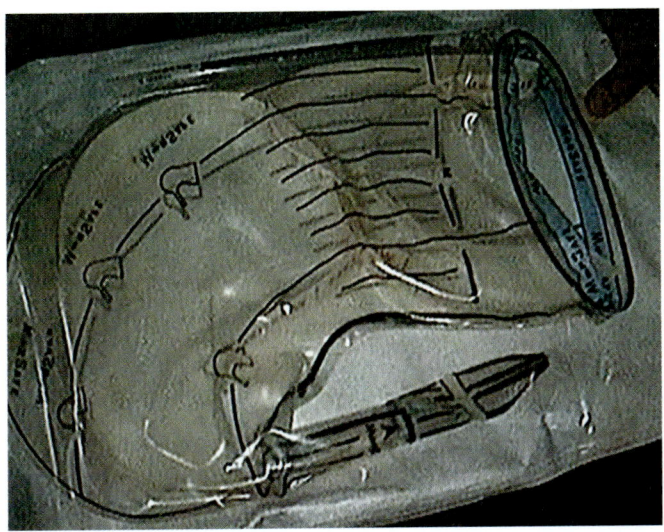

Fig. 12.1: A medium-size strong plastic bag.

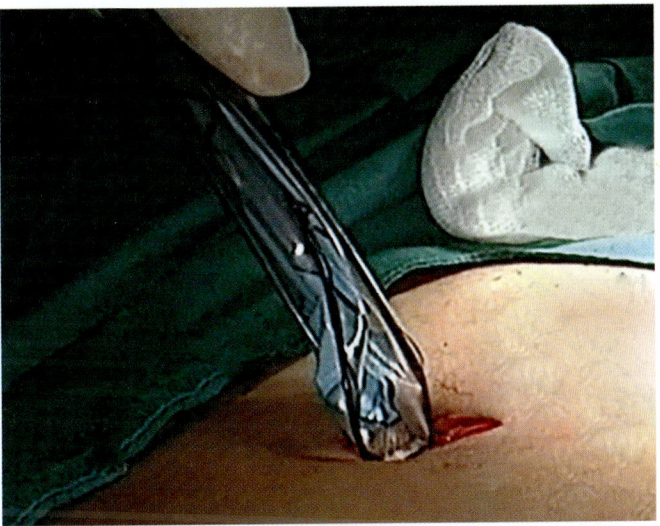

Fig. 12.2: Wide opening of the bag is folded and introduced.

10 mm trocar of the optics. Care is taken to keep the right semiflexed leg low to allow free movement of the 5 mm grasper holding the ear to be easily rail-roaded inside the 10 mm trocar, which is withdrawn. Externally, this part of the bag is seen at the umbilical region. This part of the bag which is like the ear has a 5 mm hole which is widened to introduce the 10 mm trocar which will carry the optics. Once in place, the optics is introduced and CO_2 insufflation is started. The optics and the screen clearly show opening of the bag with the specimen within and the mouth of the bag coming from the left lower port is blocked by the assistant. Once everything is in place a 12 mm morcellator handpiece with a blunt tip trocar is introduced under vision inside the bag from the left lower port. A clear vision makes you

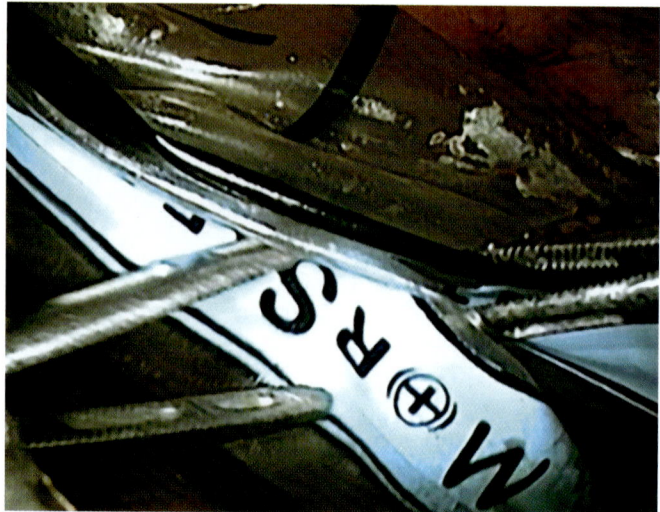

Fig. 12.3: Systematic pulling of remaining part of the mouth of the bag with atraumatic graspers.

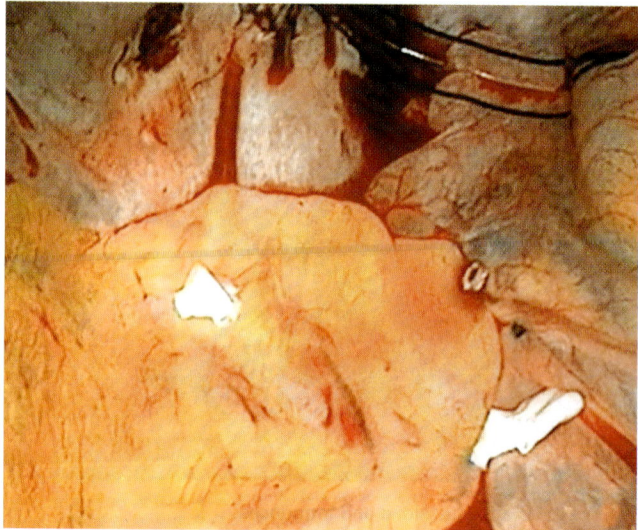

Fig. 12.4: The wide ring of the opening of the bag.

visualize that the bag has replaced practically as the peritoneal lining with all abdominal structures outside the bag but the specimen is within the bag in front of the morcellator.

The unique feature of the morcellator handle is that the sharp inner blade is not fully exposed but only a rim is seen with a hood of the morcellator handpiece. A 10 mm single tooth grasper is introduced inside the morcellator, which will hold the specimen, and morcellation is done under vision (Fig. 12.5). The projecting hood of the morcellator handpiece protects the sharp circular inner cutting blade and the specimen gets morcellated exactly in the fashion of orange peeling of 10 mm long pieces. With a series of long strips the whole specimen is morcellated. The bag now contains the small bits of morcellated remnant pieces and the blood of specimen side (Fig. 12.6). The morcellator handpiece is removed blocking the mouth of the bag to prevent unnecessary scatter of tissue or fluid on the face of surgeon or assistant. The 10 mm optics and the trocar carrying the optics are removed.

A knot is tied on the long ear-shaped plastic next from the left lower port under external vision, the bag is pulled out and one can see the knotted part of the ear getting withdrawn inside the umbilicus into the abdominal cavity and then comes out from the left lower port (Fig. 12.7).

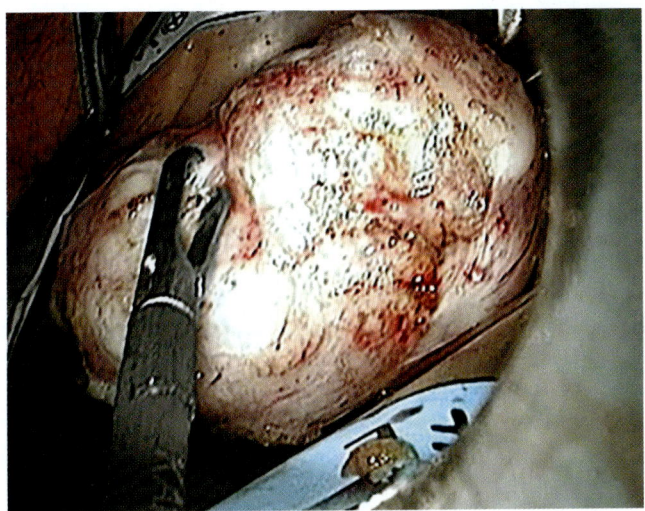

Fig. 12.5: Transferring specimen in the bag with single tooth grasper.

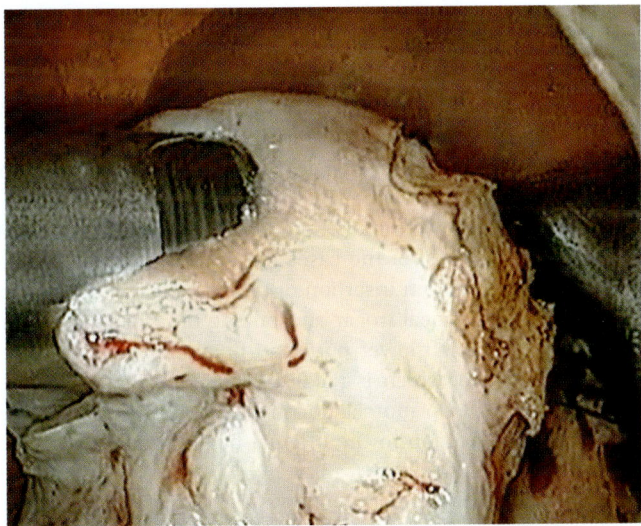

Fig. 12.6: Morcellation done under vision.

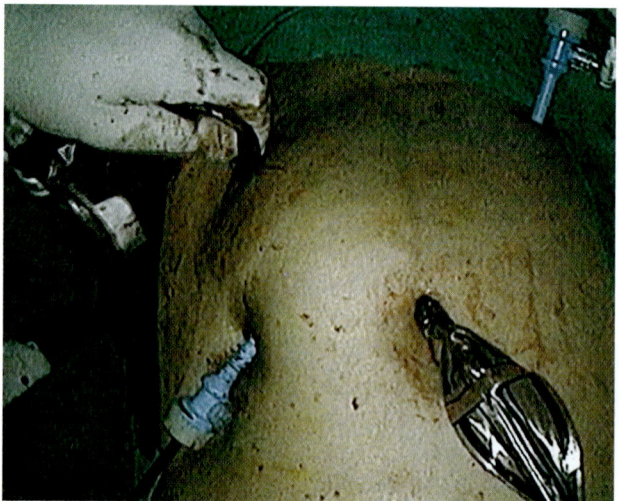

Fig. 12.7: A knot is tied and the bag is pulled out.

The optics is reintroduced from the 10 mm umbilical port and under vision with a port closure device the left lower port is closed. A good look of the entire peritoneal cavity confirms hemostasis and also clearly shows that not a drop of specimen side fluid or a small piece of the specimen is seen within the peritoneal cavity.

Technical issues:
Care has to be taken that the abdominal opening for the morcellator to enter should be adequate for free movements.

The mouth of the bag once out from lower left port and the ear has to come out from the umbilical port without any twists. Thus, the learning curve would include making sure to align the two marked parallel lines of the bag to the optics, to avoid the twist.

When faced with technical difficulty in one such case, sharp part of Rotocut was used to puncture the bag, and to our surprise complete morcellation without any spillage, in the bag itself, was possible.

From May 14th, 2015 onwards in properly indicated cases of laparoscopic myomectomy and total laparoscopic hysterectomy for large uterus, a total of 142 cases were done back-to-back with uterus as big as 1.8 kg of about 28 weeks with huge fibroids of 17 cm and multiple fibroids like eight fibroids of 4–5 cm in size (Figs. 12.8 to 12.10).

Barring in two cases were in two parts where technical difficulty due to twisting of the back with the specimen inside. Rest of the cases there were no major difficulty found and currently on an average the time from insertion of the bag, putting the specimen in the bag and taking the eye from the umbilical trocar and pulling the closed bag with the specimen and mouth of the bag from the left lower port, and finally introducing the trocar with the 10 mm optics to the small hole, which is made in the eye and starting the pneumoperitoneum and inserting the blunt tip morcellator inside the bag on an average was over in 18 minutes. Few further modification in the original bag are made to make the procedure easy and patient friendly.

Emphasis would again be on the technique, which is simple, dependable, and achieves all the functions of no spillage of any tissue material from the specimen into the peritoneal cavity.

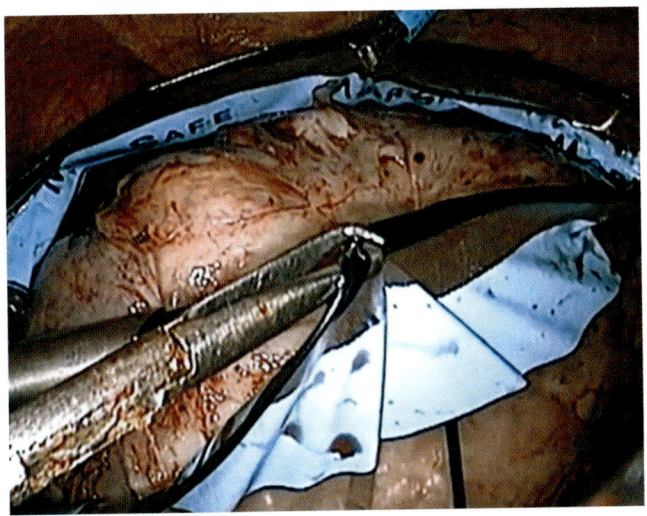

Fig. 12.8: Endobag opened inside the abdominal cavity.

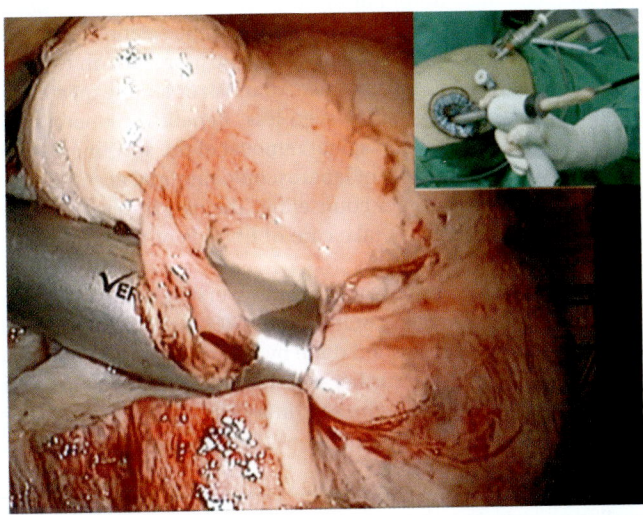

Fig. 12.9: Morcellation of fibroid inside the endobag (inset picture of bag mouth outside the abdomen).

Recent statistics regarding clinical characteristics and management experience of unexpected uterine sarcoma stated that among 4,248 patients who underwent myomectomy for presumed leiomyoma, 9 (0.2%) had unexpected uterine sarcoma [1 (<0.1%) had leiomyosarcoma; 8 (0.2%) endometrial stromal sarcoma]. The malignancy was identified in 5 (0.2%) of 3,068 women who were treated by laparoscopy with power morcellation and 4 (0.3%) of 1,180 who underwent laparotomy (P = 0.274). Thus, the overall incidence of unexpected uterine sarcoma after myomectomy was low and incidental power morcellation of unexpected uterine sarcoma seemed to cause no increase in sarcoma dissemination.

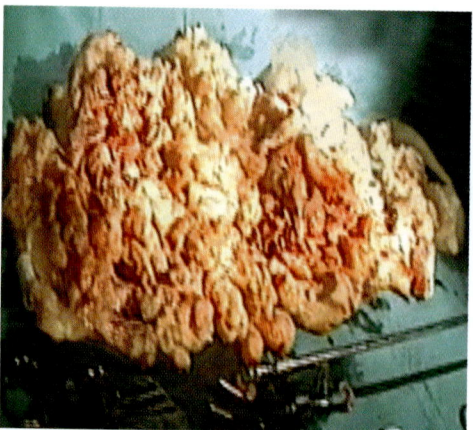

Fig. 12.10: Morcellated fibroid.

TAKE-HOME MESSAGE

The controversy of morcellating a fibroid or uterus, which may have unsuspected malignancy or leiomyosarcoma, is voiced and overhyped beyond genuine scientific proportion. We have a few groups of patients and activists who put laparoscopic morcellation to a total disrepute, in contrary to recent meta-analysis suggesting the actual risk of an unexpected leiomyosarcoma not more than 1 in 2,000 cases or probably even less. Benefits of laparoscopic morcellation should be given as an option along with vaginal removal of the specimen, especially in young and deserving patients, wherein benefits of laparoscopic minimal access surgery with a quick recovery should be extended after proper counseling. The new in-bag morcellation technique as described by the author would easily take care of fibroids or uterus up to 26 weeks in size or weighing up to 2 kg.

The most interesting scientific aspect of this controversy is that even if a leiomyosarcoma is removed by an open en bloc surgery, still there is 50% risk of spread or already residual existing disease compared to 60% risk when done by laparoscopic morcellation, that is, only a 10% risk reduction with open surgery. Further with the in-bag morcellation, the risk of spread drops down drastically unless originally the sarcoma or cancer was already spread.

CONCLUSION

The in-bag morcellation technique appears to handle the issue of ULMS and allows laparoscopic myomectomy and hysterectomy possible with fair safety. The scientific focus should be directed toward diagnosing leiomyosarcoma or a malignancy prior to surgery far more accurately with methods, which are yet not totally identified.

It is likely that much innovation will take place in this area in the coming months. Endobags that are specifically designed for contained morcellation will greatly facilitate this process and make it easier for surgeons to incorporate this into their practice.

Completely automatic tissue extraction devices are also being developed and may become commercially available in the next 1–2 years. These devices enable automatic morcellation in a contained environment without the need for a rotating blade or bag insufflation.

Ultimately, as innovation enters this arena, future patients will benefit as surgeons become better equipped to offer minimally invasive options for their conditions.

BIBLIOGRAPHY

1. AAGL Advancing Minimally Invasive Gynecology Worldwide. AAGL practice report: Morcellation during uterine tissue extraction. J Minim Invasive Gynecol. 2014;21(4):517-30.
2. Cucinella G, Granese R, Calagna G, et al. Parasitic myomas after laparoscopic surgery: an emerging complication in the use of morcellator? Fertil Steril. 2011;96(2):e90-6.
3. Goto A, Takeuchi S, Sugimura K, et al. Usefulness of Gd-DTPA contrast-enhanced dynamic MRI and serum determination of LDH and its isozymes in the differential diagnosis of leiomyosarcoma from degenerated leiomyoma of the uterus. Int J Gynecol Cancer. 2002;12(4):354-61.
4. Isakov A, Murdaugh KM, Burke WC, et al. A new laparoscopic morcellator using an actuated wire mesh and bag. ASME J Med Devices. 2014;8(1):011009.
5. Leibsohn S, d'Ablaing G, Mishell DR Jr, et al. Leiomyosarcoma in a series of hysterectomies performed for presumed uterine leiomyomas. Am J Obstet Gynecol. 1990;162(4):968-74.
6. Leung F, Terzibachian JJ. Re: The impact of tumor morcellation during surgery on the prognosis of patients with apparently early uterine leiomyosarcoma. Gynecol Oncol. 2012;124(1):172-3.
7. Levitz J. (2013). Doctors eye cancer risk in uterine procedure: popular technique to remove growths comes under question. [online] Available from http://online.wsj.com/news/articles/SB10001424052702304173704579264673929862850. [Accessed June, 2018].
8. Milad MP, Milad EA. Laparoscopic morcellator-related complications. J Minim Invasive Gynecol. 2014;21(3):486-91.
9. Parker WH, Fu YS, Berek JS. Uterine sarcoma in patients operated on for presumed leiomyoma and rapidly growing leiomyoma. Obstet Gynecol. 1994;83(3):414-8.
10. Pritts EA, Vanness DJ, Berek JS, et al. The prevalence of occult leiomyosarcoma at surgery for presumed uterine fibroids: a meta-analysis. Gynecol Surg. 2015;12(3):165-77.
11. Rivard C, Salhader A, Kenton K. New challenges in detecting, grading, and staging endometrial cancer after uterine morcellation. J Minim Invasive Gynecol. 2012;19(3):313-6.
12. Seidman MA, Oduyebo T, Muto MG, et al. Peritoneal dissemination complicating morcellation of uterine mesenchymal neoplasms. PLoS One. 2012;7(11):e50058.
13. Shibley KA. Feasibility of intra-abdominal tissue isolation and extraction, within an artificially created pneumoperitoneum, at laparoscopy for gynecologic procedures. J Minim Invasive Gynecol. 2012;19(6):S75.
14. The American Congress of Obstetricians and Gynecologists. Power morcellation and occult malignancy in gynecologic surgery. [online] Available from http://www.acog.org/Resources_And_Publications/Task_Force_and_Work_Group. [Accessed June, 2018].
15. Wiser A, Holcroft CA, Tulandi T, et al. Abdominal versus laparoscopic hysterectomies for benign diseases: evaluation of morbidity and mortality among 465,798 cases. Gynecol Surg. 2013;10(2):117-22.
16. Zhang J, Dai Y, Zhu L, et al. Clinical characteristics and management experience of unexpected uterine sarcoma after myomectomy. Int J Gynaecol Obstet. 2015;130(2):195-9.

Medical Management of Fibroids

13

Poonam Loomba, Poonam Goyal

INTRODUCTION

One out of four women visiting a gynae clinic is found to be having these benign tumors of variable size, number, location, and consistency. The detection may be incidental finding or after the woman is symptomatic as with abnormal uterine bleeding, pressure symptoms, dysmenorrhea or infertility. Not every woman needs to be cured and suggested to get rid of these benign masses. There should be a scientific reason and patient prerogative while taking decisions on prescribing therapy for a fibroid. Thus it would not be wrong to say that treatments need to be tailor-made for each woman preceded by counseling and followed with reassurance.

We would be discussing all types of currently available medical therapies based on literature review. Very few good randomized trials are there, in fact, US Food and Drug Administration (FDA) does not approve all medical options which are currently available. The benign nature of the tumor should be confirmed with ultrasonography (USG) or fine-needle aspiration cytology (FNAC) before starting medical treatment.

OBJECTIVES

- Attaining a substantial reduction in size of the tumor.
- Relief from abnormal bleeding pattern.
- Relief from pressure symptoms.
- Postpone surgical treatment for duration till woman is ready for it.
- Improve quality of life in women unfit for surgery.
- Young women coming for first time with infertility till their reproductive performance is established without interventions.
- Smooth transition of a symptomatic perimenopausal woman to menopause.

SELECTION OF WOMEN FOR MEDICAL THERAPY

Prior to selecting any treatment modality, it is very essential to calculate the risk–benefit scores and cost-effectiveness for the same along with long time effects of drugs vs. surgery. Patient preferences need to be taken care of, provided there are no risks. Keeping all this in mind we try to select following categories for medical therapy:
- Young unmarried girls with single or multiple myomas, asymptomatic or presenting with symptoms like minimal to mild menorrhagia, dysmenorrhea, and pressure symptoms. Treatment is suggested till the time the girl and family are prepared for surgical removal.

- In women who are complaining of infertility, surgical implications are sometimes risky like bleeding during surgery leading to hysterectomy, wound dehiscence, intrauterine and abdominal adhesions, so medical management is best for them.
- Patients who are unfit for surgery and anesthesia due to anemia or any other medical disease.
- Some clinics offer medical treatment to women with large myomas before taking them for laparoscopic removals so as to shrink size of the tumor.
- When there is desire to preserve uterus due to any reason.
- Recurrence or new development of a tumor after myomectomy and the patient is apprehensive about repeat surgery.
- In a perimenopausal lady having symptoms.
- In fact, drug treatment was first started for preoperative purpose to achieve amenorrhea; later it was noted that reduction in size occurs, so trials started for this.

COUNSELING BEFORE MEDICAL MANAGEMENT

Counseling is very important before we put her on medical management as she may have unrealistic expectations. Patients should be clearly told about objective of treatment as well as the fact that fibroid will shrink not disappear.

MEDICAL TREATMENT OPTIONS (FLOWCHART 13.1)

Our aim here is to discuss the drugs which actually affect the size of the tumors not the drugs which only provide symptomatic relief. One should be clear about the fact that nothing will make the fibroid disappear from the scene. The responsiveness of fibroids to hormones and presence of active hormone receptors in them makes them amenable to drugs. They can be targeted by manipulation of hormonal environment.

Drugs

- Gonadotropin-releasing hormone analogs
- Progesterone receptor modulators (PRMs)
- Selective progesterone receptor modulators (SPRMs)
- Aromatase inhibitors (AIs)
- Selective estrogen receptor modulators (SERMs).

Gonadotropin-releasing Hormone

Gonadotropin-releasing hormone agonists: Gonadotropin-releasing hormone agonists (GnRHa) are the most established successful therapy for medically managing the fibroids.
Mechanism of action: They effectively downregulate GnRH receptors at the level of pituitary and cause profound reduction in the levels of gonadotropins and also ovarian steroids, thus producing hypoestrogenic state. This results in pronounced reduction in size of fibroid. As such all myomas are heterogeneous in nature and this demonstrates a variable response to GnRHa. These suppress the expression of aromatase P450, an estrogen synthetase found in myoma cells resulting in in situ reduction of estrogen production. Symptoms like bleeding, pelvic pressure, and distortion of adjacent organs improve considerably in response to reduction in fibroid size.

Side-effects: The benefits of drug, however, are tempered by hypoestrogenic effects like:
- Hot flashes
- Headache

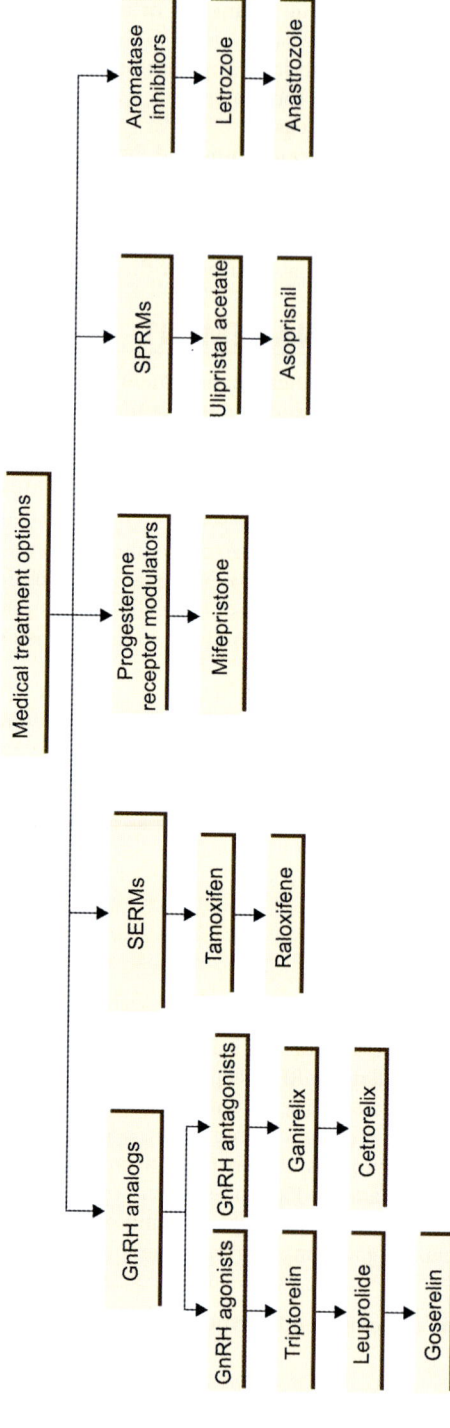

Flowchart 13.1: Drugs available for the medical treatment of fibroids.

(GnRH: Gonadotropin-releasing hormone; SERMs: Selective estrogen receptor modulators; SPRMs: Selective progesterone receptor modulators)

- Vaginal dryness
- Depression—occurs due to suppression of estrogen to the castration level and at times they are really very disturbing for the patient. There is initial flare effect also. Later on bone demineralization starts.
- All these side-effects limit their use for 6 months maximum.

The side-effects may be alleviated by the use of "add-back" therapy using estrogen, progestins or both.

Other details: A single injection of GnRHa produces an initial stimulation of pituitary gonadotropins, resulting in increased secretion of follicle-stimulating hormone (FSH) and luteinizing hormone (LH) and the expected gonadal response called flare effect. However, continuous or repeated administration of GnRHa in a continuous nonpulsatile fashion or administration of supraphysiological doses ultimately produces inhibition of the pituitary-gonadal axis. This happens because the newer receptor formation is relatively slow and existing ones are already blocked. Now with prolonged use agonist starts behaving like an antagonist.

Gonadotropin-releasing hormone agonists undoubtedly induce fibroid tumor shrinkage, the degree of which has been shown to be directly proportional to the percentage of cells that are estrogen receptor positive, thus implicating estrogen as a major effector of tumor growth and its reduction as the central mechanism of fibroid shrinkage with GnRHa therapy. Chegini et al. found evidence of suppression of signal transduction pathways involving growth factors, ovarian steroids, and adhesion molecules with a resulting decrease in DNA synthesis, cell proliferation, and production of transforming growth factor-beta.

They found that medical treatment causes altered regulation in a number of genes involved in the regulation of cell growth, signal transduction, transcription factors, and cell structures. Therapy with leuprolide acetate has been associated with hyalinization of leiomyomata and decreases in uterine or tumor arterial size and blood flow variables.

A Cochrane systematic review to evaluate the role of GnRHa prior to either hysterectomy or myomectomy showed that pre- and postoperative hemoglobin and hematocrit were improved significantly by the use of GnRHa prior to surgery. Uterine volume and size, fibroid volume, and pelvic symptoms were all reduced. Hysterectomy was rendered easier, with reduced operating time. Blood loss and rate of vertical incision were reduced for both myomectomy and hysterectomy. Duration of hospital stay was also reduced.

Remarks: The disadvantages of GnRHa include cost, menopausal symptoms, and with prolonged therapy, bone demineralization. In addition, smaller fibroids may be overlooked at the time of surgery, only to recur once GnRHa is discontinued, thereby increasing the apparent risk or recurrence of fibroids following myomectomy. GnRHa cannot be used as long-term standalone therapies for fibroid disease because of the rapid rebound growth of the fibroids upon cessation of therapy.

Dosage: Can be used as 3.6 mg goserelin and/or 3.75 mg depot per month of leuprolide or triptorelin. A 3-month depot of 10.8 mg or 11.25 mg of these two can also be used.

Gonadotropin-releasing hormone antagonists:
Unlike the agonists, there is no flare effect, antagonists block pituitary GnRH receptors immediately causing decline in gonadotropins with immediate effect. The rapid effect enables shorter duration of treatment and related side-effects. Pituitary function normalizes on cessation of treatment.

About the drug: Ganirelix Acetate and cetrorelix Acetate have been used for this purpose; with daily dose 29–43% reduction has been noted. Higher cost and daily dose requirement has made it unfavorable for use. However, shorter duration course treatment can be used prior to surgery for shrinkage of myoma.

Remarks: GnRH antagonists can be used before surgery.

Dosage: The dose used 0.25 mg/day of cetrorelix acetate is enough to create iatrogenic temporary fully reversible hypogonadotropic hypogonadism inducing fibroid shrinkage in volume as well as diminution of vascularization to ease the surgical procedure. 3 mg depot injection can also be tried for this.

Progesterone Receptor Modulators

Mifepristone:

History: Early reports of the use of mifepristone for the treatment of fibroids date back to 2002, when De Leo et al. used doses ranging from 12.5 mg to 50 mg daily and reported reduction in uterine as well as fibroid volume of 40–50% associated with amenorrhea in most subjects. This report was corroborated by a paper a year later from a group who used mifepristone at a dose of 5 or 10 mg per day for 1 year, and found that it was effective in decreasing mean uterine volume by 50%, while amenorrhea occurred in 40–70% of the subjects.

Mechanism of action: It has antiprogesterone and antiglucocorticoid activities. High concentrations of progesterone receptors (PRs) have been identified in myomas compared to the surrounding myometrium. This class of medication targets and reduces the number of PRs and blocks them. It effectively produces amenorrhea. Further, mifepristone decreases the number of PRs in myoma also as in the normal myometrium. It results in inhibiting ovarian cyclicity, maintaining hormonal status similar to early follicular phase, and decreasing vascular supply of myomas, thus reduction in size.

Side-effects: Prolonged treatment is associated with unusual endometrial hyperplasia in some women on mifepristone which limited the long-term use of this drug. This has not been seen previously with other drugs. There is formation of cystically dilated endometrial glands, which is different from cystic endometrial hyperplasia. It has low or nil mitotic activity, no atypia. However there is potential difficulty in monitoring as on ultrasound endometrium appears thick. Moreover, being an antiprogesterone in nature, it promotes unopposed milieu of estrogens and its prolonged use will ultimately cause hyperplastic endometrium with atypia. If endometrium is persistently thick on USG or more than 10 mm, biopsy should be done.

Other details: Drug is available in Indian market as 10 mg and 25 mg tablets. It is yet not approved by US FDA for this indication. The apparent effectiveness of mifepristone, however, in reducing myoma volume and improving fibroid-related symptoms and quality of life, and the minimal side effects, all point to a need for a large randomized controlled trial (RCT) with sufficient power to define its true place in the medical management of uterine fibroids.

A combination of mifepristone and the levonorgestrel intrauterine system (LNG-IUS) could prove especially useful as the IUS would obviate the development of endometrial hyperplasia while also promoting a reduction in menstrual flow. In another RCT, 100 women were assigned to mifepristone 5 or 10 mg daily for 3 months without a placebo group; with both doses, there were equivalent reductions in fibroid and uterine volumes and symptomatic improvements.

Till further research clarifies the drug status, it would be wise to use 10 mg OD for a period of 3 months and if required more it should be given again after a gap of 1 month.

Dosage: Various clinical trials have been done from 5 mg to 50 mg dose and for a period of 3–12 months, but exact dose and duration is not clearly determined.

As of now lesser dose for a lesser duration is judicious recommendation. 10 mg or 25 mg to be used once daily at the same time, over a period of 3 months. If required, it can be started again after a period of 1 month. 1 month gap is given to prevent too much of endometrial hyperplasia. Proper patient counseling and follow-up is a must.

Selective Progesterone Receptor Modulators

The effects of progesterone on target tissues are mediated via the PR, which belongs to the nuclear receptor family.

Progesterone has dual actions on fibroid growth:
- It stimulates growth:
  - By upregulating epidermal growth factor (EGF) and Bcl-2.
  - By downregulating the expression of tumor necrosis factor-alpha.
- While it inhibits growth:
  - By downregulating insulin-like growth factor-1 (IGF-1) expression.

While it has long been established that estrogen promotes fibroid growth, recent biochemical and clinical studies have suggested that progesterone and the PR may also enhance proliferative activity in fibroids. These observations have therefore raised the possibility that antiprogestins and agents or molecules that modulate the activity of the PR could be useful in the medical management of uterine fibroids (Fig. 13.1). Since the emergence of mifepristone (RU-486), the first PR antagonist, more than 25 years ago, hundreds of steroidal as well as nonsteroidal compounds displaying progesterone antagonist (PA) or mixed agonist or antagonist activity have been synthesized. Collectively, they are known as SPRMs. Some of the PRMs as well as SPRMs which have been the subject of recent clinical trials or research studies in relation to fibroid treatment include mifepristone, CDB-4124 (telapristone), CP-8947, J867 (asoprisnil), and CDB-2914 (ulipristal acetate).

Ulipristal acetate (UPA): It is a SERM, a new progesterone receptor ligand which displays tissue-selective agonist/antagonist activity on target cells (Figs. 13.2A and B).

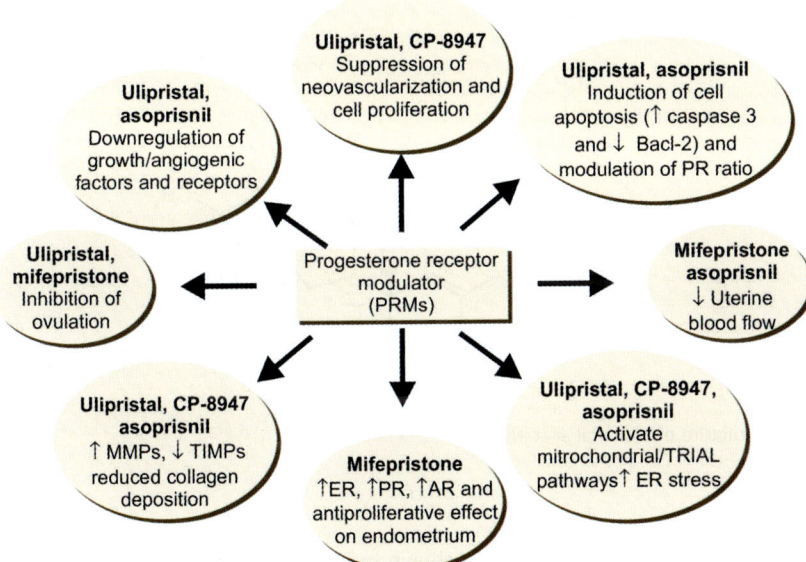

Fig. 13.1: Mechanism of action of progesterone receptor modulators on uterine fibroids. A number of clinical trials have established the potential of SPRMs in the treatment of uterine fibroids. They are associated with a reduction in pain, bleeding, size of fibroids, and overall improvement in quality of life. Unlike long-acting GnRH analogs, they do not have the drawbacks of profound estrogen deficiency and decrease in bone mineral density.

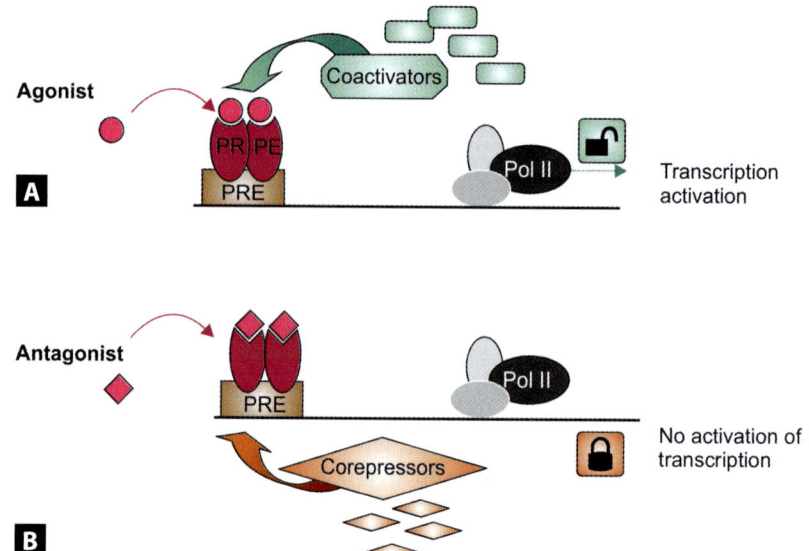

Figs. 13.2A and B: Mechanism of action of progesterone receptor ligands. (A) Ligand-agonist binds to the progesterone receptor and induces activation of transcription by coactivators; (B) Ligand antagonist binds to the receptor and prevents recruitment of coactivators. Corepressors are involved and the transcription processes are not activated.
Source: N. Chabbert-Buffet, et al. Molecular and Cellular Endocrinology. 2012;358:232-43.

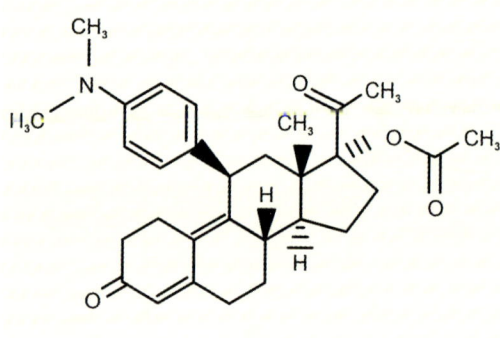

Fig. 13.3: Structure of ulipristal acetate.

Chemical structure of ulipristal acetate:
The chemical structure of UPA has been shown in Figure 13.3.

About the drug:
- A first class effective SPRM specifically designed for uterine fibroids.
- It is well-tolerated.
- It has a partial antagonist effect on progesterone receptors.
- It binds with PRs but not with estrogen receptors.
- It blocks or delays ovulation by inhibiting FSH or LH levels.

- There is no bad effect on bone density.
- It causes endometrial thickening.
- It leads to amenorrhea due to antiproliferative action on endometrium.
- Acts only on leiomyoma cells not on normal myometrial cells.
- It has antiproliferative action on myoma.
- It leads to induction of apoptosis and cell death ways in myoma.
- Usually 25–30% reduction in size has been noted, even 68–90% reduction in fibroid volume has been reported.

All this translates into clinically evident reduction in fibroid size as well as volume of uterus and effective control of bleeding and pain.

Facts about research on drug: A study recently done and published by the name of "PREMYA" has concluded positive outcome of UPA. It was done on 1,473 patients with symptomatic fibroid disease who were to be taken for surgery. A dose of 5 mg per day was given for 3 months. Incidence of surgery was reduced by 38.8% even after stopping treatment, patients were symptom-free.

Dosage: UPA is given in 5 mg dose per day after meals preferably at the same time. It is to be started just after periods on day 4 or 5 and is to be given for 13 weeks or 3 months. Then a stop of one menstrual cycle or 4 weeks is given followed by 13 weeks of drug intake again. Thus prolonged use of drug is safe. This much dose comes out to be sufficient for achieving fibroid shrinkage as well as symptomatic relief. Compliance with intermittent course of treatment is good.

Safety analysis: Side-effects are usual like—
- Headache
- Pain
- Upper gastrointestinal symptoms like bloating, acidity, gastritis
- Breast discomfort or tenderness
- Generalized sensation of bloating
- Hot flashes in less than 3% of patients
- No bad effect on bone
- No bad effect on liver and renal profile
- No bad effect on ovarian profile
- Endometrial thickening have to be watched.

Facts to be remembered: Clinician detecting endometrial thickening in women treated with UPA needs to be aware that administration of the drug for longer than 3 months may lead to endometrial thickening. This is related to cystic glandular dilation. It is not endometrial hyperplasia, and pathologists need to be aware of PRM-associated endometrial changes (PAEC) and avoid misclassifying the appearance as hyperplasia. This is the probable reason to give a gap of one menstrual cycle after three cycles; the drug's clinical effect is maintained during this gap.

It is also important to consider the limitations of the current data while describing the effects of SPRMs on the endometrium. Most existing studies have described the endometrial changes over short periods (months) of follow-up and atypical hyperplasia and possibly malignant changes take years to develop. Long-term studies are therefore necessary to evaluate such outcomes.

Before prescribing the drug, it is recommended to check her liver function.

Drug can be started again after 1 month and given for further 3 months.

Current status of drug: This is the only SPRM recommended and available for treating fibroids. It has been approved by Ministry of Health and Family and is available in India since 2016. Around 1,15,000 patients have already been treated with the drug in India. Current status of drug worldwide has been discussed in separate chapter.

Asoprisnil: It is a SPRM. It significantly represses both duration and intensity of uterine bleeding as well as the uterine volume, consequently reducing the volume of fibroids. 5 mg/10 mg/25 mg per day dose of asoprisnil have been tried in various studies. Both higher doses gave better results. Drug tolerance was good. It is quite a promising drug but still not available in India. Reduction in size of fibroids was seen up to 80%.

Selective Estrogen Receptor Modulators

Selective estrogen receptor modulators are nonsteroidal estrogen receptor ligands that display tissue-specific agonist or antagonist estrogenic actions. They are most commonly used in the treatment and prevention of estrogen receptor-positive carcinoma of the breast; well-known examples being tamoxifen and raloxifene. In patients receiving raloxifene, decrease in size of myoma was observed in 6–12 months. The treatment has no effect on normal myometrium. 60–180 mg of raloxifene has been tried in various studies. There was no adverse effect on bone density even after 18 months of use. This is also at present an off-label drug for treatment of myoma.

Aromatase Inhibitors

Aromatase inhibitors significantly block both ovarian and peripheral estrogen production within 1 day of treatment. The underlying mechanism is the inhibition of the aromatase enzyme, an enzyme that catalyzes the conversion of androgenic substances into estrogens. Recent reports have suggested that aromatase is expressed to a greater extent in uterine leiomyoma tissues of African–American women compared to Caucasian women, which may contribute to the higher incidence of fibroids in African–American women. Aromatase inhibitors have been shown to be effective against fibroids in limited short-term studies with dosing regimens that included 2.5 mg per day of letrozole and 1 mg per day of anastrozole. One of the major concerns with the use of AIs is the reported bone loss with prolonged use, which necessitates the concomitant use of oral contraceptive pills or progesterone. Need of contraception is also to be addressed. A recently published RCT compared the effects of 3 months of AI (letrozole) to that of 3 months of GnRHa (triptorelin) on uterine leiomyoma volume and hormonal status. The results showed an advantage of the rapid onset of action of AIs in addition to the avoidance of the flare-ups that initially occur with GnRHa. Both treatment options induced significant shrinkage of the uterine fibroids and improvement in leiomyoma-associated symptoms. The mean reduction of leiomyoma volume with 3-month use of anastrozole is 55.7%. Several RCTs are underway that would hopefully add to our understanding of the potential promising role of AIs in the treatment of uterine leiomyomas. Further research on AIs as a therapy, specifically in reproductive age women, is advocated. These are still off-label for use in treatment of myomas.

Others:
- *Cabergoline*: A preliminary study published in 2007 favored the use of cabergoline as a medical treatment of uterine fibroids. The authors reported a volume reduction of about 50% with 6 weeks' use.
- *Combined oral contraceptives*: They do not affect the size of fibroid; nevertheless they are very frequently used for management of heavy menstrual bleeding. They are neutral on fibroid growth.
- *LNG-IUS*: Originally the drug was developed for long-term contraception and is in the market for two decades. It considerably reduces the blood loss and has been used in noncavity distorting symptomatic myomas. It is neutral in terms of effect on the fibroid. There is no reduction in volume or number of fibroids.

Limitation of Medical Treatment

Fibroids typically regrow after stopping the treatment. Patient should be kept under watch during the treatment phase to monitor for size of fibroid, regression of bleeding issues, and relief of pressure symptoms. Medical treatment thus gives a temporary reduction in volume of fibroids with sensible improvement in symptoms.

CONCLUSION

Heavy menstrual bleeding is key symptom of uterine fibroids and a major reason for patient to seek treatment. Current evidence indicates that progesterone and estrogen are key growth factors in pathogeneses of fibroids therefore, current myoma therapies used hormone modulating strategies to achieve fibroid regression and control of bleeding. We have options like GnRHa, mifepristone, and UPA which can be used with good safety profile but at the same time, further studies are indicated to note the long-term effects and side-effects of these drugs. Patient counseling is a must; she must understand that fibroid would not vanish. As such all patients are not for medical therapy. In the end, a careful patient selection and individualized treatment goes a long way in patient's satisfaction and clinician's appreciation.

BIBLIOGRAPHY

1. Arici A. Myomas. Obstetrics and Gynecology Clinics of North America. 2006;33(1):1-232.
2. Chwalisz K, Parker RL, Williamson S, et al. Treatment of uterine leiomyomas with the novel selective progesterone receptor modulator (SPRM). J Soc Gynecol Investig. 2003;10(2 Suppl):Abstract 30IA.
3. Coccia ME, Comparetto C, Bracco GL, et al. GnRH antagonists. Eur J Obstet Gynecol Reprod Biol. 2004;115(Suppl):S44-56.
4. De Leo V, Morgante G, La Marca A, et al. A benefit risk assessment of medical treatment for uterine leiomyomas. Drug Saf. 2002;25(11):759-79.
5. Donnes J, Tomaszewski J, Vázquez F, et al. Ulipristal acetate versus leuprolide acetate for uterine fibroids. New Engl J Med. 2012;366:421-32.
6. Englund K, Blanck A, Gustavsson I, et al. Sex steroid receptors in human myometrium and fibroids: changes during the menstrual cycle and GnRH treatment. J Clin Endocrinol Metab. 1998;83(11):4092-6.
7. Felberbaum RE, Germer U, Ludwig M, et al. Treatment of uterine fibroids with slow release formulation of the GnRH Antagonist Cetrorelix. Hum Reprod. 1998;13(6):1960-8.
8. Fernandez H, Schmidt T, Powell M, et al. Real world data of 1473 patients treated with ulipristal acetate for uterine fibroids: Premya study results. Eur J Obstet Gynecol Reprod Biol. 2017;208:91-6.
9. Fibroids. Segars JH (Ed). In: Gynecology in Practice Series. Arici A (Ed). UK: Wiley Blackwell; 2013.
10. Flierman PA, Oberye JJ, Van der Hulst VP, et al. Rapid reduction of leiomyoma volume during treatment with GnRH antagonist ganirelix. BJOG. 2005;112(5):638-42.
11. Gonzalez-Barcena D, Alvarez RB, Ochoa EP, et al. Treatment of uterine leiomyomas with luteinizing hormone-releasing hormone antagonist cetrorelix. Hum Reprod. 1997;12(9):2028-35.
12. Iveson TJ, Smith IE, Ahern J, et al. Phase I study of the oral non-steroidal aromatase inhibitors CGS 20267 in postmenopausal patients with advanced breast cancer. Cancer Res. 1993;53(2):266-70.
13. Manyonda I, Sinthamoney E, Belli AM. Controversies and challenges in modern management of uterine fibroids. BJOG. 2004;111(2):95-102.
14. Monleón Sancho J, Romaguera E, Romero A, et al. Ulipristal acetate, 5 mg: a new alternative. Med Clin (Barc). 2013;141(Suppl 1):40-6.
15. Murphy AA, Kettel LM, Morales AJ, et al. Regression of uterine leiomyomata in response to the antiprogesterone RU 486: dose-response effect. Fertile Steril. 1995;64(1):187-90.
16. Murphy AA, Kettel LM, Morales AJ, et al. Regression of uterine leiomyomata in response to the antiprogesterone RU 486. J Clin Endocrinol Metab. 1993;76(2):513-7.
17. Nowak RA. Fibroids: pathophysiology and current medical treatment. Baillieres Best Pract Res Clin Obstet Gynaecol. 1999;13(2):223-38.

18. Olive DL, Lindheim SR, Pritts EA. Non-surgical management of leiomyoma: impact on fertility. Curr Opin Obstet Gynecol. 2004;16(3):239-43.
19. Palomba S, Russo T, Orio Jr F, et al. Effectiveness of combined GnRH analogue plus raloxifene administration in treatment of uterine leiomyomas: a prospective, randomized, single blind, placebo controlled clinical trial. Hum Reprod. 2002;17(12):3213-9.
20. Palomba S, Russo T, Orio Jr F, et al. Long term effectiveness of GnRH Agonists plus Raloxifene administration in women with uterine leiomyomas. Hum Reprod. 2004;19(6):1308-14.
21. Shozu M, Sumitani H, Segawa T, et al. Inhibition of in situ expression of Aromatase P450 in leiomyoma of the uterus by leuprorelin acetate. J Clin Endocrenol Metab. 2001;86(11):5405-11.
22. Steinaur J, Pritts EA, Jackson R, et al. Systematic review of mifepristone for the treatment of uterine leiomyomata. Obstet Gynecol. 2004;103(6):1331-6.
23. Wallach EE, Vlahos NF. Uterine myomas—An overview of development clinical features and management. Obstet Gynecol. 2004;104(2):393-406.

Newer Nonsurgical Treatment Options for Fibroids

14

Shalu Gupta, Meenu Handa

INTRODUCTION

For many years, surgery has been the most common treatment offered to patients but now effective alternative treatments are available. These treatments are effective in decreasing both morbidity and mortality associated with surgery. They also help in preserving fertility of patients desiring future pregnancy.

For optimal outcome, we need to individualize the treatment depending on:
- Understanding symptom(s) affecting patient's quality of life.
- Which specific treatments offer best benefit to the patient?
- Minimally invasive therapy should be offered to treat the symptom(s) and preserve fertility if needed.

Treatment modality offered depends on factors such as:
- Patient age
- Type and severity of symptoms
- Size of the fibroid(s)
- Location of the fibroid(s)
- Reproductive plans and obstetrical history.

NEWER NONSURGICAL TREATMENT OPTIONS AVAILABLE
- Uterine artery embolization (UAE)
- Magnetic resonance-guided focused ultrasound (MRgFUS)
- Transvaginal uterine artery occlusion
- Endometrial ablation—refer to chapter on AUB due to fibroids.

Uterine Artery Embolization
- It was first introduced in 1995.
- Most widely used treatment as an alternative to surgical management.

Mode of Action

Embolization causes transient ischemia of endometrium and myometrium for 48–72 hours. This causes irreversible infarction in the fibroid and may damage endometrium. The uterus recovers this ischemia but endometrium remains affected.

Indications

- Women who wish to preserve their uterus but are not interested in future pregnancies
- Women with poor surgical risks
- Women who will not accept blood transfusions
- Severely anemic women requiring immediate intervention.

Contraindications

- Pregnancy
- Infertility (or desire for future pregnancy)
- Genitourinary malignancy
- Comorbidities like pelvic inflammatory disease and salpingitis (increased risk for infection)
- Presence of an adnexal mass
- Desire to avoid a hysterectomy as under any circumstances, there is a small (1%) risk of hysterectomy because of procedure-related complications
- Contraindicate any endovascular procedure:
  - Impaired renal function
  - Coagulopathy
  - Allergy to contrast material.

Pretreatment

- Clinical assessment to ensure symptoms are due to fibroid
- MRI—to confirm diagnosis
- Remove intrauterine contraceptive device (IUCD), if present
- Single dose prophylactic antibiotic
- Low molecular weight heparin in high-risk patients
- Gonadotropin-releasing hormone (GnRH) agonist—optional.

Procedure

Uterine artery embolization is a percutaneous, image-guided procedure, and should be done by experienced interventional radiologist.

An angiographic catheter is introduced into the common femoral artery and directing it into the uterine arteries. Once the catheter is in place, embolic agents (polyvinyl alcohol particles or tris-acryl gelatin microspheres) are then introduced to slow down the blood flow to the fibroid (Figs. 14.1A and B).

Advantages

- Shrinkage of myomas of approximately 30–70%
- Symptomatic relief ranged from 85% to 95% on short and midterm follow-up (5 years)
- Shortened hospital stay, less pain, and a quicker return to work than those undergoing hysterectomy or myomectomy.

Disadvantages

- Unscheduled visits and readmissions.
- Larger uteri and/or more leiomyomas at baseline are at greater risk of failure.
- Relatively high rate of reintervention for treatment failure.
- One reported randomized trial (Table 14.1).

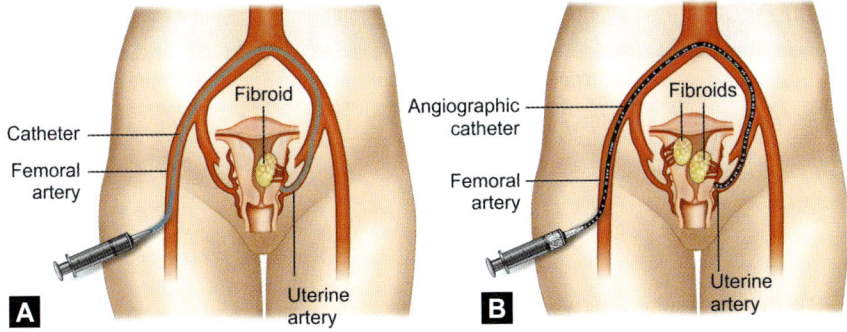

Figs. 14.1A and B: Uterine artery embolization.

Table 14.1: Randomized controlled trial for uterine artery embolization (UAE).

	Uterine artery embolization	Hysterectomy
Minor complications	58%	40%
Readmission for repeat UAE	11%	0%
Major complications	4.9%	2.7%

Complications

Complication rates are low in UAE. The FIBROID registry (largest prospective study published) reported an in-hospital complication rate of 2.7%, with 0.6% rate of major adverse effect.

Immediate complications (During procedure):
- Local complication—hematoma, thrombosis, dissection, and pseudoaneurysm
- Spasm of uterine artery—use vasodilators or microcatheters
- Nontargeted embolization—rare.

Early complications (Within 30 days):
- Moderate ischemic pain—settle down with parenteral analgesia in 12-14 hours postoperative
- Postembolization symptoms:
  - Generalized malaise, fatigue, nausea, and low-grade fever settling in 8-14 days.
  - Prolonged symptoms more than 10 days—suspect infection.
- Readmission for analgesia and fluid resuscitation
- Others:
  - Urinary tract infection
  - Deep vein thrombosis.

Late complications (More than 30 days):
- Vaginal expulsion of an infarcted fibroid (up to 10%)
- Vaginal discharge—self-limiting
- Hysterectomy in 2.9% cases
- Ovarian failure 1-2% patient especially older age group, more than 45 years of age.
- Intrauterine infection, though rare (<1%), increase risk in patients with:

Table 14.2: Comparison of pregnancy outcomes between uterine artery embolization and myomectomy.

	Uterine artery embolization	Myomectomy
Pregnancy rates	50%	78%
Miscarriage rate	64%	23%
Delivery rate	19%	48%

- Pre-existing genitourinary infections
- Adnexal pathology.
- Clinical UAE failure in 5–9% cases—growth of new fibroids.
- Technical UAE failure causes—embolization of only one uterine artery as for a successful treatment bilateral UAE is required.
- Rarely uterine necrosis
- Amenorrhea—Less than 1% in under 40 years.

Effects of UAE or Uterine Fibroid Embolization on Fertility

- Difficult to interpret as studies are small and heterogeneous.
- More adverse pregnancy outcomes than after myomectomy (Table 14.2).
- Studies also suggest that UAE is associated with loss of ovarian reserve, especially in older patients (Evidence level-III).
- Transient or permanent amenorrhea in 5% of women.
- The incidences of cesarean section and postpartum hemorrhage were found to be higher following UAE (66% vs. 48.5% and 13.9% vs. 2.5%, respectively) than in control pregnancies matched for age and fibroid location.

Recommendations by RCOG

- Proper selection of patients
- Uterine artery embolization should be given as treatment options in patient seeking treatment for fibroids
- Proper counseling, consent, and information should be given
- Good results up to 5 years post-UAE
- Only one-thirds of women requires reintervention after 5 years
- Due to lack of solid evidence, it is difficult to make recommendations for women who wish for future pregnancy
- To be done under supervision of multidisciplinary team comprising competent interventional radiologist and gynecologist.

Transvaginal Temporary Uterine Artery Occlusion

- Transvaginal uterine artery occlusion is one of the minimally invasive methods of reducing blood flow in the uterine arteries causing transient ischemia to the fibroids.
- A Doppler ultrasound-enabled transvaginal clamp (Flostat, Vascular Control Systems, San Juan Capistrano, CA, USA) is placed temporarily in the vaginal fornices. The clamp occludes the uterine arteries by mechanical compression against the cervix and is left in place for 6 hours and then removed (Fig. 14.2).

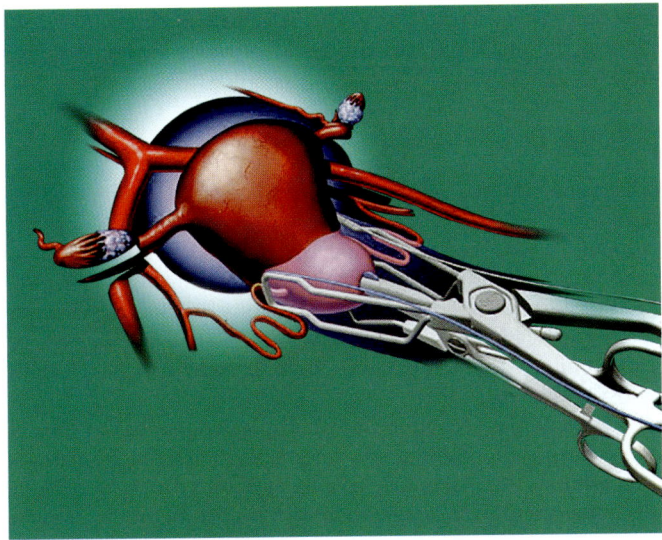

Fig. 14.2: Transvaginal temporary uterine artery occlusion.

Table 14.3: Comparison between uterine artery occlusion and uterine artery embolization.

	Uterine artery occlusion	Uterine artery embolization
Advantages		
Radiation exposure	No	Yes
Risk of non-target embolization	No	Yes
Post-procedure pain	Less	More
Short-term results	Same	Same
Disadvantage		
Long-term benefits	Less	More

- Comparison between transvaginal uterine artery occlusion with UAE is given in (Table 14.3).

Magnetic Resonance-guided Focused Ultrasound

- Approved by US FDA in 2004
- Recent option for the treatment of uterine leiomyomas in premenopausal women who have completed childbearing.

Mode of Action

Uterine fibroid tissue is destroyed by coagulative (thermal) necrosis through heating tissue to over 70°C. This is achieved by converging multiple high frequency ultrasound beams and focusing on small volumes of target tissue.

Magnetic resonance imaging (MRI) is used to direct ultrasound beams to a focal point within a fibroid, resulting in tissue necrosis with minimal damage to surrounding tissue.

122 Fibroids

The MRI gives best resolution, accuracy, and sensitivity to detect uterine fibroids. It gives good visualization of the anatomic structures and provides real-time thermal monitoring during procedure.

Procedure (Fig. 14.3)

- The patient lies prone upon a gel pad coupled to a water tank that is used to propagate the ultrasound beam.
- Prior to treatment, T2-weighted MR is used to identify target fibroids and assess proximity to critical structures including the bowel, spine, and neurovascular bundles.
- The fibroid is then outlined and a sonication plan is developed. After a low-energy test dose, therapeutic sonications are begun.
- MR is used to monitor tissue temperature to ensure adequate power delivery and avoid surrounding tissue damage.
- At treatment completion, repeat contrast MR is repeated to measure area of nonperfusion volume (NPV), which is represented as a volume and percentage ablation of the targeted fibroid and determines the percentage of area of fibroid destruction (Fig. 14.4).
- The patient is subsequently discharged home with postoperative instructions.

Advantages

- Outpatient procedure
- Symptomatic improvement in first 3 months and maintained up to 3 years. Thirty percent patient may require reintervention after 3 years
- Reduction in myoma volume of approximately 37–40%
- Short-term morbidity is low
- Recovery is rapid
- Procedure to be cost-effective.

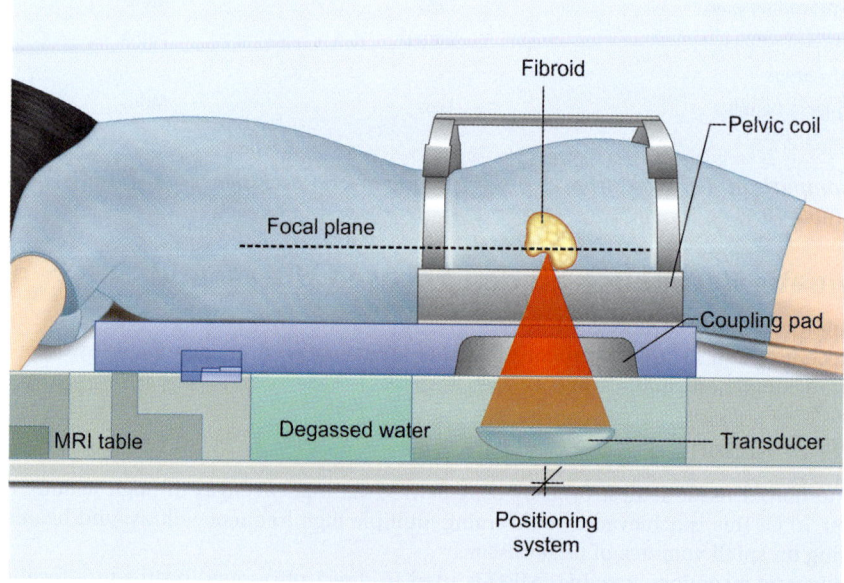

Fig. 14.3: Procedure for magnetic resonance-guided focused ultrasound.

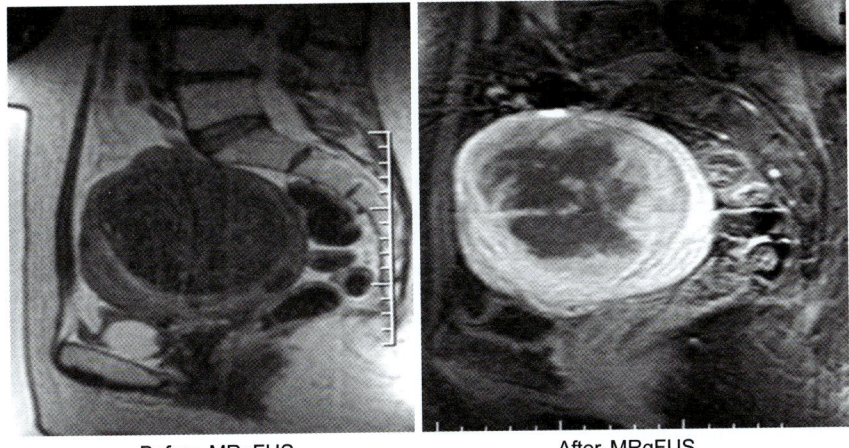

Fig. 14.4: MRI image showing perfusion before and after procedure.
Source: Hindley J, Gedroyc WM, Regan L, et al. MRI guidance of focused ultrasound therapy of uterine fibroids: early results. Am J Roentgenol. 2004;183(6):1713-9.

Disadvantages

- The maximum size of a leiomyoma for this procedure is uncertain.
- Size, vascularity, and access are limiting factors.
- According to a survey, fibroids more than 10 cm are not an absolute contraindication. MRgFUS can be considered after counseling. Further study is needed to determine the optimal fibroid size.
- Time-consuming and costly.

Contraindications

The clinical and technical ineligibility for MRgFUS has been described in Table 14.4.

Relative contraindication: Desire for future pregnancy was originally a contraindication for this therapy, now can be treatment modality in women considering future pregnancy following counseling.

Table 14.4: Contraindications of magnetic resonance-guided focused ultrasound.

Clinical ineligibility	Technical ineligibility
Fibroid—large (>10 cm), multiple, pedunculated, high vascular index, or degenerated or calcified	Patient not able to lie in prone position for long time
Postmenopausal	Obese
Pelvic inflammatory disease	Metallic implants incompatible with MRI
Suspected malignancy	Nonenhancement with gadolinium
Adenomyosis	Sensitive to MRI contrast
Undiagnosed vaginal bleeding	Intervening bowel or bladder could be damaged by treatment
Fibroids resectable with a hysteroscope	

Effects of MRgFUS on Fertility

There are several case reports and one case series of pregnancy following MRgFUS. A series of 50 cases from all centers doing MRgFUS was observed and followed. 54 uneventful pregnancies were achieved in 50 patients. Mean birth weight was 3.3 kg and there was 64% vaginal delivery rate. There was no specific pattern of complications. 9% of women had placentation problems, but in this series, all had prior uterine surgery as a risk factor for this complication.

Regarding pregnancy, there are only 35 published reports of live birth following MRgFUS and the heterogeneity of these data is great. Although 53% of pregnancies resulted in vaginal delivery, the power of this case series is too low.

Drawbacks

- No large scale studies
- Data on their reproductive outcomes in patients trying to conceive are insufficient to make recommendations
- Studies are needed to determine long-term outcome and optimal candidates for this procedure; comparative studies are also needed.

CONCLUSION

The possibility of newer minimally invasive technologies offers a new hope to the women with symptomatic fibroids who wish to avoid surgery and who have fertility concerns. Both UAE and MRgFUS are good alternatives to surgery in symptomatic large fibroids with comparable in terms of safety and post-procedure outcome and cost-effectiveness. Though reproductive outcomes are needed to be followed with large-scale studies. The limiting factors in the routine use of these minimally invasive newer technologies are expensive set-up and good teamwork of gynecologists with interventional radiologists.

BIBLIOGRAPHY

1. Aitken E, Khaund A, Hamid SA, et al. The normal human myometrium has a vascular spatial gradient absent in small fibroids. Hum Reprod. 2006;21:2669-78.
2. Bradley LD, Gueye NA. Leiomyoma therapeutic options: is it now prime time for stratified medicine? Fertil Steril. 2016;105(5):1045-6.
3. Clarka NA, Mumfordb SL, James H. Reproductive impact of MRI-guided focused ultrasound surgery for fibroids: a systematic review of the evidence. Curr Opin Obstet Gynecol. 2014;26(3):151-61.
4. Funaki K, Fukunishi H, Sawada K. Clinical outcomes of magnetic resonance-guided focused ultrasound surgery for uterine myomas: 24- month follow-up. Ultrasound Obstet Gynecol. 2009;34(5):584.
5. Gupta JK, Sinha A, Lumsden MA, et al. Uterine artery embolization for symptomatic uterine fibroids. Cochrane Database Syst Rev. 2014;12:CD005073.
6. Hesley GK, Gorny KR, Henrichsen TL, et al. A clinical review of focused ultrasound ablation with magnetic resonance guidance: an option for treating uterine fibroids. Ultrasound Q. 2008;24(2):131.
7. Hindley J, Gedroyc WM, Regan L, et al. MRI guidance of focused ultrasound therapy of uterine fibroids: early results. Am J Roentgenol. 2004;183(6):1713-9.
8. Homer H, Saridogan E. Uterine artery embolization for fibroids is associated with an increased risk of miscarriage. Fertil Steril. 2010;94(1):324-30.
9. http://www.nice.org.uk/nicemedia/live/11349/57237/57237.pdf.
10. http://www.rcog.org.uk/files/rcog-corp/uploaded files/WPRUterineArteryEmbolisation 2009.pdf.
11. Hutchins FL, Jr, Worthington-Kirsch R, Berkowitz RP. Selective uterine artery embolization as primary treatment for symptomatic leiomyomata uteri. J Am Assoc Gynecol Laparosc. 1999;6:279-84.
12. Jacoby VL, Kohi MP, Poder L, et al. PROMISe trial: a pilot, randomized, placebo–controlled trial of magnetic resonance guided focused ultrasound for uterine fibroids. Fertil Steril. 2016;105(3):773-80.

13. Kaump GR, Spies JB. The impact of uterine artery embolization on ovarian function. J Vasc Interv Radiol. 2013;24:459-67.
14. Lichtinger M, Burbank F, Hallson L, et al. The time course of myometrial ischemia and reperfusion after laparoscopic uterine artery occlusion-theoretical implication. J Am Assoc Gynecol Laparosc. 2003;10:554-63.
15. Mara M, Maskova J, Fucikova Z, et al. Midterm clinical and first reproductive results of a randozimed controlled trial comparing uterine fibroid embolization and myomectomy. Cardiovasc Intervent Radiol. 2008;31:73-85.
16. National Institute for Health and Clinical Excellence. (2007). Current SOGC Clinical Practice Guidelines, 2005.
17. Payne JF, Haney AF. Serious complications of uterine artery embolization for conservative treatment of fibroids. Fertil Steril. 2003;79(1):128-31.
18. Pron G. Magnetic resonance-guided high-intensity focused ultrasound (MRgHIFU) treatment of symptomatic uterine fibroids: an evidence-based analysis. Ont Health Technol Assess Ser. 2015;15(4):1-86.
19. Rabinovici J, David M, Fukunishi H, et al. MRgFUS Study Group. Pregnancy outcome after magnetic resonance-guided focused ultrasound surgery (MRgFUS) for conservative treatment of uterine fibroids. Fertil Steril. 2010;93(1):199.
20. Ravina JH, Herbreteau D, Ciraru-Vigneron N, et al. Arterial embolization to treat uterine myomata. Lancet. 1995;346:671-2.
21. Smith WJ, Upton E, Shuster EJ, et al. Patient satisfaction and disease specific quality of life after uterine artery embolization. Am J Obstet Gynecol. 2004;190:1697-1703.
22. Spies JB, Ascher SA, Roth AR, et al. Uterine artery embolization for leiomyomata. Obstet Gynecol. 2001a;98:29-34.
23. Spies JB, Bruno J, Czeyda-Pommersheim F, et al. Long-term outcome of uterine artery embolization of leiomyomata. Obstet Gynecol. 2005;106(5 Pt 1):933.
24. Spies JB, Sacks D. Credentials for uterine artery embolization. J Vasc Interv Radiol. 2004;15:111-3.
25. Stewart EA. Uterine fibroids. Lancet. 2001;357(9252):293.
26. Tropeano G, Amoroso S, Scambia G. Non-surgical management of uterine fibroids. Hum Reprod Update. 2008;14(3):259-74.
27. Walker WJ, Pelage JP. Uterine artery embolisation for symptomatic fibroids: clinical results in 400 women with imaging follow-up. Br J Obstet Gynecol. 2002;109:1263-72.
28. Worthington-Kirsch R, Koller NE. Time course of pain after uterine artery embolization for fibroid disease. Medscape Womens Health. 2002b;7:4.
29. Worthington-Kirsch R, Popky GL, Hutchins FL, Jr. Uterine arterial embolization for the management of leiomyomas: quality-of-life assessment and clinical response. Radiology. 1998;208:625-9.
30. Worthington-Kirsch R, Spies JB, Myers ER, et al. The Fibroid Registry for Outcomes Data (FIBROID) for uterine embolization: short term outcomes. Obstet Gynecol. 2005;106:52-9.
31. Zupi E, Pocek M, Dauri M, et al. Selective uterine artery embolization in the management of uterine myomas. Fertil Steril. 2003;79:107-11.

15
Fibroids and Malignancy

Reeta Mahey, Venus Dalal

INTRODUCTION

Uterine leiomyoma (fibroid) is the most common benign smooth muscle uterine neoplasm among women of reproductive age. Women with a uterine mass presumed to be a leiomyoma may have a uterine sarcoma or a leiomyoma variant. Malignant transformation of benign leiomyoma to leiomyosarcoma, although a rare occurrence but can happen in certain patients like in postmenopausal with large myomas, rapid growing myomas, and in certain subset of leiomyoma.

Overall, sarcomas contribute to less than 5% of all uterine malignancies. In a recently published meta-analysis, the prevalence of uterine sarcoma in presumed uterine fibroids ranged from 0.00% to 0.49%. Sarcomas are classified into leiomyosarcoma (LMS), endometrial stromal sarcoma (ESS), and undifferentiated sarcoma (US). Of these, most common subtype is LMS. These are aggressive tumors usually seen after 40 years age with high rates of early metastasis. Median survival from the time of diagnosis is 10 months.

There are a number of leiomyoma variants in which the smooth muscle tumor manifests one histologic facet of malignancy, yet lacks all others. These include cellular leiomyoma, atypical leiomyoma, leiomyomatosis peritonealis disseminata, intravenous leiomyomatosis, and benign metastasizing leiomyomas. These are defined by their quasi-malignant capacity to metastasize while remaining histologically and clinically benign. Finally, some smooth muscle tumor variants cannot be definitely classified, and consequently are deemed to have an uncertain malignant potential like smooth muscle tumors of uncertain malignant potential (STUMP). Incidence of atypical variants (including malignancy) is about 1.2% (0.7–2.2%).

Exact malignant potential of these types is unknown but long-term follow-up is recommended due to rare risk of transformation to LMS.

Surgeries, including myomectomy and hysterectomy, are commonly performed to treat symptomatic leiomyomas. With advances in minimally invasive surgical techniques and devices, laparoscopic surgery has gained worldwide popularity. To remove large uterine masses, mechanical morcellator has been used but this power morcellation can lead to dispersion of myoma pieces in the abdomen or in the abdominal wall. Very rarely these pieces might contain atypical cells like cellular or atypical myoma, LMS. FDA estimated that risk of LMS in a presumed benign fibroid is 1 in 498. But in other studies, findings of LMS in presumed nonmorcellated hysterectomy specimens has been reported at 0.23–0.49%.

We have encountered only one case of unsuspected LMS in last 9 years following total laparoscopic hysterectomy which was done in another hospital. Histopathology of hysterectomy specimen was benign leiomyoma. Two years later, patient noticed a 10 × 8 cm swelling at the site of previous morcellation port (Fig. 15.1A). Fine needle aspiration of the mass also confirmed the features of leiomyoma. MRI abdomen revealed another mass

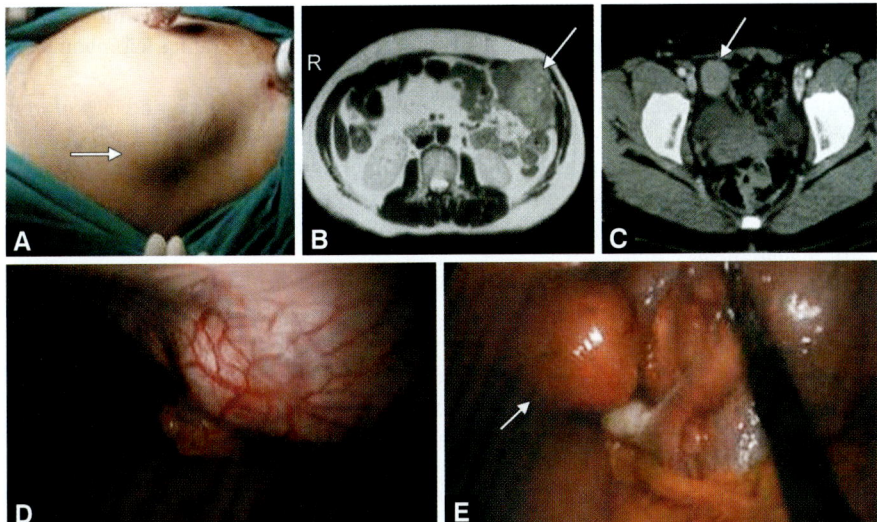

Figs. 15.1A to E: (A) Abdominal mass occupying left hypogastrium and lumbar area at previous morcellation site; (B) MRI showing hypointense lesion (10 × 8 cm) occupying left abdominal wall involving rectus sheath; (C) MRI showing hypointense mass (4 × 4 cm) in right adnexa separate from ovary; (D) Laparoscopic view showing inner side of the abdominal mass; (E) Pelvic mass (4 × 4 cm) near right infundibulopelvic ligament.

Table 15.1: Various modalities for detection of leiomyosarcoma.

Imaging	Sensitivity	Specificity
MRI	100%	96.9%
LDH (Total)	100%	87.7%
LDH 3	90%	92.3%
LDH and MRI	100%	99.2%

about 4 × 4 cm in the pelvis with similar intensity features (Figs. 15.1B and C). Patient underwent laparoscopic assisted removal of both masses (Figs. 15.1D and E) and to surprise, histopathology of both masses revealed features of LMS with high mitotic activity. Follow-up positron emission tomography (PET) scan was normal with no evidence of residual tumor and patient is under follow-up.

ROLE OF IMAGING

Unfortunately, not all uterine cancers can be diagnosed preoperatively. Further research is required as investigations are inconclusive. Sensitivity and specificity of few modalities have been evaluated (Table 15.1) in recent studies. Most sarcomas present with symptoms similar to benign fibroids such as abnormal uterine bleeding, pain or lump abdomen but signs like large myoma and rapid increase in size points toward malignancy especially in postmenopausal females. If a sarcoma is expected after ultrasound evaluation, magnetic resonance imaging (MRI) and serum lactate dehydrogenase (LDH) may be helpful in further evaluation. Uterine sarcomas often demonstrate moderate to high uptake in the fluorodeoxyglucose (FDG) PET scan, compared with very low uptake of FDG in benign leiomyomas. These findings should be interpreted with caution, however, as several reports of degenerating leiomyomas have exhibited increased uptake as well.

Hematogenous dissemination is the most common route of metastasis, and 50% of women with clinical stage I LMS have evidence of lung metastases at presentation. Total abdominal hysterectomy with or without bilateral salpingo-oophorectomy is an adequate surgical procedure for LMS. More trials are needed to address the need of adjuvant radiotherapy or chemotherapy. The 5-year survival for a stage I LMS or US is 63% compared with 14% for stage IV malignancies.

MANAGEMENT

If histopathology of LMS is given in a hysterectomy specimen, then no further intervention is required and patient can be kept on follow-up.

But if LMS report comes in a myomectomy specimen, hysterectomy with or without salpingo-oophorectomy should be done.

If report is ESS—complete surgery (hysterectomy and bilateral salpingo-oophorectomy) should be done.

As there is no confirmatory diagnostic test to detect LMS in a presumed benign myoma, following steps are advised while removing large myomas laparoscopically:
- Vigilant examination of abdomen during morcellation.
- Morcellation should be done by expert or under guidance.
- Histopathological examination of every myoma specimen should be done carefully from each centimeter of specimen. Also area of necrosis, degeneration, and hemorrhage should be taken for histopathological examination.
- Proper counseling regarding chance of atypical variants or sarcoma in the morcellated specimen leading to all the complications discussed above. Need of follow-up and need of repeat surgical intervention should be explained to these special cases.

The need of informed written consent:
With regard to all forms of tissue morcellation, the following risks should be included in the discussion:
- Dissemination of malignant tissue in the peritoneal cavity, which may worsen prognosis.
- Dissemination of benign tissue, which may result in untoward health consequences, including the need for re-operation or additional treatments.
- Rendering complete pathologic evaluation of a tissue specimen more difficult.
- Injury to adjacent organs unique to the technique of morcellation.

These risks should be weighed in the context of the benefits of a minimally invasive approach as well as the risks and benefits of expectant management or laparotomy as alternatives.

PROPOSED ALTERNATIVES

Modified morcellation techniques, i.e. minilaparotomy, vaginal morcellation, and Contained in Bag Morcellation (CIBM) are alternative methods of specimen retrieval to avoid intraperitoneal dissemination of the myoma tissue.

CONCLUSION

The risk of LMS in a fibroid is rare. Further large number trials are required to evaluate the sensitivity and specificity of different imaging and biochemical modalities to make optimal cut-offs to differentiate between benign and malignant lesions.

BIBLIOGRAPHY

1. Anupama R, Ahmad SZ, Kuriakose S, et al. Disseminated peritoneal leiomyosarcomas after laparoscopic "myomectomy" and morcellation. J Minim Invasive Gynecol. 2011;18(3):386-9.
2. Bharambe BM, Deshpande KA, Surase SG, et al. Malignant transformation of leiomyoma of uterus to leiomyosarcoma with metastasis to ovary. J Obstet Gynaecol India. 2014;64(1):68-9.
3. D'Angelo E, Prat J. Uterine sarcomas: a review. Gynecol Oncol. 2010;116(1):131-9.
4. Goto A, Takeuchi S, Sugimura K, et al. Usefulness of Gd-DTPA contrast-enhanced dynamic MRI and serum determination of LDH and its isozymes in the differential diagnosis of leiomyosarcoma from degenerated leiomyoma of the uterus. Int J Gynecol Cancer. 2002;12(4):354-61.
5. Guntupalli SR, Ramirez PT, Anderson ML, et al. Uterine smooth muscle tumor of uncertain malignant potential: a retrospective analysis. Gynecol Oncol. 2009;113(3):324-6.
6. Kanade TT, McKenna JB, Choi S, et al. Sydney contained in bag morcellation for laparoscopic myomectomy. J Minim Invasive Gynecol. 2014;21(6):981.
7. Leibsohn S, d'Ablaing G, Mishell DR, et al. Leiomyosarcoma in a series of hysterectomies performed for presumed uterine leiomyomas. Am J Obstet Gynecol. 1990;162(4):968-74; discussion 974-6.
8. Leung F, Terzibachian J-J, Gay C, et al. Hysterectomies performed for presumed leiomyomas: should the fear of leiomyosarcoma make us apprehend non laparotomic surgical routes? Gynécologie Obstétrique Fertil. 2009;37(2):109-14.
9. Parker WH, Fu YS, Berek JS. Uterine sarcoma in patients operated on for presumed leiomyoma and rapidly growing leiomyoma. Obstet Gynecol. 1994;83(3):414-8.
10. Rha SE, Byun JY, Jung SE, et al. CT and MRI of uterine sarcomas and their mimickers. Am J Roentgenol. 2003;181(5):1369-74.
11. Stein K, Ascher-Walsh C. A comprehensive approach to the treatment of uterine leiomyomata. Mt Sinai J Med N Y. 2009;76(6):546-56.
12. Wu C, Zhang X, Tao X, et al. Leiomyomatosis peritonealis disseminata: A case report and review of the literature. Mol Clin Oncol. 2016;4(6):957-8.

Recurrence and Treatment Outcomes in Fibroids

Kavitha Gautham

INTRODUCTION

Uterine myomas are the most common pelvic tumors in women. Once treated, they are notorious for recurring. Clinical studies have reported a recurrence rate of 5–30%. Malone followed up to 125 cases over a period of 5–10 years and noted a recurrence rate of 47%. This wide range seems to be because of discrepancies in long-term follow-up and different criteria used in diagnosis. Significance factors for nonrecurrence seem to be occurrence of term pregnancies after treatment, number of myomas removed, and the period of observation, not significant ones seem to be the age of the patient at the myomectomy and the site of myomas.

Candiani et al. did a study on the 10 years probability of recurrence. They showed that women who gave birth to a child after myomectomy had a 10-year recurrence rate of 15% against 30% for those who did not. Incidence of recurrence was more, if two or more fibroids had been removed.

INCIDENCE OF FIBROID RECURRENCE

The most significant complication related to the treatment of uterine fibroids is regrowth and associated return of bothersome symptoms. Myomectomy is associated with persistence, regrowth, or de novo development of fibroids and return of symptoms following surgery in up to 50% of cases. Even women undergoing hysterectomy can have resurgence of symptoms 8% of the time following surgery. There are essentially no studies of uterine artery embolization (UAE) and long-term outcome. Broder and colleagues (2002) found that 20% of patients who underwent UAE required further invasive therapy between 3 years and 5 years following the procedure. Options following treatment failures include repeat conservative surgery versus hysterectomy.

RECURRENCE VERSUS NEW OCCURRENCE OF FIBROIDS

Recurrence is the regrowth of the same fibroid. Mostly happens with medical management and with radiological intervention.

Reoccurrence or new occurrence—this is new occurrence of fibroids or growth of new fibroids and it happens with surgical management.

PROGNOSTIC FACTORS FOR RECURRENCE
Age
There is considerable debate about the effect of age. No relationship was found in two studies. The risk of recurrence tended to increase with age in the study by Fedele on the contrary it dropped in patients operated after age of 35 in another study. For Bonney, the younger the woman undergoing myomectomy, the higher the risk of recurrence. These conflicting results were explained by two phenomena working in opposite directions. On one hand, population of women free of disease until then. The incidence rate was 4.3 per 1,000 women—years for the age group 25-29 years, and 22.5 per 1,000 women-years for the age group 40-44 years. On the other hand, the subpopulation of women presenting clinically significant myomata at a young age is probably more at risk than the other of having more active "myometrial disease" and thus recurrence after myomectomy.

Number of Myomata
The risk of recurrence increases distinctly with the number of myomata removed. Two explanations can be found for this relationship; one is that the more myomata there are in the myometrium the more difficult it is to obtain comprehensive exeresis; the other is that it is likely that a large number of myomata in the myometrium mean that the "myometrial disease" is more evaluative.

GnRH Agonists
Gonadotropin-releasing hormone (GnRH) agonists seem to increase the risk of recurrence after myomectomy. Two studies have given contradictory results. A first randomized clinical trial found no link between the use of agonists preoperatively and the risk of recurrence, but this study is not broad enough. Another randomized clinical trial found an increased risk of recurrence in the group treated preoperatively. It is possible that because the small interstitial myomata are made even smaller by the agonists they might not be detected during the operation.

Conversely, sequential use of agonists postoperatively (3 months per year) could reduce the long-term risk of recurrence in women who have had complete surgical exeresis. The analogs probably act on the growth of small intraclinical myomatous nuclei. If the results of this pilot study are confirmed by randomized clinical trials, preventive measures for postoperative recurrence could be proposed in certain particular cases with a high risk of recurrence (young and motivated women, and removal of a large number of myomata).

Property of the Surgical Procedure
It is essential that exeresis be as complete as possible. Taken on its own, this is not enough to limit the risk of recurrence because many cases of myomatous uterus include small nuclei, which are undetectable perioperatively and will be left behind. It does, however, avoid the early reappearance of clinically significant myomata. Several steps needed in order to diagnose all the myomatous nuclei peri- and preoperatively; transvaginal and suprapubic ultrasound investigation by a highly experienced ultrasound operator, diagnostic or preoperative hysteroscopy; meticulous palpation of the myometrium; and opening of the cavity when there is the slightest doubt.

Laparoscopic Approach

Only one study has been devoted especially to the risk of recurrence after laparoscopic myomectomy. The cumulative rate at 5 years is considerably higher than that observed in the series of myomectomy by laparotomy and the recurrences occur more quickly. In our institution, we are carrying out a study at present into recurrence and our preliminary not permit correct palpation into recurrence and our preliminary results are quite similar. Because the laparoscopic approach does not permit correct palpation of the myometrium, small interstitial myomatous nuclei could be overlooked, meaning exeresis would be incomplete more frequently than when laparotomy is used, if these results are confirmed then extreme caution should accompany the use of the laparoscopic route in cases of multiple myoma. In particular, preoperative detection of myomata needs to be extremely thorough.

Parity after Myomectomy

Several studies have found that pregnancy after the myomectomy is associated with a lower risk of recurrence. Similarly, the fact of pregnancy loss is associated with a higher risk of recurrence. To our mind, these results simply demonstrate the fact that the myomata themselves are probably factors for infertility or loss of pregnancy. The persistence or recurrence of myomata would thus reduce the likelihood of conception or taking a pregnancy full term after the myomectomy.

RECURRENCE AFTER MEDICAL MANAGEMENT

Medical therapy avoids complications associated with surgery and permits uterine preservation.

Medical management therapies, which are available in reducing the symptoms and size of the fibroids, are:
- *Long-acting progesterone*: Depo-Provera 150 mg/month for 6 months.
  - Volume of the fibroid is reduced but the effect is temporary.
- *Antiprogestin (mifepristone, RU486)*: 25 mg daily for 3 months resulted in 50% reduction in size, but recurred after stopping the treatment.
- *Selective progesterone receptor modulator (SPRM)*: Ulipristal.
- *Selective estrogen receptor modulator (SERM)*: Raloxifene.
  - In postmenopausal women results in reducing the size.
- *Aromatase inhibitors*:
  - *Gestrinone* reduces up to 40% reduction
  - *Danazol* is an isoxazole derivative of 17-alpha ethinyl-testosterone (ethisterone). It reduces volume by 23.6%.

Pretreatment with GnRH Analogs

The GnRH analogs decrease uterine muscle size and numbers, hence, fibroid size. There is a 50% reduction in fibroid size with GnRH analogs. It also causes a reduction in blood flow and hence less blood loss during surgery. The disadvantage is its cost and the fact that fibroids regrow within 2–3 months of stopping treatment. Besides it causes vasomotor symptoms and bone loss.

Pretreatment with GnRH analogs did not affect the recurrence rate nor the myoma-related symptoms. Study done by Friedman et al. found that the critical factor seems to the number of myomas seen initially. If it was less than three then the chances of recurrence were 9 in 10 patients.

Gonadotropin-releasing hormone is associated with increased risk of recurrence of fibroids after myomectomy.

The use of GnRH agonist preoperatively is highly likely to influence "recurrence" rates. Smaller fibroids would tend to shrink and not be seen, or be ignored as too small to remove, at time of surgery, only to reappear and grow even more rapidly after withdrawal of GnRH agonist. No wonder then that preoperative use of GnRH agonists has been reported as high-risk factor for recurrence of fibroids.

GnRH Antagonists

Daily injection shows 29% reduction in volume within 3 weeks. Medical treatment is indicated mainly for temporary control of symptoms and preoperative status of the patients. The symptoms and size of the fibroid usually recurs once the medical treatment is stopped.

The aim is to reduce the size of the fibroid and improve the hematological states of the patient.

Medical management definitely causes certain percentage of reduction in fibroid size. But recurrence is seen once the treatment is stopped. Hence, medical management for reduction of size of fibroid is advised only during the preoperative period.

Radiological Therapy

Uterine Artery Embolization

Uterine artery embolization (UAE) has been found to provide good short-term relief of bulk-related symptoms and reduction in menorrhagia associated with uterine fibroids. Its impact on future fertility and future pregnancy outcome as well as long-term efficacy is currently unknown and therefore desire for future fertility is relative contraindication to this procedure. In treating fibroid-related symptoms, it is similar to the response symptoms; it is similar to the response rate seen following myomectomy (87.5% for UAE vs 93.3% for myomectomy).

Although those are more minor complications related to UAE, there were no significant differences in serious or long-term complications between myomectomy and UAE. However, there is an increased likelihood of requiring further surgical intervention within 2–5 years of UAE.

Magnetic Resonance Imaging-guided Focused Ultrasound

Image-guided therapy (IGT) is a rapidly developing field in a less invasive alternative.

According to clinical outcomes, magnetic resonance guided focused ultrasound (MRgFUS) treatment is feasible, reproducible, and significantly reduces symptoms in more than 75% of women treated with fibroids. The rate of side effects is generally low. Rabinovici et al. have reported on safe and successful outcomes of pregnancies after MRgFUS. Evaluate the efficacy and safety of MRgFUS for the enhancement of fertility in women with uterine fibroids who are diagnosed with unexplained infertility.

RECURRENCE AFTER MINIMAL INVASIVE SURGERY

Depending on size and location, myomectomy can be performed through a laparoscope or hysteroscope, or via a laparotomy incision. Aside from the surgical risks including bleeding, infection, and organ injury, there is a significant 10–27% risk of fibroid recurrence following abdominal myomectomy, with similar recurrence figures for hysteroscopic resection.

Recurrence of fibroids following laparoscopic myomectomy, however, can reach as high as 50% by some reports. Significant hemorrhage as a complication of myomectomy can result in emergent hysterectomy in a small number of cases.

- *Myomectomy by laparotomy*: Abdominal myomectomy by laparotomy is associated with longer surgical time and greater blood loss when compared with hysterectomy and is associated with a 15% recurrence rate for uterine fibroids. 10% of women undergoing myomectomy through an abdominal incision will subsequently undergo hysterectomy within 5–10 years for persistent symptoms. The usual surgical risks apply, including bleeding, infection, contiguous organ injury, and unintended hysterectomy. Cases of uterine rupture in pregnancies subsequent to myomectomy have been reported in the literature. Some authorities recommend managing patients with history of myomectomy as you would for vaginal birth after cesarean candidates. Patients should be counseled regarding this low risk of uterine rupture in subsequent pregnancies following myomectomy, regardless of route of removal.
- *Myomectomy by laparoscopy:* This minimally invasive surgery is completed through a number of small abdominal incisions. Careful patient selection based on size, location, and number of fibroids is important in deciding whether the patient is a candidate for laparoscopic myomectomy. If the mass is between 5 cm and 7 cm in diameter, the laparoscopic approach may be more appropriate and recovery is more rapid than with the abdominal approach. However, risk of recurrence is higher; it has been reported to be 33% by 27 months following surgery and can reach as high as 50%.
- *Myomectomy by hysteroscopy*: This is the first-line procedure for intracavitary fibroids when preservation of fertility is desired. Preoperative sonohysterography is mandatory to determine the location of the fibroid in relation to the uterine wall and extent of protrusion into the uterine cavity. Hysteroscopic myomectomy carries additional risks related to the requirement for use of high-flow distention media, which can cause hyponatremia, coma, and death from fluid overload. Rare but significant complications include electrical burns to genital organs and bowel as well as heavy bleeding, which may require emergent hysterectomy. Guidelines published in 2011 provide information on developments in hysteroscopic equipment and techniques, as well as the use of pharmacological agents.

Risk of Recurrence of Leiomyomata after Myomectomy

Abdominal myomectomy (by laparotomy or by laparoscopy) aims to obtain total exercises of the myomata while preserving reproductive function.

The optimism of the pioneers of this technique was based on the fact that they believed recurrence were in fact the reappearance of myomata left behind during the first surgical treatment.

Role of Reoperation and Hysterectomy

The crude rate of reoperation varies from one study to the next. However, it can be estimated that on average one patient out of two presenting with recurrence (evaluated clinically) had to be reoperated.

The crude rate of hysterectomy after myomectomy by laparotomy varies from 4.3% to 16.8% for studies with a maximum follow-up over 8 years. One study shows a high rate of hysterectomy (26.7%) after myomectomy with no particular explanation apart from a long follow-up period. The hysterectomy rate after *leiomyomata* (LM) differed little (6.1–13.8%) from that observed after laparotomy but the study follow-up was shorter. It can be estimated that on average one patient out of three presenting with a reoccurrence needs a hysterectomy.

Risk of Malignancy Recurrence

Laparoscopic power morcellation poses the risk of spreading unsuspected cancerous tissues, most notably uterine sarcomas, beyond the uterus. Based on currently available information, the Food and Drug Administration (FDA) discourages the use of laparoscopic power morcellation during a hysterectomy or myomectomy for uterine fibroids.

Brohl et al. found the risk of unexpected uterine sarcomas (UUSs) varied significantly across age groups, and the risk of uterine sarcoma ranged from a peak of 10.1 cases per 1,000 for patients. A retrospective analysis of 10,248 cases of myomectomy and hysterectomy for uterine fibroids and found that 48 cases of UUSs, which was 04.7%.

A number of studies have shown that the incidence of UUSs ranges from 0.09% to 0.49% among women undergoing benign hysterectomy or myomectomy.

Obstetric Consideration following Surgery

Uterine rupture occurred at 34 weeks of gestation or later in 85.7%, and during labor in 14.3% of cases.

There was no uterine rupture during the trials of labor and also spontaneous uterine rupture seems to be rare after LM. This risk should not deter the use of LM, if needed. When performing LM, particular care must be given to the uterine closure.

Bhandari S et al. in her studies states that intrauterine adhesions were seen in 11 out of 51 (21.57%) cases.

FUTURE RESEARCH

Although LM were more numerous and large in women with a preoperative history of LM, the prevalence of myomata diagnosed by fine histological section was no higher than in uteri removed for reasons other than myoma. The true question is therefore to establish which factors are at the origin of the growth of small residual myomatous nuclei (after myomectomy). It is thus essential to identify and clarify the role played by the various factors encouraging myoma growth, i.e. estrogen, progesterone, and cytokines; chromosomal abnormalities associated with individual myomata and family predisposition to myomata.

Use of these factors in clinical practice could then benefit from more suitable treatment strategies or drug treatment to prevent recurrence.

CONCLUSION

Abdominal myomectomy (by laparotomy or by laparoscopy) enables all the myomata to be excised while maintaining reproductive function. A cumulative risk of clinically significant recurrence of approximately 10% at 5 years for myomectomy by laparotomy. After laparoscopic myomectomy, there appears to be a greater risk of recurrence. In one-third of cases, recurrence becomes the reason for a hysterectomy. The risk of recurrence increases when there is more than one myoma. The use of GnRH agonists preoperatively could increase the risk of recurrence. Persistence or recurrence of the myoma thus reduces the chances of conception or taking a pregnancy full term after the myomectomy. It is essential to obtain the most complete exeresis possible in order to reduce the risk of recurrence to a minimum. However, it is inevitable that small and undetectable nuclei will remain within the myometrium whatever approach is used (laparoscopy or laparotomy). It would be an advantage to know what the growth factors are and how to identify groups at high risk of recurrence, so that the treatment strategies could be better adapted and appropriate prophylactic methods developed.

BIBLIOGRAPHY

1. American Congress of Obstetrician and Gynecologists. ACOG committee opinion: Uterine artery embolisation. Obstet Gynecol. 2004;103:403-4.
2. Andersen J. Growth factors and cytokines in uterine leiomyomas. Semin Reprod Endocrinol. 1996;14:269-82.
3. Bajekal N, Li TC. Fibroids, infertility and Pregnancy wastage. Hum Reprod Update. 2000;6:614-20.
4. Berkeley AS, DeCherney AH, Polan ML. Abdominal myomectomy and subsequent fertility. Surg Gynecol Obstet. 1983;156:319-22.
5. Bonney V. The technique and results of myomectomy. Lancet. 1931;220:171-3.
6. Broder MS, Goodwin S, Chen G, et al. Comparison of long-term outcomes of myomectomy and uterine artery embolisation. Obstet Gynecol. 2002;100:864-8.
7. Brohl AS, Li L, Andikyan V, et al. Age-stratified risk of unexpected uterine sarcoma following surgery for presumed benign leiomyoma. Oncologist. 2015;20:433-9.
8. Brosens I, Deprest J, Dal Cin P, et al. Clinical significance of cytogenetic abnormalities in uterine myomas. Fertili Steril. 1998;69:232-5.
9. Brown AB, Chamberlain R, Te Linde RW. Myomectomy. Am J Obstet Gynecol. 1956;71:759-63.
10. Brown WW III, Coddington CC III. Expectant and medical management of uterine fibroids. In: Tulandi T (Ed). Uterine fibroids: Embolization and other treatments. Cambridge University Press: London; 2003.
11. Buttram VC, Reiter R. Uterine leiomyomata: etiology, symptomatology and management. Fertil Steril. 1981;36:433-45.
12. Candiani GB, Fedele L, Parazzini F. Risk of recurrence after myomectomy. Br Obstet Gynecol. 1991;98:385-9.
13. Cramer SF, Patel A. The frequency of uterine leiomyomas. Am J Clin Pathol. 1990;94:435-8.
14. Dadak C, Feiks A. Organ-sparing surgery of leiomyomas of the uterus in young females. Zentralbl Gynecol. 1988;110:102-6.
15. De Leo V, LaMarca A, Morgante G. short term treatment of uterine fibroymomas with danazol. Gynecol Obstet Invest. 1999;47:258.
16. Di Spiezio Sardo A, Mazzon I, Bramante S, et al. Hysteroscopic myomectomy: a comprehensive review of surgical techniques. Hum Reprod Update. 2008;14:101-19.
17. Eisinger SH, Meldrum S, Fiscella K, et al. Low dose mifepristone for uterine leiomyomata. Obstet Gynecol. 2003;101:243-50.
18. Fauconnier A, Chapron C, Babaki-Fard K, et al. Recurrence of leiomyomata after myomectomy. Hum Reprod Update. 2000;6:595-602.
19. Fedele L, Parazzini F, Luchini, et al. Recurrence of fibroids after myomectomy: a transvaginal ultrasonographic study. Hum Reprod. 1995;10:1795-6.
20. Fedele L, Vercellin P. Treatment with GnRH agonist before myomectomy and the risk of short-term myoma recurrence. Br J Obstet Gynecol. 1990;97:393-6.
21. Finn WF, Muller PF. Abdominal myomectomy: special reference to subsequent pregnancy and to the reappearance of fibromyomas of the uterus. Am J Obstet Gynecol. 1950;60:109-14.
22. Flierman PA, Oberye JJ, vander Hulst VP, et al. Rapid reduction of leiomyoma volume during treatment with the GnRH antagonist ganirelix. BJOG. 2005;112:638-42.
23. Frenandaz H, Sefrioui O, Virelizer C, et al. Hysteroscopic resection of submucosal myomas in patients with infertility. Hum Reprod. 2001;16:1489-92.
24. Friedman AJ, Daly M, Juneau-Norcross M, et al. Recurrence of myomas after myomectomy in women pretreated with leupride acetate depot or placebo. Fertil Steril. 1992;58:205-8.
25. Gavrilova-Jordan LP, Rose CH, Traynor KD, et al. Successful term pregnancy following MR-guided focused ultrasound treatment of uterine leiomyoma. J Perinatol. 2007;27:59-61.
26. Graebe K, Garcia-Soto A, Aziz M, et al. Incidental power morcellation of malignancy: a retrospective cohort study. Gynecol Oncol. 2015;136:274-7.
27. Gupta JK, Sinha A, Lumsden MA, et al. Uterine artery embolisation for fibroids is associated with an increased risk of miscarriage. Fertil Steril. 2010;94:324-30.
28. Iversen RE Jr, Chelmow D, Strohbehn K, et al. Relative morbidity of abdominal hysterectomy and myomectomy for management of uterine leiomyomas. Obstet Gynecol. 1996;88:415-9.
29. Jin C, Huy, Chen XC, et al. Laparoscopy versus open myomectomy: A meta-analysis of randomized controlled trails. Eur J Obstet Gynecol Reprod Biol. 2009;145:14-21.

30. Johnson N, Fletcher H, Raid M. Depo Medroxy Progesterone Acetate (DMPA) therapy for uterine myomata prior to Surgery. Int J Gynaecol Obstet. 2004;85:174-6.
31. Kongnyuy EJ, Van den Brock N, Weysonge CS. A systematic review of randomized controlled trails to reduce hemorrhage during myomectomy for uterine fibroids. Int Gynecol Obstet. 2008;100:4-9.
32. La Marca A, Giulini S, Vito G, et al. Gestrinone in the treatment of uterine leiomyomata: Effects on uterine blood supply. Fertil Steril. 2004;82:1694-6.
33. Lefebvre G, Vilos G, Allaire C, et al. The Management of uterine leiomyomas. J Obstet Gynaecol Can. 2003;128:1-10.
34. Lethaby A, Vollenhoven B. Fibroids (uterine myomatosis, leiomyomas). Clin Evid. 2002;7:1666-78.
35. Loeffer FE, Noble AD. Myomectomy at the Chelsea hospital for women. J Obstet Gynecol Br Commonw. 1970;77:167-70.
36. Malone LG. Myomectomy: recurrence after removal of solitary and multiple myomas. Obstet Gynecol. 1969;34:200-3.
37. Marshall LM, Spiegelman D, Barbieri RL, et al. Variation in the incidence of uterine leiomyoma among premenopausal women by age and race. Obstet Gynecol. 1997;90:967-73.
38. Morita Y, Ito N, Ohashi H, et al. Pregnancy following MR-guided focused ultrasound surgery for a uterine fibroid. Int J Gynecol Obstet. 2007;99:56-7.
39. Murphy AA, Kettel LM, Morales AJ, et al. Regression of uterine leiomyomata in response to the antiprogesterone RU486. J Clin Endocrinol Metab. 1993;76:513.
40. Mussey RD, Randall LM, Doyle LW. Pregnancy following myomectomy. J Am Assoc Gynecol. 1945;49:508-12.
41. Nezhat FR, Roemisch M, Nezhat CH, et al. Recurrence rate after laparoscopic myomectomy. J Am Assoc Gynecol Laparosc. 1998;5:237-40.
42. Palomba S. Long-term effectiveness and safety of GnRH agonist plus Raloxifene administration in women with uterine leiomyomas. Hum Reprod. 2004;6:1308-14.
43. Parker WH, Fu YS, Berek JS. Uterine sarcoma in patients operated on for presumed leiomyoma and rapidly growing leiomyoma. Obstet Gynecol. 1994;83:414-8.
44. Rabinovici J, David M, Fukunishi M, et al. MR guided focused ultrasound pregnancies: pregnancy outcome following magnetic resonance guided focused ultrasound surgery (MRgFUS) for conservative treatment of uterine fibroids. Fertil Steril. 2010;93:199-209.
45. Reich H, Thompson KA, Nataupsky LG, et al. Laparoscopic myomectomy: an alternative to laparotomy or hysterectomy? Gynecol Endosc. 1997;6:7-12.
46. Rein MS, Powell WL, Walters FC, et al. Cytogenetic abnormalities in uterine myomas are associated with myoma size. Mol Hum Reprod. 1998;4:83-6.
47. Rice JP, Kay HH, Mahomey BS. The clinical significance of uterine leiomyomas in pregnancy. Am J Obstet Gynecol. 1989;160:212-6.
48. Roenfield DL. Abdominal myomectomy for otherwise unexplained infertility. Fertil Steril. 1986;46:328-30.
49. Ross RK, Pike MC, Vessey MP, et al. Risk factors for uterine fibroids: reduced risk associated with oral contraceptives. Br Med J. 1986;293:359-62.
50. Roth TM, Gustilo-Ashby T, Barber MD. Effects of race and clinical factors on short-term outcomes of abdominal myomectomy. Obstet Gynecol. 2003;101:881-4.
51. Royal College of Obstetricians and Gynaecologists (RCOG); British Society for Gynaecological Endoscopy. Best practice in outpatient hysteroscopy (Green–top guideline; No. 59). RCOG: London (UK); 2011.
52. Sankaran S, Manyonda IT. Medical management of fibroids. Best Pract Res Clin Obstet Gynaecol. 2008;22:655-76.
53. Sirjusingh A, Bassaw B, Roopnarinesingh S. The results of abdominal myomectomy. West Ind Med J. 1994;43:138-9.
54. Stewart EA, Faur AV, Wise LA. Predictors of subsequent surgery for uterine leiomyomata after abdominal myomectomy. Obstet Gynecol. 2002;90:426-32.
55. Sudik R, Husch K, Steller J, et al. Fertility and pregnancy outcome after myomectomy in sterility patients. Eur J Obstet Gyn Reprod Biol. 1996;65:209-14.
56. Takamizawa S, Minakami H, Usui R, et al. Risk of complications and uterine malignancies in women undergoing hysterectomy for presumed benign leiomyomas. Gynecol Obstet Invest. 1999;48:193-6.

57. Theben JU, Schellong AR, Altgassen C, et al. Unexpected malignancies after laparoscopic-assisted supracervical hysterectomies (LASH): an analysis of 1,584 LASH cases. Arch Gynecol Obstet. 2013;287:455-62.
58. Vavala V, Lanzone A, Monaco A, et al. Postoperative GnRH analog treatment for the prevention of recurrences of uterine myomas after myomectomy. A pilot study. Gynecol Obstet Invest. 1997;43:251-4.
59. Venkatachalam S, Bagratee JS, Moodley J. Medical management of uterine fibroids with medroxyprogesterone acetate (DepoProvera): A pilot study. J Obstet Gyneacol. 2004;24:798-800.
60. Vercellini P, Maddalena S, Giorgi OD, et al. Abdominal myomectomy for infertility: a comprehensive review. Hum Reprod. 1998;13:873-9.
61. Verkauf BS. Myomectomy for fertility enhancement and preservation. Fertil Steril. 1992;58:1-15.
62. Vikhlyaeva EM, Khodzhaeva ZS, Fantschenko ND. Familial predisposition to uterine leiomyomas. Int J Gynaecol Obstet. 1995;51:127-31.
63. Walker CL. Role of hormonal and reproductive factors in the etiology and treatment of uterine leiomyoma. Recent Prog Hormone Res. 2002;57:277-94.
64. Wallach EE, Viahos NF. Uterine myomas: an overview of development, clinical features, and management. Obstet Gynecol. 2004;104:393-406.
65. Wright JD, Tergas AI, Cui R, et al. Use of electric power morcellation and prevalence of underlying cancer in women who undergo myomectomy. JAMA Oncol. 2015;1:69-77.
66. Wu T, Chen X, Xie L. Selective Estrogen Receptor Modulators (SERMS) for uterine leiomyomas. Cochrane Database Syst Rev. 2007;(2):CD005287.
67. Zhang J, Zhang J, Dai Y, et al. Clinical characteristics and management experience of unexpected uterine sarcoma after myomectomy. Int J Gynaecol Obstet. 2015;130:195-9.

Fibroids and Sexual Dysfunction

Mohit Rajendra Saraogi

INTRODUCTION

Sexual dysfunction is a term that broadly encompasses problems involving sexual desire, arousal, orgasm, and sex pain disorders such as vaginismus and dyspareunia. The usual etiological factors for female sexual dysfunction include medical diseases, depression, psychological factors, medications, prior history of sexual abuse and gynecological ailments such as fibroids and endometriosis.

Fibroids or leiomyomas are benign smooth muscle tumors, which usually arise from the smooth muscles and connective tissue of the uterus although occasionally they can arise from other sites as well. The prevalence of fibroids is quoted to be 21.4% globally in the age group of 30–60 years, but varies from place to place.

Statistics show that 20–50% of uterine fibroids are symptomatic and subsequently these women seek treatment and surgical intervention to improve their quality of life.

Most women suffering from fibroids remain asymptomatic and do not suffer from sexual dysfunction. However, a large number of women on the other hand suffer from sexual dysfunction due to fibroids as can be quantified and established by the female sexual function index. The consequences of fibroids and sexual dysfunction are far reaching as they have socioeconomic and psychological implications on a couple.

Can Fibroids affect Sex Life?

The answer is most definitely yes. Symptomatic fibroids can have various manifestations, which can most certainly affect a couple's sex life. This is illustrated in the Flowchart 17.1.

Menorrhagia and Menstrual Irregularities

The most common symptom associated with fibroids is menorrhagia or excessive menstrual bleeding. In severe cases, a woman can continue bleeding for the entire month. This itself can be a predominant cause of female sexual dysfunction, as it often interferes with both desire and arousal in a woman. Most women will not allow intercourse at the time of menstruation.

Dyspareunia and Dysmenorrhea

Symptomatic fibroids can present with both dysmenorrhea and dyspareunia. The pain associated with menses often creates a psychological blockage, which leads to decreased arousal and decreased sexual desire in women. Women with large fibroids presenting with dyspareunia are often aversive to sex. In a study carried out in Italy, it was proven beyond

Flowchart 17.1: Various manifestations of symptomatic fibroids.

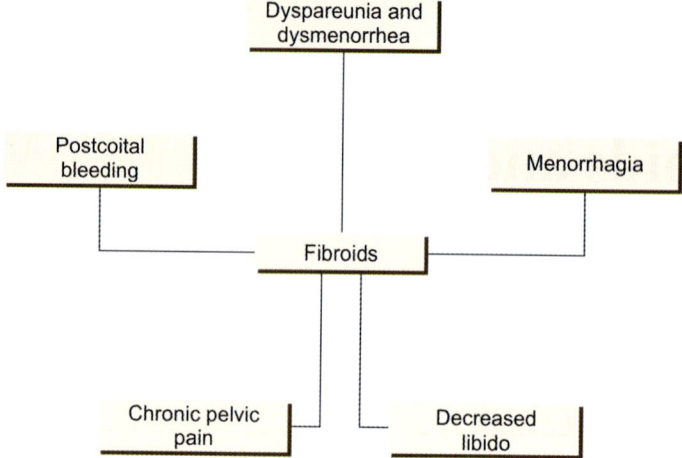

doubt that women having fibroids are more likely to report moderate-to-severe dyspareunia and moderate-to-severe noncyclical pelvic pain as compared to women without fibroids (statistically significant).

Chronic Pelvic Pain

Women with symptomatic fibroids often suffer from moderate to severe noncyclical pelvic pain. This interferes with all aspects of sexual functioning and well-being.

Decreased Libido

According to a study carried out by Lawrence and Vollenhoven, women with fibroids reported an incidence of 32%, 27%, and 12% for mood changes (decreased sexual desire), vaginal dryness, and decreased libido. As will be illustrated in the Flowchart 17.2 below all of the above can be inter-related as one symptom can lead to the other.

Postcoital Bleeding

Cervical fibroids can often present with postcoital bleeding besides acting a mechanical impedance to coitus. This postcoital bleeding can be a major turn off and can seriously impair the sex life of a couple. Also a large cervical fibroid can occupy a large part of the vagina and can limit sexual intercourse.

CYCLE OF FEMALE SEXUAL DYSFUNCTION

As depicted in the Flowchart 17.2, all aspects or components of sexual functioning such as desire, arousal, orgasm, and absence of pain are inter-related. Abnormality in any of the components can subsequently lead to disruption of the other components as well. Hence, the presenting complaint of a woman suffering from sexual dysfunction need not be the original problem but may be a consequence of some other underlying pathology.

Fibroids can affect desire, arousal, orgasm, and can cause dyspareunia. Then these symptoms tend to have a positive feedback reaction and seem to be self propagating.

Flowchart 17.2: Cycle of female sexual dysfunction.

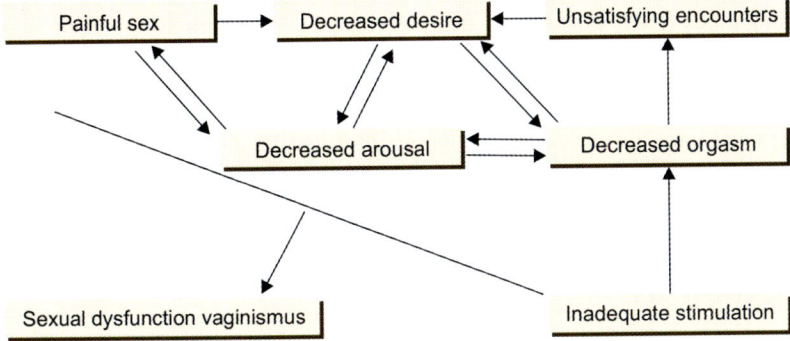

TREATMENT OPTIONS FOR SYMPTOMATIC FIBROIDS

A number of interventional procedures are available for the treatment of fibroids such as:
- Myomectomy—i.e. removal of only the fibroid either laparoscopically or as an open procedure
- Subtotal abdominal hysterectomy—i.e. supracervical hysterectomy
- Total abdominal hysterectomy
- HIFU or high-intensity focused ultrasound therapy
- Uterine artery embolization.

OUTCOME AND COMPARISON OF INTERVENTIONAL PROCEDURES FOR FIBROIDS ON SEXUAL DYSFUNCTION

- *Comparison of total and subtotal hysterectomy*: A number of studies conducted by Kupperman et al. and other investigators in UK and Denmark have reached the same consensus. Both total and subtotal hysterectomy resulted in a significant improvement in the quality of sex life of women suffering from fibroid induced sexual dysfunction. However, between the procedures there is no difference in outcomes either immediately or on a 12-month follow-up.
- *Comparison of HIFU and conventional myomectomy*: According to a study carried out both myomectomy and HIFU led to an improvement in sexual functioning in women suffering from fibroids. However, the improvement was only marginal in both groups and not statistically significant when comparing the two treatment modalities.
- *Sexual functioning and well-being after uterine artery embolization in women with symptomatic fibroids*: According to a study, there was a statistically significant increase ranging from 20% to 22.5% 3 months after uterine artery embolization indicating that sexual function improved. 34% and 37% women reported and increase in sexual activity and desire. 68% had an increase in the total score for sexual functioning.

CONCLUSION

Fibroids are a frequent cause of female sexual dysfunction although sexual dysfunction is usually not the presenting symptom associated with fibroids. Due to the high incidence and prevalence of fibroids globally, its impact on a woman personal well-being and health cannot be underestimated. Also sexual dysfunction being a relatively taboo topic in India, women do not come out with complaints of sexual dysfunction easily. Being healthcare providers for women, we must ask women diagnosed with fibroids about their sexual life and look for signs of sexual dysfunction on questioning. Using objective scoring systems like the female sexual functioning index (FSFI) can simplify this process. In women with symptomatic fibroids, all modalities of treatment are known to improve the FSFI. However, we need to remember that sexual dysfunction has a psychosomatic component as well and is self propagating, which is why in addition to interventional procedures; there may be need for counseling as well. Although there have been isolated case reports of worsening of sexual dysfunction following interventional procedures—these are usually secondary to complications and are an infrequent occurrence. All in all intervention is recommended for women suffering from sexual dysfunction secondary to symptomatic fibroids.

BIBLIOGRAPHY

1. Bizjak T, Turkanovic AB, But I. Prevalence and risk factors of uterine fibroids in North-East Slovenia. Gynecol Obstet (Sunnyvale). 2016;6:350.
2. Kuppermann M, Summitt RL Jr, Varner RE, et al. Sexual functioning after total compared with supracervical hysterectomy: A Randomized trial. Obstet Gynaecol. 2005;105:1309-18.
3. Lippman SA, Warner M, Samuels S, et al. Uterine fibroids and gynecologic pain symptoms in a population-based study. Fertil Steril. 2003;80:1488-94.
4. Louie AR, Armstrong JA, Findeiss LK, et al. Comparison of sexual dysfunction using the female sexual function index following surgical treatments for uterine fibroids. Case Rep Obstet Gynecol. 2012;2012:368136.
5. Phillips NA. Female Sexual Dysfunction: Evaluation and Treatment. Wellington School of Medicine. [online] Available from http://citeseerx.ist.psu.edu/viewdoc/download?doi=10.1.1.472.6936&rep=rep1&type=pdf. [Accessed June, 2018].
6. Vollenhoven BJ, Lawrence AS. Uterine Fibroids: A clinical review. BJOG. 1990;97:285-98.
7. Voogt MJ, De Vries J, Fonteijn W, et al. Sexual functioning and psychological well being after uterine artery embolization in women with symptomatic uterine fibroids. Fertil Steril. 2009;92:756-61.
8. Zimmermann A, Bernuit D, Gerlinger C, et al. Prevalence, symptoms and management of uterine fibroids: an international internet-based survey of 21,746 women. BMC Womens Health. 2012;12:6.

Fibroids and Gastrointestinal Symptoms

18

Sunita Chandra, Poonam Goyal

INTRODUCTION

Fibroids are made of the muscle tissue found in the uterus, but their location is not limited to inside the uterine cavity. They can also grow on the outside of the uterus, and within the uterine walls, and can even attach themselves to the uterus by a stem. They are well circumscribed but noncapsulated and have varying degree of fibrous connective tissue. They can at times attain massive size and can truly become giant tumors.

Size can be typically given by comparing with gravid uterus:
- *Large fibroids:* Those, which are 3–4 months gestation size
- *Massive fibroids:* More than 4 months to term size
- *Giant fibroids:* Those, which have size of 25 lbs and above.

TYPES OF FIBROIDS DEPENDING ON LOCATION

- Intramural
- Submucosal
- Subserosal
- Cervical.

In women whose fibroids are growing to large size in the uterus or outside the uterus, other organs are affected due to pressure effects.

Apart from pelvic symptoms like pain, heavy bleeding, and possibly infertility, fibroids can also cause problems with bladder, bowel, and pelvic vasculature.

This chapter deals with the symptoms produced when fibroids cause pressure and affect the gastrointestinal (GI) system.

SYMPTOMS OF UTERINE FIBROIDS

Most women with small fibroids have no pressure symptoms, but those who have huge size fibroids will experience some pressure GI symptoms.

Gastrointestinal symptoms:
- Upper GI discomfort
- Bloating sensation
- Heaviness in abdomen
- Backache
- Indigestion

- Diarrhea
- Constipation
- Tenesmus
- Hemorrhoids
- Bowel obstruction
- Irritable bowel syndrome (IBS).

Upper Abdomen

Pressure symptoms of fibroids include feeling like having a full stomach. A fibroid can push up stomach creating early satiety. It gives a feeling fullness faster and may not be able to eat as much as previously, sometimes leading to weight loss. Early feeling of satiety can lead to loss of weight in due course of time. If the fibroid grows big enough, abdomen can look enlarged, as though female is pregnant.

Lower Abdomen

A large enough fibroid can push down on the rectum, and making bowel movements difficult. If the fibroid is on the underside of the uterus, one can have constipation or pain when defecating. Hemorrhoids can be another unpleasant result of rectal pressure and difficulty moving bowels.

Irritable bowel syndrome or other digestive problems if are present earlier, they usually get worsen and sometimes treating clinician thinks them to be asymptomatic.

DIAGNOSIS OF FIBROIDS

In the most cases, the symptoms of fibroids are rarely felt, and the patient does not know she has them, they are usually discovered during a vaginal examination.
- Clinical examination will reveal a large uterus in the absence of pregnancy.
- Ultrasound—can detect fibroids and eliminate other possible conditions, which may have similar symptoms, an ultrasound can be used over the abdomen or transvaginally. It can also give evidence of central necrosis in large fibroids.
- Magnetic resonance imaging (MRI) can be done for exact size mapping and number of fibroids.
- For GI symptoms, upper GI endoscopy and colonoscopy may be needed.

TREATMENT FOR FIBROIDS

If the women have no symptoms and the fibroids are not affecting her day-to-day life, she may receive no treatment at all. Even women who have heavy periods but whose lives are not badly affected by this symptom may also opt for no treatment.

During menopause, fibroids usually shrink and symptoms will often become less apparent or disappear altogether.

When treatment is necessary, it may be in the form of medication or surgery.
- Medical management
- Surgical management.

Medical Treatment

- Gonadotropin releasing hormone (GnRH) agonist injection
- LNG-IUS (levonorgestrel intrauterine system)

- Selective progesterone receptor modulators (SPRMs)—ulipristal and asoprisnil
- Mifepristone.

Anti-inflammatory Drugs

Response to medical treatment is variable. Medical treatment may not work for large fibroids. (Details of medical treatment covered elsewhere in book).

Surgical Management

Depending on symptoms and whether therapy has failed, the patient may have to undergo surgery. The following surgical procedures may be considered:
- Hysterectomy
- Myomectomy to relieve pressure.

Nonsurgical Newer Options

- UAE (uterine artery embolization)
- Magnetic resonance-guided percutaneous laser ablation
- Magnetic resonance-guided focused ultrasound surgery. This will not relieve pressure symptoms immediately and not recommended for massive tumors.

Symptomatic Treatment

To improve digestive problems, drugs like bloating sensation gastritis proton pump inhibitors (PPIs) can be used empty stomach in the morning.

For constipation, lactulose, isabgol can be used.

For hemorrhoids, stool softeners and local application of calcium dobesilate and capsule of the same can be used.

CONCLUSION

Large fibroids cause various GI symptoms due to the bulky nature. Even small fibroid pressing on rectum can cause tenesmus, constipation, or even diarrhea. Medical treatment may not be successful for big fibroids and surgery may be needed. Specific treatment may be given to the GI symptoms caused by pressure effects of fibroid. Need is of proper judgment, to zero down on fibroid as the culprit and treat accordingly. Surgery is very rewarding in these cases.

BIBLIOGRAPHY

1. Buttram VC Jr, Reiter RC. Uterine leiomyomata: etiology, symptomatology, and management. Fertil Steril. 1981;36:433-45.
2. Cantuaria GH, Angioli R, Frost L, et al. Comparison of bimanual examination with ultrasound examination before hysterectomy for uterine leiomyoma. Obstet Gynecol. 1998;92:109-12.
3. Mulayim N, Gucer F. Borderline smooth muscle tumors of the uterus. Obstet Gynaecol Clin North Am. 2006;33(1):171-81.
4. Segars JH. Fibroids. In: Arici A (Ed). Gynaecology in Practice. Wiley Blackwell: UK; 2013.
5. Weekes LR. Massive fibroid. J Natl Med Assoc. 1977;69(1):17-22.

Genitouriary Dysfunction in Uterine Fibroids

19

Rutvij Dalal

INTRODUCTION

Leiomyomas are benign smooth muscle neoplasms of the uterus that typically originate from the myometrium. They are often referred as uterine myomas and incorrectly called as fibroids because of their fibrous consistency due to considerable amount of collagen contained in them. Their incidence among women is generally cited as 20-25%. During the reproductive years, the incidence of this tumor increases with age. They are rare before 20 and most commonly seen between 30 years and 40 years and have been reported to be nearly 70% in Caucasians and over 80% in African-American women in a study conducted by D Baird and colleagues. After menopause, the leiomyomas shrink in size, and new tumor development is uncommon. Thus it seems that most risk or protective factors depend on circumstances that chronically alter estrogen or progesterone levels or both. Other hormones such as growth hormone and prolactin are also thought to promote fibroid growth, but their role is less defined. More recently, growth factors have shown to mediate the growth promoting effects of estrogen and play an important role in development of fibroid. Potentially important factors include transforming growth factor, epidermal growth factor, insulin-like growth factor, and platelet-derived growth factor.

SYMPTOMS ASSOCIATED WITH FIBROIDS

Most of the women with leiomyomas are asymptomatic. However, symptomatic women typically complain of bleeding, pain, pelvic discomfort, dysmenorrhea, leukorrhea, dyspareunia, infertility and pregnancy wastage, lower urinary tract symptoms and rare ones like myomatous erythrocytosis syndrome which is seen in less than 0.5% women. Symptoms correlate with size, site, number, and degenerative changes within the tumor and range from abdominal mass, menorrhagia, dysmenorrhea, pain, and recurrent abortions to constipation and tenesmus. As pathophysiology and management of other symptoms are covered elsewhere in the book, this chapter shall focus primarily on the urinary complaints associated with fibroids.

GENITOURINARY DYSFUNCTION

Urinary complaints as a result of uterine fibroid(s) are rare and usually due to a fibroid in the lower uterine body or a large cervical fibroid. The urinary symptoms that arise are usually due to pressure effects directly on the bladder or associated neurovascular effects. For example, a large fibroid in the lower uterine area pressing the bladder fundus can cause incomplete filling leading to frequency and/or urgency. A posterior wall fibroid can also lead to retroverted uterus that gets impacted in the pouch of Douglas leading to urinary retention or pressure effects on the bladder neck or urethra. A large anterior cervical fibroid can cause similar symptoms or it can press onto the urethra causing acute retention of urine. Rarely, an anterior large fibroid can also cause genuine stress incontinence or urge incontinence. Fibroids, depending on their location and size, can also cause sexual problems including dyspareunia and loss of libido.

URINARY RETENTION

Urinary retention is not so common in females, and when they occur they usually have very predictable reasons depending on the age of the patient and her history. A detailed history, physical examination as well as simple investigations like pelvic ultrasound and urinalysis, is usually enough to nail the diagnosis, but certainly the help of cystoscopy, urodynamic studies, and an MRI are very useful where the reason is not very obvious. Leiomyomas appear as well-defined solid masses with a whorled appearance but sometimes may be hypoechoic as well. Areas of calcification may be seen as echogenic foci with shadowing; and there may be cystic areas suggestive of necrosis or degeneration within the tumor. Doppler ultrasonography (USG) usually shows circumferential vascularity which may be absent in necrotic fibroids. CT scan is not the investigation of choice for diagnosing uterine leiomyomas; however, magnetic resonance imaging can accurately characterize pelvic masses and differentiate submucosal, intramural, and subserosal fibroids. The delay in diagnosing uterine leiomyomas presenting with acute urinary retention further complicates the management (Figs. 19.1A and B).

Cervical fibroids form 1% to 2% of all the fibroids. They could arise from the anterior, posterior or the lateral wall of the cervix or it could be central involving the whole of the cervix. Depending on the size as well as the site of the tumor, it may cause symptoms like urinary frequency, urinary retention, constipation, lower abdomen pain, menstrual abnormalities, dyspareunia, and postcoital bleeding. Urinary retention usually leads to episodes of recurrent urinary tract infections and pyuria. It is imperative that such infections are treated promptly and effectively with suitable antibiotics depending on the culture or sensitivity reports to prevent serious consequences like acute pyelonephritis and renal failure (Fig. 19.2).

Operative management of cervical fibroids poses important challenges. Bigger cervical fibroids arising from the anterior or posterior wall of the cervix causing pressure symptoms need special care due to proximity to the various important structures as well as increase in the vascularity. To avoid injury to the important surrounding structures, mainly the ureters, it is always advisable to do intracapsular dissection and proceed with the hysterectomy when the tissues are more or less in the normal anatomical positions. Some surgeons prefer double J stenting of the ureters to prevent intraoperative injury to the ureters, although this is debatable.

There are only a few published papers about uterine fibroids causing acute urinary retention. A recent review of literature by Wu et al., revealed a total of 37 cases only in literature of uterine leiomyomas causing acute urinary retention (16 case reports and 5 case series); this included their own case series of 6 patients with acute urinary retention. Various mechanisms have been postulated by which acute urinary retention may occur due to a leiomyoma. The most common theory is that the proximal urethra and bladder neck compression may be caused by anterior and superior displacement of the cervix due to the impacted fibroid. In normal voiding, the cervix is rotated away from the urethra or bladder neck; this movement is hindered by the impacted uterine fibroid. Other proposed mechanisms include pelvic congestion due to premenstrual hormonal induced factors, detrusor muscle ischemia due to vascular steal effect of the fibroid, and stretching of nerves that innervate the bladder, i.e. the pudendal and sacral nerves by the fibroid.

148 *Fibroids*

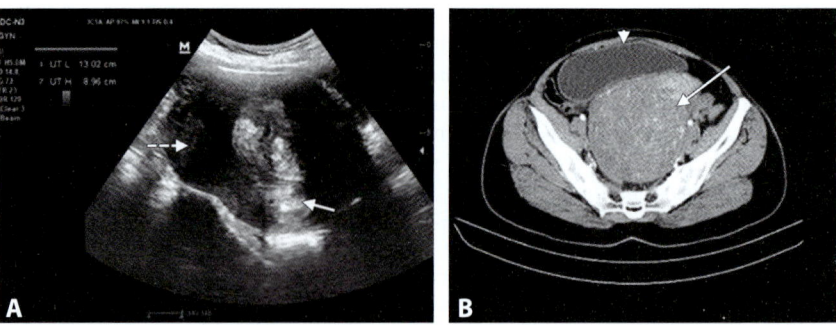

Figs. 19.1A and B: (A) Transabdominal ultrasonography showing large cervical fibroid (arrow) measuring 9.3 × 9.2 cm with normal sized uterus (dashed arrow) seen on top; (B) Contrast enhanced computed tomography—large homogenously enhancing solid myoma mass (arrow) measuring 11 × 10.5 cm seen posterior to the bladder (arrow head).

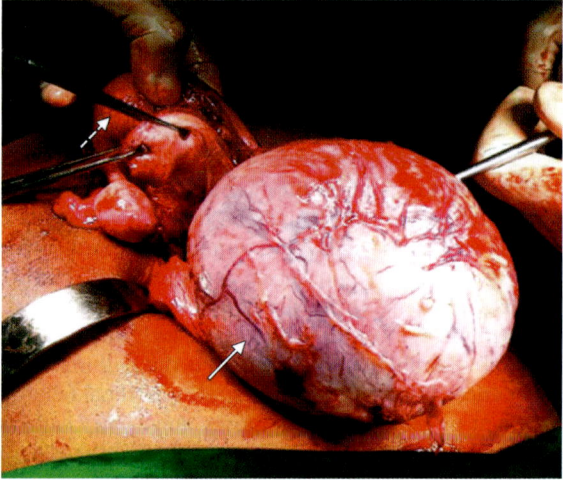

Fig. 19.2: Intraoperative photograph showing normal sized uterus (dashed arrow) and large cervical fibroid (arrow) measuring 15 × 10 cm, for which myomectomy was done.

Rather than the actual size, impaction or incarceration of a leiomyoma or the uterus in the hollow of the sacrum may also be a critical factor for the development of acute urinary retention in the majority of cases. This is borne out by the fact that very large uterine leiomyomas often do not cause acute retention of urine as they grow out of the sacral promontory freely without entrapment into the hollow of the sacrum. A large pedunculated submucous tumor may fill and distend the vagina and press the urethra, against the symphysis causing urinary retention.

In the absence of neurological disorders, urodynamic studies or neuromuscular testing are apparently noncontributory in either diagnosis or management of patients presenting with acute retention of urine due to uterine leiomyomas. It is important to document the renal function as urinary obstruction may cause hydronephrosis with derangement of renal parameters. Intravenous pyelography can effectively diagnose associated hydroureter and hydronephrosis. Post-surgery, the hydronephrosis and hydroureter usually reverts to normal. Chronic bladder obstruction from the leiomyoma can be severe enough to cause increase in the thickness of the bladder wall and enlargement of the bladder resembling that seen in men with urethral obstruction from the prostatic enlargement. Indeed in these neglected cases, the bladder may fill the entire lower abdominal wall so that an incision above the umbilicus is required to enter the peritoneal cavity to remove the tumor without injury to the bladder.

There is no current consensus on the management of urinary retention in patients with uterine leiomyomas. Wu et al., have proposed an algorithm for the management of patients with acute urinary retention due to leiomyoma. They suggest that short-term management of acute urinary retention due to uterine leiomyoma (size ≥5–6 cm) is bladder decompression by catheterization, while long-term management is based on either uterus preserving options (in whom fertility is desired) or hysterectomy in those who are menopausal. Pre- or perimenopausal women may be tried with hysterectomy or gonadotropin-releasing hormone agonists, aromatase inhibitors or ulipristal acetate (selective progesterone receptor modulator). An interesting management option was published by Arleo EK et al. in which they did uterine artery embolization (UAE) for fibroid-induced acute urinary retention. 24 hours after the procedure, they removed the Foley catheter and there was negligible post-void residual. Although the post-procedure MRI revealed negligible change in the size of the fibroid, there was no urinary retention seen in the follow-up. The authors suggest a "vascular steal theory" which is responsible for the success of the procedure in spite of no significant change in the size of the fibroid.

URGENCY, FREQUENCY, AND OTHER VOIDING DISTURBANCES

Although these symptoms are rare in women with uterine fibroids, they can all occur depending the exact location and size of the fibroid(s). The myoma with its sheer volume can impinge upon the bladder fundus leading to a sense of fullness with volumes as low as 100 cc, leading to urgency and frequency. Postural changes associated with sleep can give rise to nocturnal frequency and even urge incontinence in some women. Bladder neck irritation can lead to urge incontinence whereas disturbances with the urethrovesical angle can lead to genuine stress incontinence.

In a prospective study published by Langer R et al., 14 patients with large uterine fibroids and urinary symptoms were treated with monthly injections of [D-Trp6]-luteinizing hormone-releasing hormone microcapsules. The average uterine size before treatment was 728 mL; it dropped to 323 mL (a drop of 55%) after treatment. Urinary symptoms of diurnal frequency disappeared in 11 of 12 patients (P less than 0.005) after the reduction of uterine size. Urgency decreased in 11 of 13 (P less than 0.005) and nocturia in 8 of 10 (P less than 0.02). No differences were found before and after treatment in the symptoms of urge incontinence and stress incontinence in the cystometric and urethral pressure profile measurements. They concluded that symptoms of urge incontinence and stress incontinence deserve a more specific treatment as they are not related to uterine size.

There are very few papers that highlight the role of fibroids in causing incontinence. However in a detailed review of 145 women with anterior myoma, Ekin M et al. found that the frequency of genitourinary symptoms was significantly higher in women with myomas, including stress urinary incontinence (SUI), urgency, frequency, urge urinary incontinence (UUI), and dyspareunia. SUI and mixed urinary incontinence (MUI) were the most common symptoms associated with myoma size. In one cross-sectional study involving 78 women with fibroids, Parker-Autry C used the validated Bristol Female Lower Urinary Tract Symptom-Scored Form (BFLUTS-SF) questionnaire to ascertain the various symptoms associated with fibroids. They found that the most prevalent lower urinary tract symptoms (LUTS) were nocturia (91%), urgency (59%), and urinary incontinence (45–54%). Women with moderate and severe urinary urgency had significantly larger uterine volumes

(P = 0.017). There is good evidence that women with uterine fibroids have a significantly higher incidence of stress urinary incontinence. Rarely a fibroid presents itself with complaints like dyspareunia.

The bowel is less apt to show symptoms from pressure than the bladder, but constipation can be caused and aggravated by the pressure of the leiomyoma against the rectum. The small intestines may be entwined causing small bowel obstruction. Pressure of a large broad ligament leiomyoma can cause pressure on the ureter and result in hydroureter and hydronephrosis. Repeated infection is commonly associated with pyelonephritis.

SUMMARY

A large uterine fibroid or a cervical fibroid because of their size or site can impinge on the urine outflow tract and can lead to any or all of the above symptoms like acute retention, urgency, frequency, and incontinence in varying permutations. A thorough evaluation by a gynecologist or urologist keeping a high degree of suspicion and aided by a thorough clinical examination including a per vaginal and/or per rectal exam and ancillary tools like abdominal or transvaginal ultrasound goes a long way in clinching the diagnosis which when timely managed can prevent serious sequelae like acute renal failure from developing. It is desirable to have a close collaboration among peers of different specialties like urology/gynecology/radiology to have a multidisciplinary approach that these patients often require. Urologists may look for nongynecologic causes of retention more commonly, and delay pelvic examinations. As pelvic organ etiologies are common causes of retention in women, this delay can lead to unnecessary invasive tests and patient suffering.

The choice of approach for the management of uterine myomas depends on many factors, both medical and social, including age, parity, childbearing aspirations, extent and severity of symptoms, size, location and number of myomas, associated medical condition(s), possibility of malignancy, and desire for uterine preservation. The preferred surgical procedures are to perform myomectomy or hysterectomy. The major problem associated with myomectomy is heavy operative blood loss and postoperative adhesion formation. Technically resection of cervical fibroids is challenging due to the vascularity and proximity to vital structures like the ureters. Hysterectomy is a reasonably safe procedure offering the best result in terms of relieving the symptoms of bleeding, pressure, or pain caused by fibroids in the patients diagnosed with multiple myomas who do not desire to retain fertility.

BIBLIOGRAPHY

1. Andrada AO, De Vicente JM, Cidre MA. Pelvic plexus compression due to a uterine leiomyoma in a woman with acute urinary retention: a new hypothesis. Int Urogynaecol J. 2014;25:429-31.
2. Arleo EK, Tal MG. Fibroid-induced acute urinary retention: treatment by uterine artery embolization. Int Urogynecol J Pelvic Floor Dysfunct. 2008;19(1):161-5.
3. Baird DD, Harmon QE, Upson K, et al. A prospective, ultrasound-based study to evaluate risk factors for uterine fibroid incidence and growth: methods and results of recruitment. J Womens Health (Larchmt). 2015;24(11):907-15.
4. Bidzinki M, Siergiel M, Pudkiewiez J, et al. Acute urinary retention due to cervical myoma - a case report and review of the literature. Ginekol Pol. 2015;86(1):77-9.
5. Dagur G, Suh Y, Warren K, et al. Urological complications of uterine leiomyoma: a review of literature. Int Urol Nephrol. 2016;48(6):941-8.
6. Ding DC, Hwang KS. Female acute urinary retention caused by anterior deflection of the cervix which was augmented by an uterine myoma. Taiwan J Obstet Gynaecol. 2008;47:350-1.
7. Dragomir AD, Schroeder JC, Connolly A, et al. Uterine leiomyomata associated with self-reported stress urinary incontinence. J Womens Health (Larchmt). 2010;19(2):245-50.

8. Dutton S, Hirst A, McPherson K, et al. UK multicentre retrospective cohort study comparing hysterectomy and uterine artery embolisation for the treatment of symptomatic uterine fibroids (HOPEFUL Study): main results on medium term safety and efficacy. BJOG. 2007;114(11):1340-51.
9. Ekin M, Cengiz H, Öztürk E, et al. Genitourinary symptoms and their effects on quality of life in women with uterine myomas. Int Urogynecol J. 2014;25(6):807-10.
10. Ezeama C, Ikechebelu J, Obiechina NJ, et al. Clinical presentation of uterine fibroids in Nnewi, Nigeria: a 5 year review. Ann Med Health Sci Res. 2012;2:114-8.
11. Kjerulff KH, Langenberg PW, Rhodes JC, et al. Effectiveness of hysterectomy. Obstet Gynecol. 2000;95(3):319-26.
12. Langer R, Golan A, Neuman M, et al. The effect of large uterine fibroids on urinary bladder function and symptoms. Am J Obstet Gynecol. 1990;163(4 Pt 1):1139-41.
13. Mavromatidis G, Dinas K, Mamopoulos A, et al. Acute urinary retention due to a uterine fibroid in a non-pregnant woman. Clin Exp Obstet Gynecol. 2009;36:62-3.
14. Mihmanli V, Cetinkaya N, Kilickaya A, et al. Giant cervical myoma associated with urinary incontinence and hydroureteronephrosis. Clin Exp Obstet Gynecol. 2015;42(5):690-1.
15. Narmada, Hameed J, Radhika, et al. Interesting cases of different types of cervical fibroids. JEMDS. 2014;3(18):4775-80.
16. Okolo S. Incidence, aetiology and epidemiology of uterine fibroids. Best Pract Res Clin Obstet Gynaecol. 2008;22(4):571-88.
17. Parker-Autry C, Harvie H, Arya LA, et al. Lower urinary tract symptoms in patients with uterine fibroids: association with fibroid location and uterine volume. Female Pelvic Med Reconstr Surg. 2011;17(2):91-6.
18. Sethi P, Devi S, Vivekanand A. Acute urinary retention secondary to a cervical leiomyoma -a case report. IJCST. 2014;12(1):182-3.
19. Stovall DW. Clinical symptomatology of uterine leiomyomas. Clin Obstet Gynecol. 2001;44:364-71.
20. Wallach EE, Vlahos NF. Uterine myoma: an overview of development, clinical features and management. Obstet Gynecol. 2004;104:393-406.
21. Wegienka G, Baird DD, Hertz-Picciotto I, et al. Self-reported heavy bleeding associated with uterine leiomyomata. Obstet Gynecol. 2003;101:431-7.
22. Wu CQ, Lefebvre G, Frecker H, et al. Urinary retention and uterine leiomyomas: a case series and review of literature. Int Urogynecol J. 2015;26(9):1277-84.
23. Wu JM, Stinnett S, Jackson RA, et al. Prevalence and incidence of urinary incontinence in a diverse population of women with noncancerous gynecologic conditions. Female Pelvic Med Reconstr Surg. 2010;16(5):284-9.
24. Xin J, Lai HP, Lin SK, et al. Bladder leiomyoma presenting as dyspareunia: Case report and literature review. Medicine (Baltimore). 2016;95(28):e3971.
25. Yang JM, Huang WC. Sonographic findings of acute urinary retention secondary to an impacted pelvic mass. J Ultrasound Med. 2002;21:1165-9.
26. Yazdany T, Bhatia NN, Nguyen JN. Urinary retention and voiding dysfunction in women with uterine leiomyoma: a case series. J Reprod Med. 2012;57(9-10):384-9.

20
Infrequent or Atypical Fibroid Syndrome

Neha Priyadarshini

INTRODUCTION

Leiomyomas (fibroids) are the most common gynecological and uterine neoplasms. Clinical manifestations of uterine leiomyoma are in approximately 20–30% women older than 35 years.

DEFINITION

Presence of leiomyoma in an unusual location or with unusual growth pattern is termed as infrequent or atypical fibroid syndrome.

CLASSIFICATION OF ATYPICAL OR INFREQUENT FIBROIDS

Classification summary is given in Flowchart 20.1.

TYPES

Benign Metastasizing Fibroid or Leiomyoma (BML)
- Rare condition, first described by Steiner in 1939.
- Characterized by presence of well-differentiated leiomyoma at sites away from uterus.

Flowchart 20.1: Classification of infrequent or atypical fibroid syndrome.

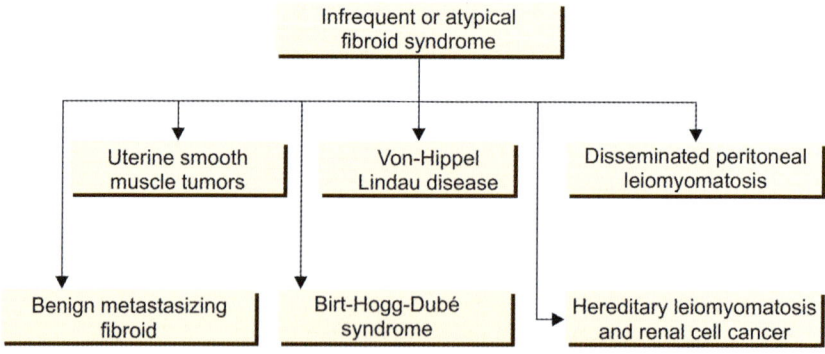

- Most commonly affected sites according to frequency of involvement are:
  - Lungs
  - Heart
  - Brain
  - Lymph node
  - Skin.

Clinical Presentation

Presence of multiple pulmonary nodules in middle-aged women with history of hysterectomy for leiomyoma or presence of concurrent leiomyoma.

Signs or Symptoms
- Chest pain
- Shortness of breath
- Cough.

Pathogenesis

Two hypotheses:
- Hematogenous
- Multiple independent foci of smooth muscle origin, classified as smooth muscle tumor of unknown malignant potential (STUMP).

Associated with:
- Diffuse peritoneal leiomyomatosis
- Intravenous leiomyomatosis
- Diffuse uterine leiomyomatosis.

Diagnosis

Radiological examination:
- Presence of pulmonary nodules, appearance may be solitary subcentimetric lesions or multiple lesions mimicking metastasis from malignant tumors (Figs. 20.1A to C).
- Cavitation or miliary pattern is occasionally associated. Rarely, calcification or pneumothorax may be present.
- CT or MRI can also depict the same findings.

Differential diagnosis of BML:
- Metastasis from malignant tumors
- Infectious granulomas
- Sarcoidosis
- Rheumatoid nodules
- Amyloidosis.
  Definitive diagnosis by image-guided core biopsy.

Management

No standard management guidelines have been formulated with regards to BML treatment but the widely accepted protocol is:
- Careful observation
- Surgical resection
- Hysterectomy with bilateral oophorectomy
- Use of progestins or aromatase inhibitors or medical therapy
- Medical castration using GnRH-RH analogs.

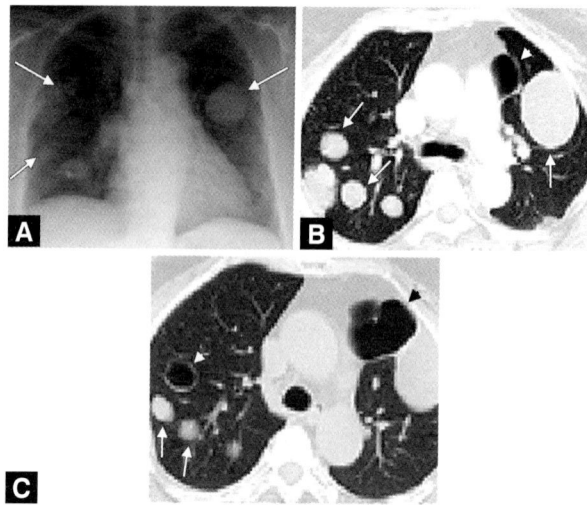

Figs. 20.1A to C: Benign metastasizing leiomyoma in a 50-year-old woman 10 years after a hysterectomy for treatment of uterine fibroids. The condition was diagnosed at open lung biopsy at another institution. (A) Frontal chest radiograph demonstrates multiple lung masses (arrows) indistinguishable from metastases; (B) Axial unenhanced CT image depicts bilateral pulmonary masses (arrows) and a bulla in the left lung (arrowhead); (C) Axial unenhanced CT image, obtained 4 years after the initial diagnosis, shows stability in the size of the nodules (arrows) and some evidence of cavitation (white arrowhead). The bulla (black arrowhead) has enlarged. The patient remained asymptomatic at the most recent follow-up evaluation.

Follow-up

Small subcentimetric lesions can be followed by surveillances scans but large tumors need surgical resection.
- A combination of medical or surgical is the ideal approach for progressive or symptomatic lesions.

Prognosis

Benign metastasizing fibroid or leiomyoma may naturally decrease following menopause. Majority remain same, some may turn aggressive.

Individualization is the key mode of therapy.

Uterine Smooth Muscle Tumors

Smooth uterine muscle of uncertain malignant potential indicates a group of tumors that cannot be diagnosed unequivocally as benign or malignant (WHO classification) (Fig. 20.2).
- Term STUMP was coined by Kempson in 1973.
- WHO classifies STUMP as uterine smooth muscle tumor not diagnosed benign or malignant.
  Stanford criteria of histological diagnosis of malignant smooth muscle tumor (Leiomyosarcoma) by Bell et al. includes at least two of the following:
- Diffuse moderate to severe atypia
- Mitotic count of at least ten mitotic figures (MF) or ten high power fields (HPFs)
- Tumor cell necrosis.

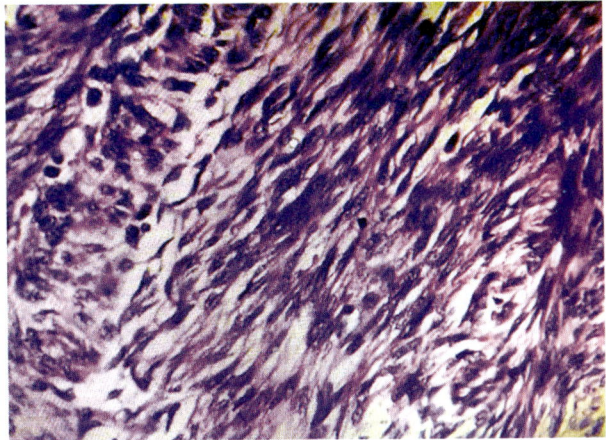

Fig. 20.2: Uterine smooth muscle tumor.

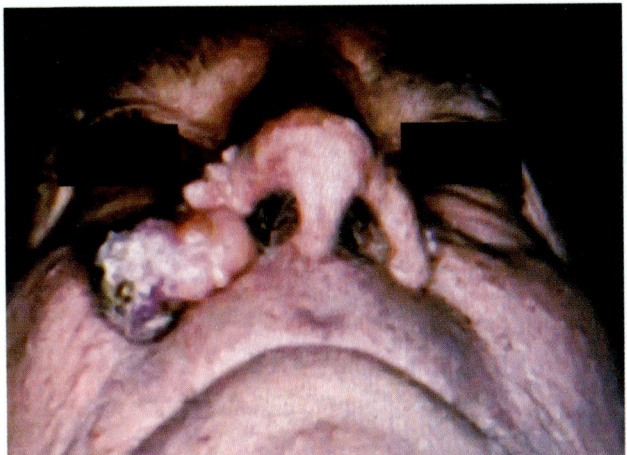

Fig. 20.3: Birt-Hogg-Dubé syndrome.

Clinical Signs and Symptoms:
- Abnormal vaginal bleeding
- Symptoms of anemia
- Rapidly growing pelvic mass
- Pressure symptoms
- Pelvic pain.
  Treatment—no standard protocol.
  If STUMP diagnosed in myomectomy patients, then hysterectomy is advised.

Birt-Hogg-Dubé Syndrome

Clinical characteristics include:
- Cutaneous manifestation (fibrofolliculomas, trichodiscomas or angiofibromas, perifollicular fibromas or acrochordons) (Fig. 20.3)

- Pulmonary cysts or history of pneumothorax
- Various types of renal tumors. Common in third or fourth decade of life, inherited as autosomal dominant pattern.

Diagnosis

- Dermatological diagnosis in individuals who have five or more facial or truncal papules with at least one histologically confirmed fibrofolliculoma.
- Lung cyst or spontaneous pneumothorax: Most individuals (89%) with Birt-Hogg-Dubé syndrome (BHDS) have multiple bilateral lung cysts, identified by high-resolution chest CT. It is likely to develop in periacinar region.
- *Renal tumors*: They are usually bilateral and multifocal. Histological tumor types are:
  - Hybrid oncocytic renal cell carcinoma, oncocytoma, chromophobe renal cell carcinoma, minority of clear cell renal cell carcinoma.

Differential Diagnosis

- *Cutaneous lesions*:
  - Acrochordons
  - BHDS-associated hamartomas should be distinguished from tuberous sclerosis complex (TSC), familial trichoepithelioma
  - Multiple endocrine neoplasia type 1 (MEN1)
  - Cowden syndrome.
- *Pulmonary manifestation*:
  - Differential diagnosis:
    - Marfan syndrome
    - Ehlers-Danlos syndrome
    - Tuberous sclerosis complex
    - Alpha-1 antitrypsin deficiency
    - Cystic fibrosis
    - Langerhans cell histiocytosis
    - Pulmonary lymphangioleiomyomatosis (LAM).
- *Renal tumor*:
  - *Differential diagnosis*:
    - Von-Hippel-Lindau syndrome
    - Hereditary papillary renal cancer (HPRC)
    - Hereditary leiomyomatosis and renal cell cancer (HLRCC).

Management

- Detailed dermatological examination or punch biopsy of suspected cutaneous lesion
- High resolution computed tomography (HRCT) or CT of chest
- Baseline abdominal or pelvic CT scan
- Clinical genetics consultation.

Treatment

Fibrofolliculomas and trichodiscomas—no treatment required.

For cosmetic reasons, Erbium-YAG or fractional CO_2 laser ablation can be used. Treatment of pneumothorax—same as general population.

Renal tumors—if size of BHDS associated kidney cancer.

Tumors less than 3 cm—conservative management; tumors more than 3 cm—partial nephrectomy.

Prognosis and Follow-up

- Yearly MRI of kidneys
- Low aggressiveness of kidney tumors and rule of 3 cm used by surgeons in treated renal tumors (Povlorich et al. 2005). Affected individuals who have two or three consecutive annual MRI examination without detection of kidney lesion may be screened every 2 years
- If suspicious lesion less than 1 cm, annual MRI done
- Renal tumors less than 3 cm—periodic screening
- Largest renal tumor more than 3 cm—nephron sparing surgery is needed
- Rapidly growing lesions, signs or symptoms including pain, blood in urine
- Atypical presentation requires individualization approach
- PET-CT scan is an option for evaluation of such lesions.

Von Hippel–Lindau Disease

Introduction

Von Hippel-Lindau disease is an uncommon autosomal dominant syndrome caused by germline mutation in the VHL gene that has been mapped to chromosome 3p25.
    Incidence: 1 in 36,000 birth.
    Common age group: 10–40; average age—26.

Signs and Symptoms

Symptomatic VHL can include vision loss.
    Retinal capillary hemangioblastomas are red–orange, well-circumscribed vascular tumors with a large feeder vessel and a large draining vessel. They can be endophytic or exophytic.
    Vitreous hemorrhage, iris neovascularization with glaucoma or cataract may be also seen.
    Extraocular sign and symptoms are—headache, vomiting, and ataxia with cerebellar hemangioblastomas, constant or transient hypertension seen with pheochromocytomas and hearing loss with endolymphatic sac tumors.

Differential Diagnosis

- Coats disease
- Wybuch Mexan syndrome
- Vasoproliferative tumors of retina
- Retinal cavernous hemangioma and racemose hemangioma.
  Diagnosis: Definitely by gene analysis.
  Screening: To be done in individuals.
- Blood relatives of someone diagnosed with VHL by positive gene analysis.
- Those who have VHL-like lesion and a positive family history of someone with VHL syndrome.
- Those with two or more VHL-like lesions.

Treatment

- Small lesion—photocoagulation
- Large lesions—cryotherapy.

Prognosis
- Life expectancy of 50 years
- Systemic morbidity is mainly due to pheochromocytoma.

Hereditary Leiomyomatosis and Renal Cell Cancer

Introduction
It is a disorder in which affected individuals tend to develop benign tumors containing smooth muscle tissues in the skin and in fundus, in uterus.

Appropriately 10–15% of such patients develop renal cell cancer. Average age of HLRCC is in fourth decade of life.

Signs and Symptoms
- Lower backache
- Hematuria
- Mass in kidney palpable on examination
- Autosomal dominant in inheritance.

Also known as—multiple cutaneous leiomyomatosis (MCL) or multiple cutaneous and uterine leiomyomatosis when it appears with renal cell cancer.

Three main symptoms are:
- Red skin papules called cutaneous piloleiomyomas
- Multiple early onset uterine leiomyomas
- Susceptibility to type 2 papillary renal cell carcinoma.

Diagnosis
Patients who have histologically confirmed multiple cutaneous piloleiomyoma or any two of the following:
- Symptomatic uterine leiomyoma less than 40 years
- Type 2 papillary carcinoma less than 40 years
- A first degree relative who meets the criteria confirmed to have HLRCC. Mean age of diagnosis ~ 41 years; 15% are at risk of developing kidney cancer.

Clinical Course and Management
The HLRCC or renal tumors are usually unilateral and solitary. They are aggressive tumors so if once a tumor is found, it is promptly resected with wide surgical margins and retroperitoneal lymphadenopathy. When there is doubt with partial nephrectomy would be curative, radical nephrectomy should be performed.

Good prognosis if found early and managed surgically.

Disseminated Peritoneal Leiomyomatosis

Introduction
It is an exceedingly rare benign disorder characterized by multiple vascular leiomyomas growing close the submesothelial tissues of the abdominopelvic peritoneum.

Pathogenesis

- Hormonal
- Smooth muscle metaplasia is the subcoelomic mesenchyme.

Diagnosis

Ultrasonography and CT reveal spectrum of feature ranging from multiple solid subcentimetric nodules to large solid masses.

The MRI shows multiple with signal intensity similar to skeletal muscle and smooth muscle in both T1- and T2-weighted images.

Differential Diagnosis

- Peritoneal carcinomatosis
- Primary peritoneal mesothelioma lymphoma
- Tuberculosis desmoid tumors
- Diagnosis by exploratory laparotomy and surgical biopsy.

Treatment

Medical or surgical castration with or without resection of leiomyomatous implants.

Prognosis

Clinical course is benign but sarcomatous transformation has been reported. Therefore, close surveillance is mandatory.

BIBLIOGRAPHY

1. Abramson S, Gilkeson RC, Goldstein JD, et al. Benign metastasizing leiomyoma: clinical, imaging, and pathologic correlation. Am J Roentgenol. 2001;176(6):1409-13.
2. Abulafia O, Angel C, Sherer DM, et al. Computed tomography of leiomyomatosis peritonealis disseminata with malignant transformation. Am J Obstet Gynecol. 1993;169(1):52-4.
3. Bell SW, Kempson PC, Hendrichson MR. Problematic uterine smooth muscle neoplasms, a clinicopatrologic study of 213 cases. Am J Sury Petrol. 1994;8(5):35-58.
4. ButtramVC Jr, Reiter RC. Uterine leiomyomata: etiology, symptomatology, and management. Fertil Steril. 1981;36(4):433-45.
5. Fulcher AS, Szucs RA. Leiomyomatosis peritonealis disseminata complicated by sarcomatous transformation and ovarian torsion: presentation of two cases and review of the literature. Abdom Imaging. 1998;23(6):640-4.
6. Horstmann JP, Pietra GG, Harman JA, et al. Spontaneous regression of pulmonary leiomyomas during pregnancy. Cancer. 1977;39(1):314-21.
7. Ip PP, Tse Ky, Tan KF. Uterine smooth muscle tumors other than the ordinary leiomyomas and leiomyosarcomas with review of selected variants with emphasis on recent ovarian and unusual morphology that may cause concern for malignancy. Adv Anat Pathol. 2010;17:91-112.
8. Kempson RC. Sarcomas and related neoplasms. In: Norris HJ, Hertis AT, Abell NR (Eds). The Uterus. Baltimore: Williams and Williams; 1973.
9. Kocica MJ, Vranes MR, Kostic D, et al. Intravenous leiomyomatosis with extension to the heart: rare or underestimated? J Thorac Cardiovasc Surg. 2005;130(6):1724-6.
10. Koh DM, Burn PR, King DM. Benign metastasizing leiomyoma with intracaval leiomyomatosis. Br J Radiol. 2000;73:435-7.
11. Raspagliesi F, Quattrone P, Grosso G, et al. Malignant degeneration in leiomyomatosis peritonealis disseminata. Gynecol Oncol. 1996;61(2):272-4.

12. Shin MS, Fulmer JD, Ho KJ. Unusual computed tomographic manifestations of benign metastasizing leiomyomas as cavitary nodular lesions or interstitial lung disease. Clin Imaging. 1996;20(1):45-9.
13. Steiner PE. Metastasizing fibroleiomyoma of the uterus. Am J Pathol. 1939;15:89-110.
14. SzklarukJ, Tamm EP, Choi H, et al. MR imaging of common and uncommon large pelvic masses. RadioGraphics. 2003;23(2):403-24.
15. Tavassoli FA, Devilee P. WHO Classification of Tumors. Tumors of the Breast and Female genital organs. Lyon: International agency for research on cancer press; 2003. pp. 236-9.
16. Thomas EO, Gordon J, Smith-Thomas S, et al. Diffuse uterine leiomyomatosis with uterine rupture and benign metastatic lesions of the bone. Obstet Gynecol. 2007;109(2 pt 2):528-30.
17. Wolff M, Silva F, Kaye G. Pulmonary metastases (with admixed epithelial elements) from smooth muscle neoplasms: report of nine cases, including three males. Am J Surg Pathol. 1979;3(4):325-42.

What's New in the World of Fibroids?

Apoorva Pallam Reddy

INTRODUCTION

Leiomyoma or fibroids have been documented since antiquity. As early as the era of Hippocrates in 460–375 BC, the lesion was reported as the "uterine stone" (Fig. 21.1).

In the 18th and early 19th century fibroids, the only management options for myomas (term coined by German pathologist Virchow) was either hysterectomy or open myomectomy. Since then, there has been a linear growth in the number of treatment modalities available for dealing with fibroids and their symptoms. Despite having known fibroids for ages and invasive surgical procedures becoming progressively safe, there has been constant exploration on finding etiopathology and safer, effective noninvasive management options. This chapter aims to give you a brief update on the recent developments of "uterine stones" and how we can apply them in our day-to-day practice.

ETIOPATHOLOGY

The development of uterine fibroids involves complex interaction among genes and environment. There are two components to myoma development; overgrowth of smooth

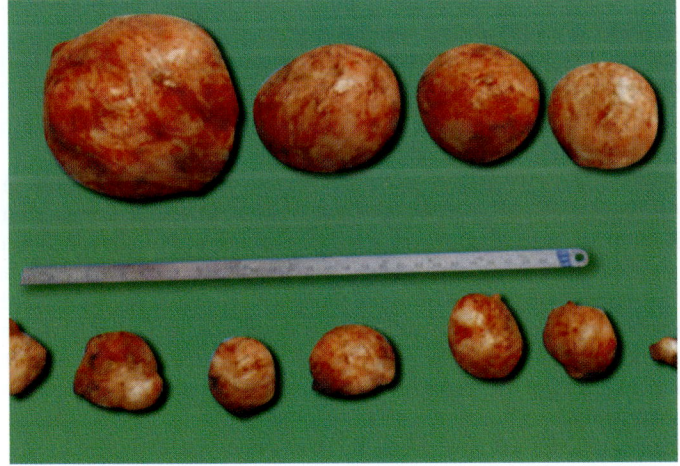

Fig. 21.1: Uterine stones/myomas.

muscle and connective tissue; first the transformation of normal myocytes to abnormal myocytes and then their growth into clinically apparent tumors. The identity of the factor(s) and molecular mechanisms involved in the cellular transformation of myometrial cells into leiomyoma, yet, remains mystique.

Update: Despite being multifactorial, latest findings suggest that up to 40% of uterine fibroids bear some chromosomal abnormalities. The most common are aberration of chromosomes 6, 7, 12, and 14 which are nonrandom and tumor-specific. These aberrations can include trisomy 12, translocation involving chromosomes (t12; 14) (q14–q15; q23–q24), deletions on chromosome 7 (q22q32), 3q and 1p, and rearrangements of 6p21, 10q22, and 13q21-q22.

The type of aberration may determine the size and location of fibroids. Intramural (35%) and subserous (29%) leiomyomas are more likely to have abnormal karyotypes than the submucous (12%) type. Large tumors carry t(12;14) abnormalities, in contrast, tumors with del (7) were found to be smaller.

Based on our current state of knowledge, one can only speculate upon the initiators of this common condition. Future research efforts may provide a better comprehension of the causes and mechanisms of uterine fibroid tumorigenesis. Understanding and uncovering of the genetic and environmental mechanisms responsible for uterine leiomyoma will aid in designing rational gene therapy protocols.

Apply: Women with a family history of fibroids should be advised against the risk factors like hyperestrogenic states, hyperinsulinemia, prolonged progesterone supplementation, obesity, high carbohydrate diet, prolonged oral contraceptive pill usage, consumption of red meat, excessive caffeine intake, etc.

DIAGNOSIS

Ultrasonography (USG) is the most widely used tool for diagnosing fibroids owing to its efficiency, cost-effectiveness, and noninvasive nature. With 2D USG, it can be a challenge to differentiate a submucosal leiomyoma from an intramural one, or to determine its relationship with the endometrial cavity. This is especially important in patients with fertility problems, recurrent pregnancy failures, and abnormal uterine bleeding. 3D USG can accurately map the exact location of leiomyomas distinguishing the borders precisely. This information is very valuable when making clinical decisions.

Three-dimensional power Doppler can also be useful in evaluating candidates for embolization by giving detailed information about collateral vessels, the presence of which decreases the chance of success of embolization.

Other approaches like MRI and invasive techniques like hysteroscopy and laparoscopy have assisted significantly in diagnosing fibroids.

Update: The two areas of conflict in investigating fibroids have been—distinguishing fibroid from adenomyosis and benign from malignant.

It is known that adenomyosis can present clinically and sonographically in a manner suggestive of fibroids. Dearth of features distinguishing localized adenomyosis from that of degenerating fibroids can lead to an increase in the number of fibroids diagnosed.

Owing to the use of power morcellators, a strategy to determine if a tumor is a leiomyosarcoma is urgently needed. At present, there is no simple, effective screening method to determine if a uterine tumor is indeed benign and not malignant, prior to treatment.

The MRI techniques demonstrate the ability to differentiate adenomyosis and fibroid and a malignant from benign tumor, but have not yet been authorized for distinguishing leiomyosarcoma from leiomyoma.

While important, this approach is clearly not cost-effective.

Elastography is a medical imaging modality that maps the elastic properties of soft tissue.

Shear wave elasticity imaging (SWEI) is a technique where a distortion is created on the soft tissue using acoustic radiation force and the response to distortion (extent of stiffness) is measured using a USG or MRI.

A prospective study of elastographic nature of normal uterine tissue, fibroids, and adenomyotic tissue has shown significant difference between the uterine fibroid, adenomyosis, and control groups. Median "lesion indices" were 2.65, 0.44 and 1.19, respectively.

There have been cases where, using shear wave elastography, a leiomyosarcoma was accurately diagnosed preoperatively, based on the degree of stiffness throughout the tumor.

However, currently we only have pilot studies and we need larger studies to confirm this to make it a major breakthrough.

Apply: If elastography is incorporated into routine sonography, benign fibroids can be distinguished from adenomyosis and malignancies with efficiency preoperatively.

MANAGEMENT

Clinical management decisions revolve around dealing of fibroid originated symptoms of the heavy menstrual bleeding, including anemia, which is often severe, chronic pain and pressure, or infertility. The constellation of choices available are conservative options like oral contraceptive pills, progesterone pills, levonorgestrel intrauterine system (LNG-IUS), selective progesterone receptor modulator, androgens, aromatase inhibitors, somatostatin analogs, gestrinone, gonadotropin releasing hormone agonists (GnRHa), GnRH antagonists, and surgical management.

Selective Progesterone Receptor Modulators

Several selective progesterone receptor modulators (SPRMs) have been tried extensively in managing fibroids in view of their promising profile (Fig. 21.2).
- *Mifepristone*: Several studies have proved the efficacy of RU 486 or mifepristone in inducing amenorrhea and reducing pictorial blood loss assessment chart (PBAC) score when used in dose ranging from 10 mg to 25 mg per day. Higher doses were more effective in reducing the size of large fibroids.

  Long-term use of the drug (6 months) at 50 mg per week doses did not result in any significant hepatotoxicity.

  However, there have been concerns on the increased incidence of endometrial hyperplasia and cystic glandular pattern in women noted in women on mifepristone (Details in Chapter 13).
- *Ulipristal acetate*: Ulipristal acetate (UA) was developed as a selective progesterone receptor modulator with pure progesterone receptor antagonistic activity and minimal antiglucocorticoid effects. 1 or 3 month course of UA has been shown to induce apoptosis and to decrease proliferation of uterine fibroid cells decreasing the volume of fibroid and eventually inducing amenorrhea. Use is safe in women seeking fertility and as it does not reduce serum estradiol levels below the 50 pg/dL levels there is no loss of bone mineral density (Details in Chapter 13).
- *Telapristone acetate (TA) (Also known as Proellex, Progenta, and CDB-4124)*: The US FDA placed a full clinical hold on telapristone in August 2009 because of elevated liver enzymes associated with drug treatment. After the hold was removed couple of months later, other routes of TA administration have been investigated extensively. A phase 2 clinical trial (ZPV-200) compared four doses of telapristone (3 mg, 6 mg, 12 mg, and 24 mg) in the form of a vaginal suppository, a gel capsule. The vaginal use of telapristone at 12 mg per day was associated with similar favorable outcomes for women with fibroids as compared to the higher oral dose. Notably, the 12 mg vaginal dose achieved a statistically significant

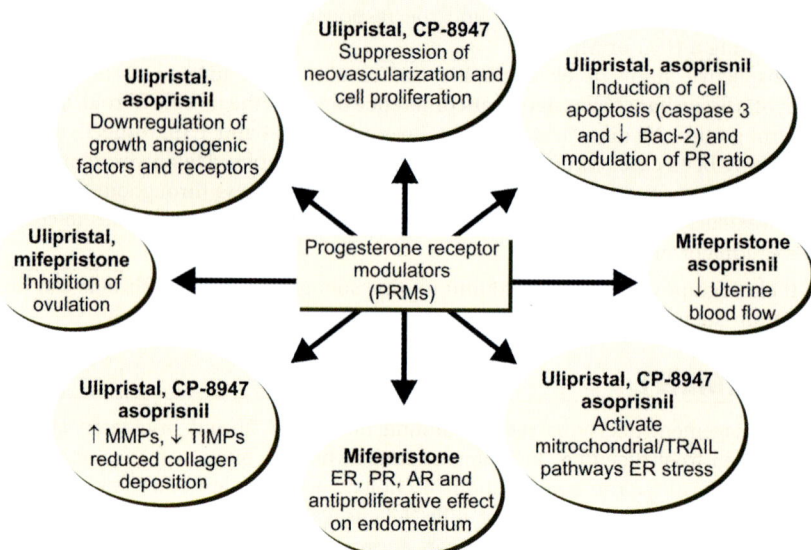

Fig. 21.2: Mechanisms of action of progesterone receptor modulators on uterine fibroids. (ER: Estrogen receptor; PR: Progesterone receptor; AR: Androgen receptor; TRAIL: TNF-related apoptosis-inducing ligand; MMP: Matrix metalloproteinases; TIMP: Tissue inhibitors of metalloproteinases)

and clinically relevant improvement in bleeding as assessed by PBAC and in tumor size as assessed by MRI with least systemic exposure at all doses tested. No evidence of hepatotoxicity was noted at the end of treatment.
- *Vilaprisan*: The phase 1 trials with vilaprisan have shown promising results with significant fall in menstrual flow and size of fibroid at doses as low as 2 mg.

The benefits over other progesterone receptor modulators (PRMs) noted were no treatment-emergent critical endometrial findings occurred, follicular growth was not suppressed, and minimum average estradiol levels remained above 40 pg/mL.

Return of menstrual bleeding was observed in all women in less than or equal to 52 days after discontinuation. Large randomized controlled trials (RCTs) are however required to validate the same.
- *Asoprisnil*: Asoprisnil is an SPRM with antagonistic effect on the endometrium, ovary and breast; partial agonistic effect on myometrium of pregnant uterus and antagonistic effect on myometrium of leiomyoma.

A randomized double-blinded placebo controlled study by Wilkens et al. showed that asoprisnil significantly reduced the fibroid size compared with placebo with either 10 mg or 25 mg dose when taken once a day for 12 weeks.

Advantages of Progesterone Receptor Modulators

In contrast to GnRHa therapy, SPRMs suppress bleeding rapidly in women with uterine leiomyomata, without suppressing estrogen secretion, with majority of women attaining amenorrhea during treatment and a noteworthy improvement in quality of life.

Further, there is emerging data to suggest that treatment with SPRMs may lower the risk for breast cancer, although further studies are necessary to investigate this potentially beneficial effect.

Concerns over Progesterone Receptor Modulators

Clinicians detecting endometrial thickening in women treated with SPRMs need to be aware that administration of SPRMs for longer than 3 months may lead to endometrial thickening and of the possible hepatotoxicity in preexisting compromised liver function. This is related to cystic glandular dilation, not endometrial hyperplasia, and pathologists need to be aware of PRM-associated endometrial changes (PAEC) and avoid misclassifying the appearance as hyperplasia

The impacts on morphology, molecular, and cellular changes with PRM administration on symptom control and long-term sequelae remain to be determined.

It is noteworthy that use of PRM may induce ovarian cyst formation and mild elevation in prolactin levels.

Despite the histological changes, Donnez et al., in their RCT of 451 patients on long-term UA (4 courses of 12 weeks each) concluded that at the end of the 4 courses, there was no any significant increase in the endometrial thickness from baseline level.

Elagolix—Orally Active GnRH Antagonist

Elagolix is a short-acting, nonpeptide, GnRH antagonist, administered orally, that unlike injectable depot GnRH agonists and antagonists, produces a dose-dependent suppression of ovarian estrogen production, that is, from partial suppression at lower doses to full suppression at higher doses. In addition, oral administration and a short half-life (~6 hours) allows for rapid elimination of elagolix from the body. It has been investigated for managing both endometriosis and fibroids as well. A phase 2, randomized, multicenter, double-blind study by Bruce et al. showed that, 150 mg once a day or 75 mg twice a day doses of elagolix treatment had minimal impact on bone mineral density (BMD) over a 24-week period similar efficacy on endometriosis-associated pain compared depot medroxyprogesterone acetate (Fig. 21.3).

Selective Estrogen Receptor Modulator

Theoretically, any agent that can block estrogen receptors should exert therapeutic effect on myoma. However, raloxifene did not shrink the size of myoma in perimenopausal women who were administered daily 60 mg doses of raloxifene over a 2-year period. There was no statistical fall in the size of the fibroids at the end of 12 weeks of treatment.

Lasofoxifene is a third generation selective estrogen receptor modulator used for managing osteoporosis and vaginal atrophy in postmenopausal women. There have been studies to evaluate its effect on myoma without demonstrating any benefits over raloxifene (Fig. 21.4).

Dietary Supplements

- *Vitamin D_3*: Sabry et al. have demonstrated significant negative correlation between vitamin D_3 levels and the size and number of fibroids. Supplementing D3 can inhibit growth and induce apoptosis in myoma resulting in diminished size (Fig. 21.5).
  - Further studies are required to determine the dose and duration of therapy required to achieve this effect.
- *Epigallocatechin gallate, green tea extract (Fig. 21.6)*: Green tea is a powerful antioxidant touted as a remedy for various symptoms including fibroids. Epigallocatechin-3-gallate

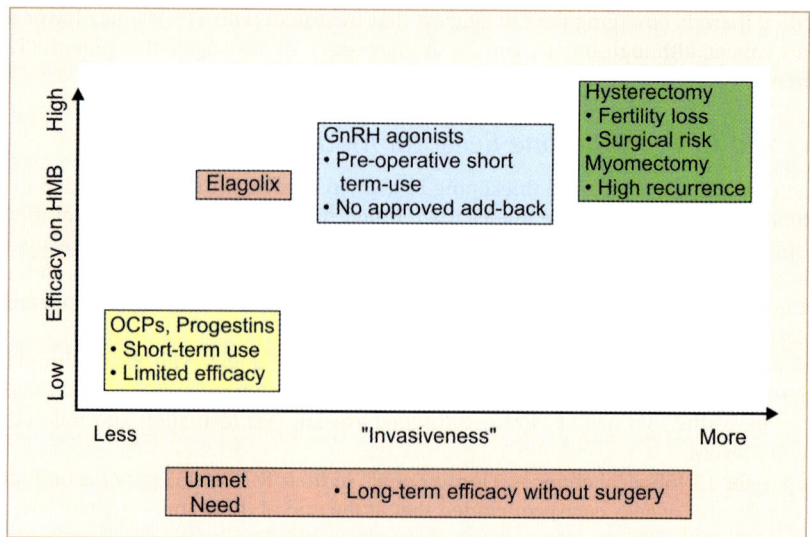

Fig. 21.3: Treatment options for heavy menstrual bleeding associated with uterine fibroids.
(HMB: Heavy menstrual bleeding; GnRH: Gonadotropin-releasing hormone; OCPs: Oral contraceptive pills)

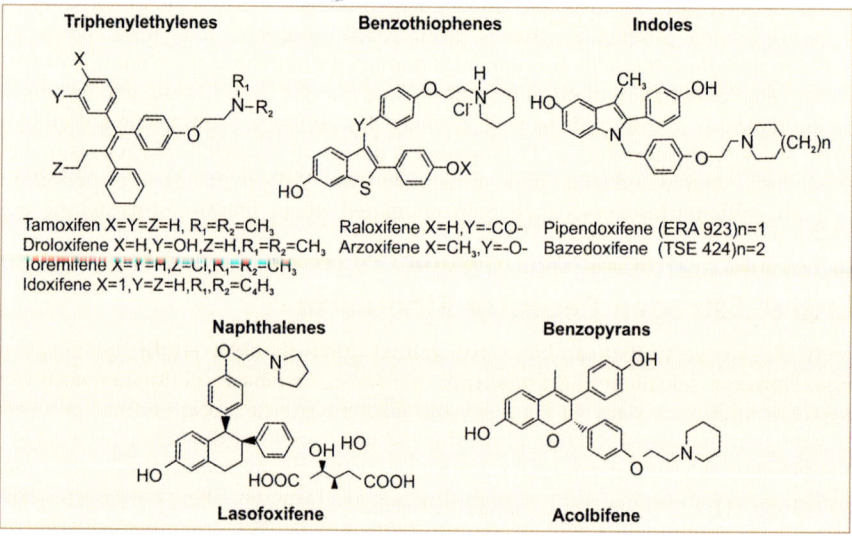

Fig. 21.4: Selective estrogen receptor modulators.

(EGCG) is the major component of catechin (>40% of the total polyphenolic mixture of green tea catechins). EGCG-induced apoptosis and inhibition of proliferation of fibroid cells is achieved by modulating signaling pathways involved in cell proliferation, transformation, inflammation, and oxidative stress.
- *Resveratrol*: A dietary phytoalexin and a component of red wine, has been shown to induce apoptosis, decrease cell viability and number, and increase the

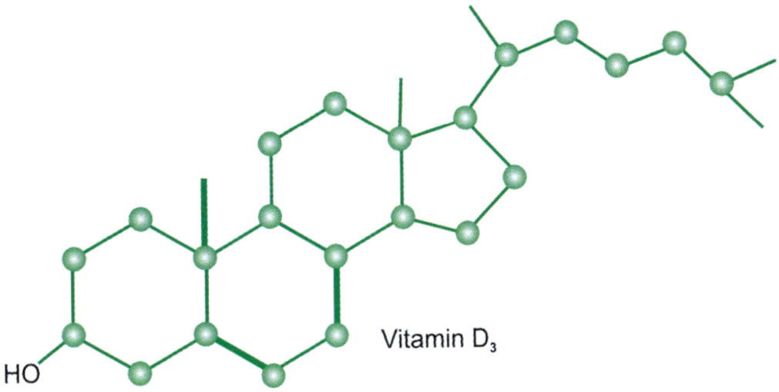

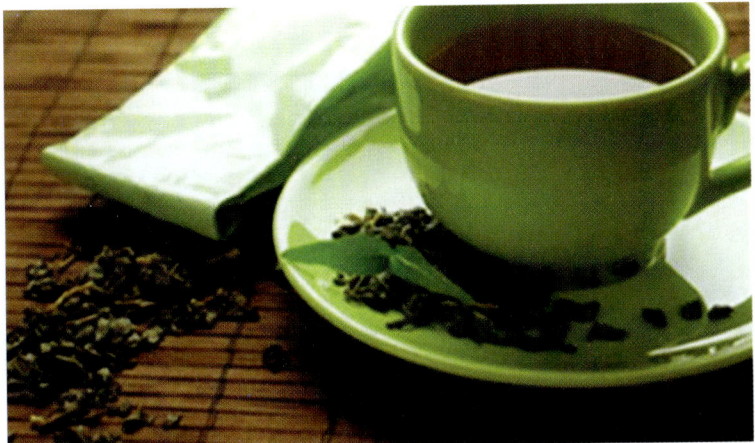

Fig. 21.5: Structure of vitamin D_3.

Fig. 21.6: Green tea extract.

percentage of cells arrested in the G1 phase in a dose-dependent manner by preventing cell cycle progression from the G1 to S phase. It is also a potent antifibrogenic effect by reducing the mRNA production and protein expression of collagen types III and I in a dose-dependent manner in vitro.

Intralesional Drug Delivering Systems

One of the main drawbacks of medical therapy for management of fibroids is the side effects exerted on the nontargeted organs. The development of nanocarriers designed to deliver drug therapeutics (e.g. antifibrotic, aromatase inhibitors, progestins, etc.) directly into the lesion is an emerging field. Over the past 50 years, nanoparticles and microspheres have been used as carriers of anticancer drugs to increase antitumor potency of the older drugs and reduce toxic side-effects. Nanocarriers (nanocapsules and nanocarriers) create a drug depot inside the fibroid by local injection. Unlike polymeric nanospheres (Fig. 21.7A), which are matrix systems of nanoparticles), nanocapsules (Fig. 21.7B) are heterogeneous vesicular systems in which the drug is confined to a cavity surrounded by a polymeric membrane.

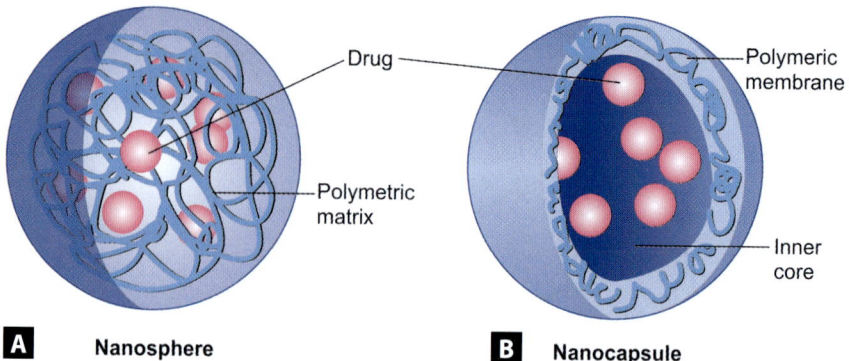

Figs. 21.7A and B: Structure of (A) A nanosphere; and (B) A nanocapsule. In a nanosphere, the drug is scattered along with the matrix system. In a nanocapsule, the drug is confined to the center of the cavity creating a "reservoir" system.

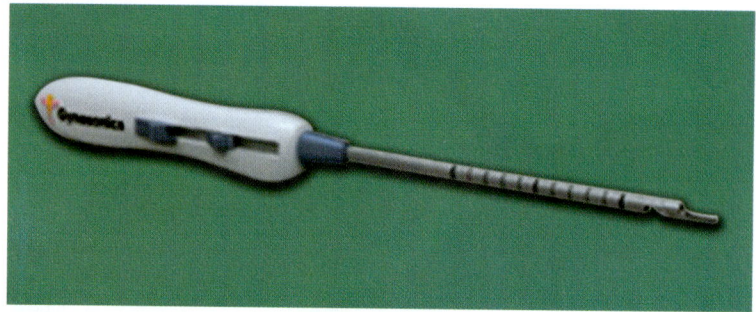

Fig. 21.8: The VizAblate treatment device (handpiece).

Radiofrequency (RF) Ablation System

The VizAblate System is a transcervical device that ablates fibroids with radiofrequency energy, guided by a built-in intrauterine ultrasound probe (Figs. 21.8 and 21.9).

Bongers et al. conducted a prospective, longitudinal, multicenter, single-arm controlled trial to evaluate the efficacy of VizAblate in reduction of fibroid size and improvement in quality of life after 3 months of therapy. 50 patients were treated, representing 92 fibroids. Perfused fibroid volumes were reduced at 3 months by an average of $68.8 \pm 27.8\%$ ($P < 0.0001$). There were no serious adverse effects recorded. VizAblate is yet to receive FDA approval.

The Halt Ablation System (Fig. 21.10)

The Halt 2000 ablation system is radiofrequency ablation system that uses laparoscopic approach with ultrasound guidance for delivery of radiofrequency waves. In a prospective, multicenter, outpatient interventional clinical trial of fibroid treatment in 124 premenopausal women, Halt significantly reduced symptom severity and improved quality of life with low surgical reintervention through 24 months of follow-up.

FDA had approved Halt in management of fibroids in 2010.

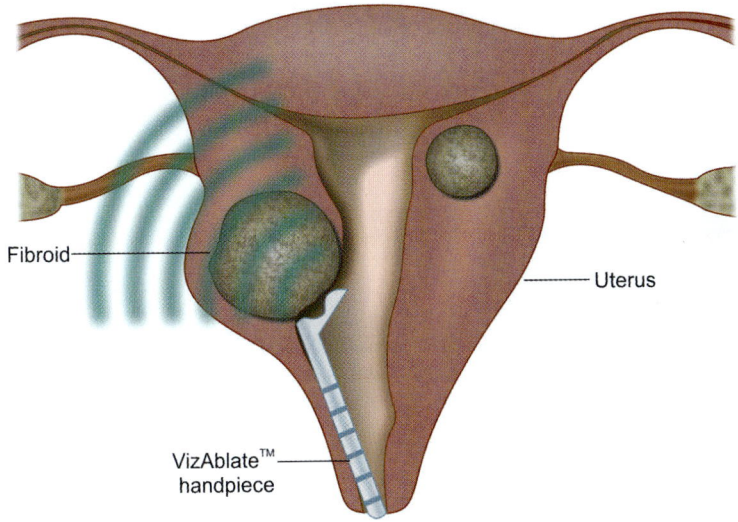

Fig. 21.9: Artistic rendition of the VizAblate system during a fibroid ablation.

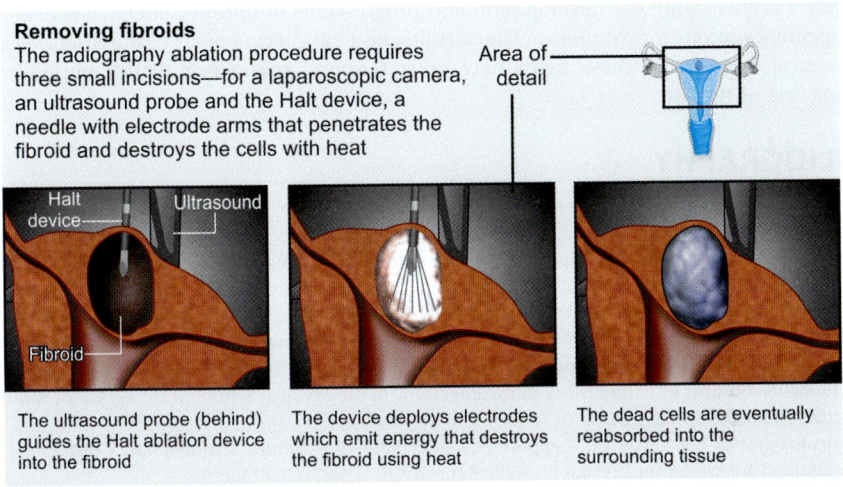

Fig. 21.10: The Halt ablation system.

Purified Bacterial Collagenase

Fibroids contain abundant and disorganized extracellular matrix (ECM). As one of the main ECM components, collagens may serve as a vulnerable nonhormonal target for treatment of fibroids. Purified *Clostridium histolyticum* collagenase (CHC), an FDA-approved drug that does not affect nerves or blood vessels, has recently shown in ex-vivo leiomyoma tissue (on hysterectomized specimen samples) to significantly degrade the altered collagen when injected into tumor (Figs. 21.11A and B).

The use of CHC, alone or with other drugs such as an SPRM, could potentially be utilized for conservative management.

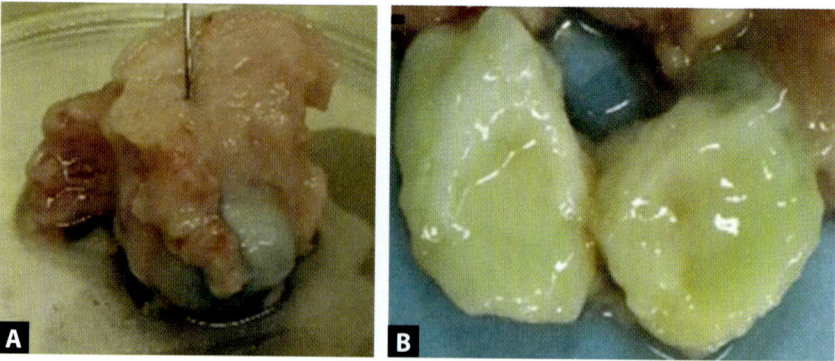

Figs. 21.11A and B: (A) Injection of *Clostridium histolyticum* collagenase into fibroid. Note the firm consistency of the fibroid; (B) Post-24-hour incubation and bisection. Note liquefaction in the center.

CONCLUSION

Understanding the etiopathology and management choices have grown leaps and bounds in the field of leiomyoma since the time of their discovery. However, there are still many more miles to go before we can call it the end. There are still many unconcluded genre like genes predisposing the development and progressions of fibroids, effective conservative management options for women seeking fertility, and long-term effects of the drugs available for medical therapy. All these fields have great scope of research and thus improvise the existing line of therapy.

BIBLIOGRAPHY

1. Becker C. Another selective estrogen-receptor modulator for osteoporosis. N Engl J Med. 2010; 362(8):752-4.
2. Bongers M, Brölmann H, Gupta J, et al. Transcervical, intrauterine ultrasound-guided radiofrequency ablation of uterine fibroids with the VizAblate® System: three- and six-month endpoint results from the FAST-EU study. Gynecol Surg. 2015;12:61-70.
3. Bouchard P, Chabbert-Buffet N, Fauser BCJM. Selective progesterone receptor modulators in reproductive medicine: pharmacology, clinical efficacy and safety. Fertil Steril. 2011;96:1175-89.
4. Bozini N, Baracat EC. The history of myomectomy at the Medical School of University of São Paulo. Clinics. 2007;62(3):209-10.
5. Brunengraber LN, Jayes FL, Leppert PC. Injectable Clostridium Histolyticum Collagenase as a potential treatment for uterine fibroids. Reprod Sci. 2014;21(12):1452-9.
6. Carr B, Dmowski WP, O'Brien C, et al. Elagolix, an oral GnRH antagonist, versus subcutaneous depot medroxyprogesterone acetate for the treatment of endometriosis: effects on bone mineral density. Reprod Sci. 2014;21(11):1341-51.
7. Catherino WH, Parrott E, Segars J. Proceedings from the NICHD conference on the uterine fibroid research update workshop. Fertil Steril. 2011;95(1):9-12.
8. Chabbert-Buffet N, Esber N, Bouchard P. Fibroid growth and medical options for treatment. Fertil Steril. 2014;102(3):630-9.
9. Donnez J, Donnez O, Matule D, et al. Long-term medical management of uterine fibroids with ulipristal acetate. Fertil Steril. 2016;105:165-73.
10. Engman M, Skoog L, Söderqvist G, et al. The effect of mifepristone on breast cell proliferation in premenopausal women evaluated through fine needle aspiration cytology. Hum Reprod. 2008;23:2072-9.
11. Flake GP, Andersen J, Dixon D. Etiology and pathogenesis of uterine leiomyomas: a review. Environ Health Perspect. 2003;111(8):1037-54.

12. Frank ML, Schäfer SD, Möllers M, et al. Importance of transvaginal elastography in the diagnosis of uterine fibroids and adenomyosis. Ultraschall Med. 2016;37(4):373-8.
13. Furukawa S, Soeda S, Watanabe T, et al. The measurement of stiffness of uterine smooth muscle tumor by elastography. Springer Plus. 2014;3:294.
14. Guido RS, Macer JA, Abbott K, et al. Radiofrequency volumetric thermal ablation of fibroids: a prospective, clinical analysis of two years' outcome from the Halt trial. Health Qual Life Outcomes. 2013;11:139.
15. Kapur A, Angomchanu R, Dey M. Efficacy of use of long-term, low-dose mifepristone for the treatment of fibroids. J Obstet Gynaecol India. 2016;66(Suppl 1):494-8.
16. Kulshrestha V, Kriplani A, Agarwal N, et al. Low dose mifepristone in medical management of uterine leiomyoma—an experience from a tertiary care hospital from north India. Indian J Med Res. 2013;137(6):1154-62.
17. Medikare V, Kandukuri LR, Ananthapur V, et al. The genetic bases of uterine fibroids: a review. J Reprod Infertil. 2011;12(3):181-91.
18. Premkumar A, Venzon DJ, Avila N, et al. Gynecologic and hormonal effects of raloxifene in premenopausal women. Fertil Steril. 2007;88(6):1637-44.
19. Sabry M, Al-Hendy A. Medical treatment of uterine leiomyoma. Reprod Sci. 2012;19(4):339-53.
20. Safety of treatment of uterine fibroids with asoprisnil. Available from: http://clinicaltrials gov/ct2/show/NCT00156208 2010.
21. Schütt B, Kaiser A. Pharmacodynamics and safety of the novel selective progesterone receptor modulator vilaprisan: a double-blind, randomized, placebo-controlled phase 1 trial in healthy women. Hum Reprod. 2016;31(8): 1703-12.
22. Taylor DK, Leppert PC. Treatment for uterine fibroids: searching for effective drug therapies. Drug Discov Today Ther Strateg. 2012;9(1):e41-e49.
23. Tristan M, Orozco LJ, Steed A, et al. Mifepristone for uterine fibroids. Cochrane Database Syst Rev. 2012;(8):CD007687.
24. Whitaker LH, Murray AA, Matthews R, et al. Selective progesterone receptor modulator (SPRM) ulipristal acetate (UPA) and its effects on the human endometrium. Hum Reprod. 2017;32(3):531-43.
25. Wiehle R, Hsu K, Wike JG. The antiprogestin telapristone shrinks fibroids when orally or as a vaginal suppository (COGI 2013). 18th World Congress On Controversies In Obstetrics, Gynecology & Infertility (COGI).
26. Wilkens J, Chwalisz K, Han C, et al. Effects of the selective progesterone receptor modulator asoprisnil on uterine artery blood flow, ovarian activity, and clinical symptoms in patients with uterine leiomyomata scheduled for hysterectomy. J Clin Endocrinol Metab. 2008;93:4664-71.
27. Wright JC, Sekar M, van Osdol W, et al. In situ forming systems (depots). In: Wright JC, Burgess DJ (Eds). Long Acting Injections and Implants. New York: Springer US; 2012. pp. 153-66.
28. Zhang D, Al-Hendy M, Richard-Davis G, et al. Antiproliferative and proapoptotic effects of epigallocatechin gallate on human leiomyoma cells. Fertil Steril. 2011;94(5):1887-93.

How Much Should She Worry? Reassuring Patients with Fibroids

22

Rakhi Singh, Seema Pandey

INTRODUCTION

"In times of stress, the best thing we can do for each other is to listen with our ears and our hearts and to be assured that our questions are just as important as our answers."

—Ferd Rogers

"But doctor my GP said, until I remove my fibroid I cannot get pregnant but my mother in-law says no surgery till I complete my family." These are common dialogues between a gynecologist and a patient, who has been diagnosed to have a myoma and now is in dilemma what is the best way to go. Counseling is an integral part of any consultation where a doctor has to make her patient understand the disease process and the various modalities of treatment available to her as a menu, along with advantages and disadvantages of each and every procedure as evidence and statistics says and let her decide. Worldwide women felt that disease-oriented counseling was inadequate and there is a need for target counseling regarding the management options, etc.

Myoma is the most common benign tumor of reproductive age group (20–40 years) arising from myometrium with an incidence of 70%. Most are asymptomatic; however pain and menorrhagia are the most common presenting symptoms. Pain is usually due to degeneration, torsion or impaction. Due to lifestyle and environmental changes, the incidence is on the rise and the women may be at different stage of her reproductive life and accordingly her priorities are different regarding the treatment part. Irrespective of her age, few questions remain same once the diagnosis is made. And as a clinician and treating doctor it is our duty to present the facts regarding all the queries she is having.

FIBROID AND ITS PROGRESSION

- Fibroids are usually very slow growing but the fibroids of less than 2 cm and more than 5 cm size will grow relatively faster.
- Intramural fibroids grow faster than submucous or subserous fibroids (Fig. 22.1).
- Parity has no relation to growth.
- Fibroids showing good vascular flow and larger feeding vessels will grow faster.
- In pregnancy fibroids tend to grow in size during first trimester but many start regressing in later half of pregnancy, especially the bigger ones.

EVALUATION OF FIBROID

- Ultrasound is the cheapest and best modality to diagnose fibroids up to the size of 4–5 cm and of 1–2 in number with relation to the position of the uterus.

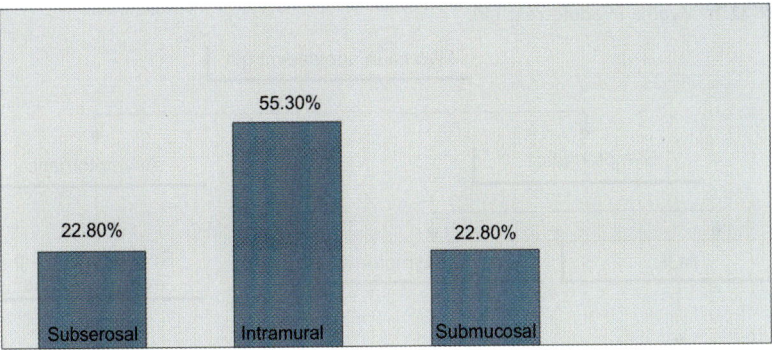

Fig. 22.1: Growth rate of the fibroid.

- Hysterosalpingography (HSG) is indicated to assess the uterine cavity and tubal patency. If a balloon catheter is used to perform the HSG, it should be deflated at the end of the procedure to allow for complete evaluation of the cavity. When HSG reveals a filling defect in the uterine cavity but HSG is obsolete these days. Sonohysterography or office hysteroscopy can more precisely define the location and attachment of the lesion(s) and determine whether a submucous myoma(s) is (are) amenable to hysteroscopic resection. Evidence indicates that sonohysterography is highly sensitive for identifying intrauterine lesions and yields results that correlate well with those obtained by hysteroscopy. Sonohysterography generally causes little discomfort and is easier to perform and less costly than office or outpatient hysteroscopy.
- Multiple fibroids are best diagnosed by MRI; site, size, and overlapping myomas are better differentiated by MRI so it is easier to make a management protocol. But the drawback is high cost and availability.
- Leiomyosarcomas are usually large heteroxenous masses containing areas of hemorrhage. They have more ill-defined irregular margins, compared to benign tumors.
- Submucous myomas are best diagnosed hysteroscopically, advantage being removal at the same sitting. However, hysteroscopy is unnecessary when the uterine cavity contour is normal on hysterosalpingography or sonosalpingography.
- Diffuse leiomyomatosis is a rare condition that consists of diffuse involvement of the myometrium by innumerable small myomas. Histologically they are benign but rarely there may be dissemination through peritoneal cavity or distant metastasis.
- Lipoleiomyomas are rare fat-containing leiomyomas with reported prevalence of 0.005–0.2%. They are detected in 0.03–0.2% of hysterectomy specimens and are benign.

MYOMA IN AN ADOLESCENT OR UNMARRIED GIRL (FLOWCHART 22.1)

- Most of the time it is an accidental finding on USG.
- The symptomatic ones present with menorrhagia and dysmenorrhea and sometimes with urinary pressure symptoms.
- Main objective is to reduce their anxiety and reassure them if the girl is asymptomatic.
- Emphasis on its benign nature and chances of extremely rare malignant transformation.
- Also emphasize on regular follow-up and diet and lifestyle modifications. Pills or progesterone only to prescribe when there is endometrial hyperplasia.

Flowchart 22.1: Myoma in adolescent girl.

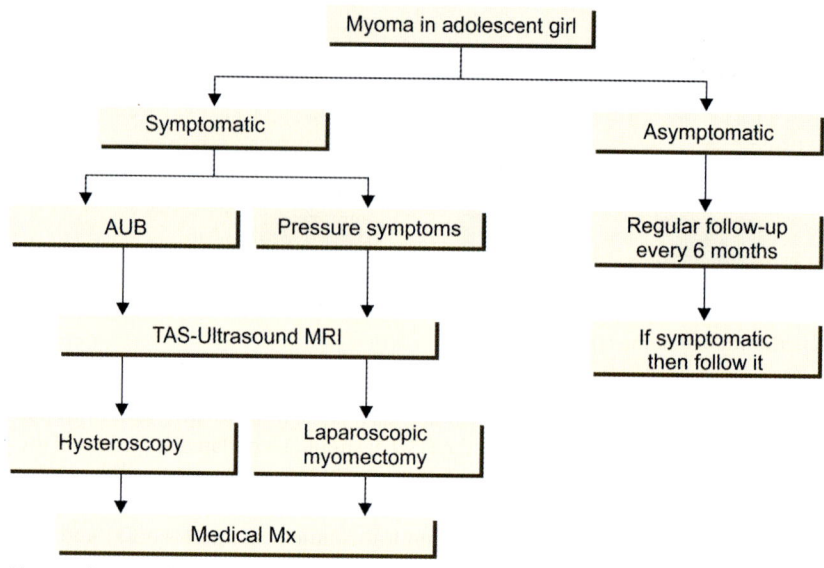

(AUB: Abnormal uterine bleeding; TAS: Transabdominal sonography; MRI: Magnetic resonance imaging)

FIBROID AND FERTILITY

This is a situation where woman is really stressed, on one hand she wants to get pregnant desperately; on the other hand she is worried about her myoma. Points she must understand before opting for any treatment are following:
- Uterine fibroids may be identified in approximately 5–10% of infertile women.
- Only 2–3% of infertility may be attributed to the effect of myoma when all other causes of infertility are excluded. However this effect may be underestimated grossly due to lack of reporting and studies included in various reviews and meta-analysis.
- Only those myomas which distort the uterine cavity (submucous myoma) and those intramural ones which are near endometrial cavity and are more than 5 cm in size may have adversely affect the fertility.
- Medical management does not improve her chances of pregnancy. Same is true for procedures like uterine artery embolization (UAE), myolysis, and MRI-guided US treatment, so these options should not be recommended for a woman with myoma seeking treatment for infertility because safety and efficacy of these treatments is not established in these cases.
- Prior to pregnancy, myomectomy can be considered especially in women with unexplained infertility and recurrent pregnancy losses (RPL), but only after thorough workup for other common causes of RPL. Whether this intervention improves her fertility potential and perinatal outcome is still a matter of debate.
- Fertility and live birth rate definitely improves post-myomectomy in cases of submucosal fibroids.
- Myomectomy is a relatively safe procedure associated with a few life-threatening complications. Due to increased incidence of adhesion formation and its complications in cases of open myomectomy, laparoscopic and hysteroscopic route is preferred.
- Evidences suggest that myoma may also adversely affect the outcome of IVF. But it is still a point of debate and consensus is divided about adverse effect of intramural myoma on IVF outcome especially for sizes less than 5 cm (Flowchart 22.2).

Flowchart 22.2: Fibroid and fertility.

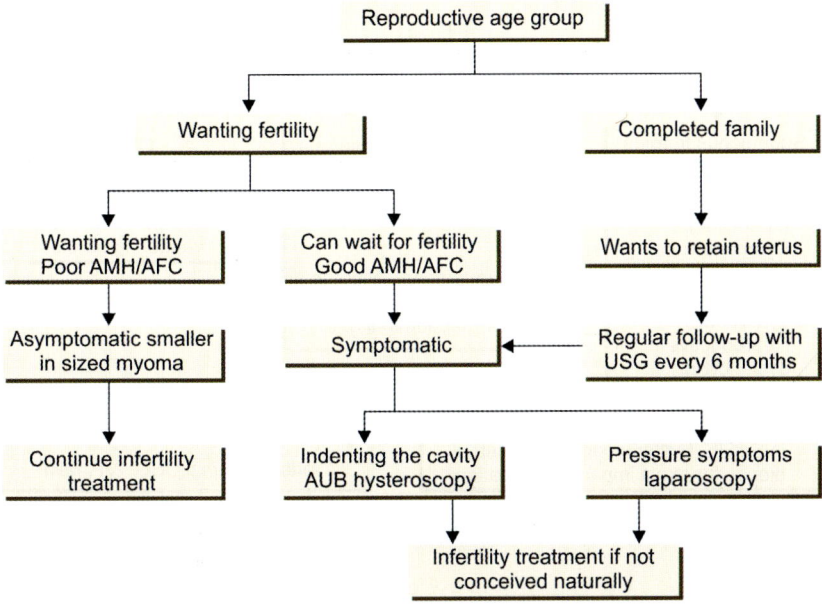

(AMH: Anti-Müllerian hormone; AFC: Antral follicle count; AUB: Abnormal uterine bleeding; USG: Ultrasonography)

FIBROIDS IN PREGNANCY

- Myomas are observed in 2.7–12.5% of pregnant women; however this data may be just the tip of iceberg due to under-reporting.
- High level of sex steroids promotes the growth of myoma in first trimester. Paradoxically larger myomas often shrink in later half of pregnancy (>5 cm size).
- The most common symptom associated with myoma in pregnancy is pain which is due to red degeneration of myoma.
- The incidence of red degeneration per say is very low in pregnancy.
- Obstetric complications are known to occur with myomas but they are not that common.
- Myoma per say is said to increase the incidence of following complications:
  - Implantation failure
  - Abortion—19%
  - Malpresentation
  - Preterm labor
  - Premature rupture of membranes
  - Abruption and abnormal placentation
  - Increased rate of C-section
  - Postpartum hemorrhage and anemia.
- Specific location of myoma is important for outcome of pregnancy. For example, a myoma adjacent to placental site is more dangerous than any other.
- Incidences of these complications came down drastically once the myomectomy was performed (19% vs. 42%) in multiple series of cases.
- Although myomectomy in early pregnancy has been successfully done, it is not recommended during pregnancy.

Flowchart 22.3: Presentation, symptoms, and diagnosis of fibroid according to its position.

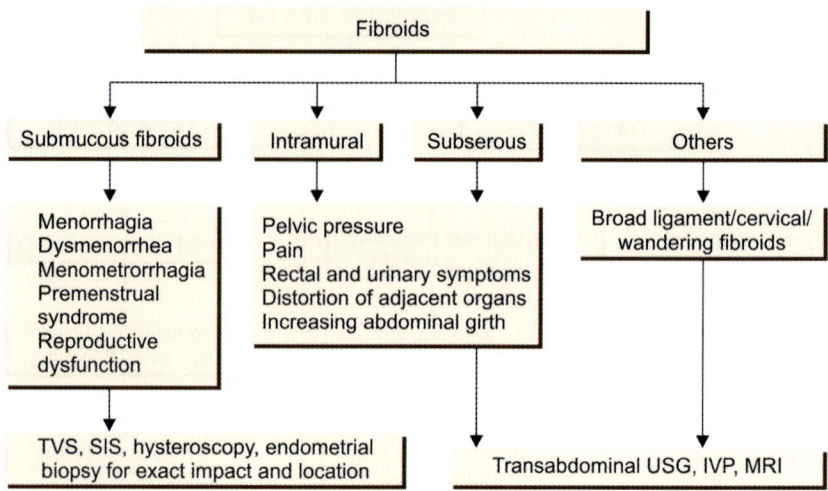

(USG: Ultrasonography; IVP: Intravenous pyelogram, TVS: Transvaginal sonography; SIS: Saline infusion sonohysterography)

- Correct route of delivery to be chosen carefully.
- If myoma happens to be in lower uterine segment it can be removed during C-section, but only after delivering the baby.
- Woman has to be reassured that although these complications are known to happen but these are not very common and emphasis on regular follow-up with her gynecologist is stressed.
- She does not need to worry unnecessarily regarding the outcome but at the same time both the doctor and patient have to be prepared to handle the worst if it ever comes.
- Puerperal sepsis (Flowchart 22.3).

FIBROIDS WITH MENORRHAGIA

- Any woman who comes to a doctor with heavy menstrual loss and or severe dysmenorrhea, first and foremost thing is her thorough clinical evaluation and complete investigations in terms of her hemoglobin status, exact number and location of the fibroids, and any comorbidity like endocrinopathy, endometriosis, pelvic inflammatory disease, etc. which may exaggerate her symptoms and sufferings.
- Next concern is her age and desire to preserve her uterus, whether her family is completed or not. Once she is reassured about her situation and she starts understanding about her disease she has to be stressed upon treating or controlling the bleeding so her health is not compromised further.
- Tranexamic acid and mefenamic acid are two good molecules which can be used to control the menstrual bleeding and pain. Many women think that taking these medicines may hamper their future fertility and may cause some side-effects so counseling about its emergency use and reassurance that it would not cause any harm is very important.
- Once the investigations are completed, if patient has endometrial hyperplasia, she can be counseled about taking oral progesterones or levonorgestrel intrauterine system (LNG-IUS) as per her preference. The importance of endometrial biopsy and histopathology has to be emphasized.

- Submucous myomas distorting the endometrial cavity have to be removed preferably by hysteroscopy to control the bleeding.
- In perimenopausal group, if follow-up is not possible then an option of hysterectomy may be given.
- Any woman having comorbidities like endometriosis should be advised to undergo laparo-hysteroscopic examination with counseling for surgical intervention at the same sitting if needed.
- Although myoma volume may be reduced approximately 50% by medical treatments, the uterus typically returns to pretreatment size after the medications are discontinued.

FIBROIDS IN PERIMENOPAUSAL GROUP (FLOWCHART 22.4)

- She usually presents with abnormal uterine bleeding (AUB).
- Even if it is a small asymptomatic myoma, her worry is about its future course if she does not take prompt action.
- She has to be reassured regarding rarity of malignant transformation and stress upon regular follow-up has to be done.
- A slowly growing intramural or subserous myoma with mild or no symptoms can be left for follow-up after thorough evaluation by transvaginal sonography and histopathological examination of endometrial tissues.

Malignant Transformation

- It is less than 1%. The incidence of leiomyosarcoma in hysterectomy specimens obtained from women receiving surgical treatment for uterine myomas increases with age, from as low as 0.1% among women of childbearing age to a high of 1.7% among women who receive surgical treatment for uterine myomas after age of 60, and is not related to uterine size or to the rate of uterine growth. These observations suggest that more women may die as a result of complications of hysterectomy performed for asymptomatic myomas during the reproductive years (1 to 1.6 per 1,000) than would be saved from death by excision of a leiomyosarcoma.
- Malignant transformation is a rarest of rare event for adolescents.

Flowchart 22.4: Fibroid in perimenopausal age.

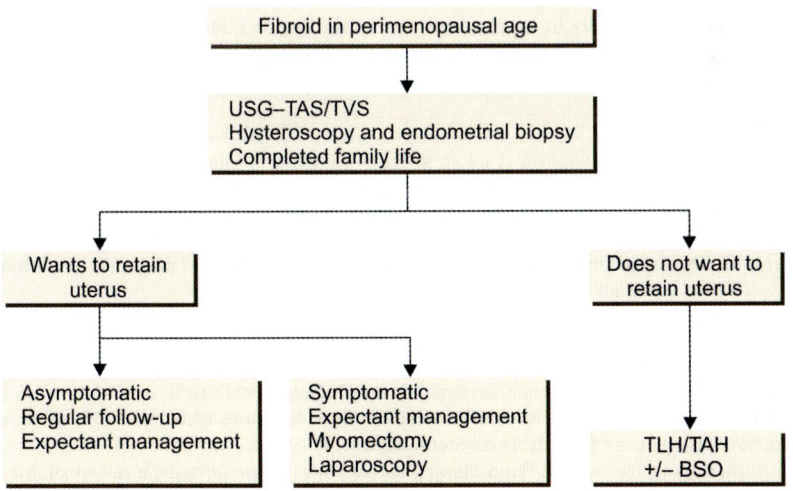

(USG: Ultrasonography; TVS: Transvaginal sonography; TAS: Transabdominal sonography; TLH: Total laparoscopic hysterectomy; TAH: Total abdominal hysterectomy; BSO: Bilateral salpingo-oophorectomy)

- Leiomyosarcomas occasionally arise from pre-existing myomas but usually occur de novo.
- Degeneration of fibroids: Most common is hyaline degeneration (present in more than two-thirds of cases). Calcification is common in older age. Red degeneration usually occurs in pregnancy.

Recurrence or Newer Myoma after Surgery

- Ideally the myomas never reoccur only the newer ones are formed if they are not removed during the previous surgery or they had regressed due to the medical management given prior to surgery.
- The chance of a newer myoma developing is only 5–10% if there were one or two myomas which were removed in the next 10 years, and in case of multiple myomas removal the chance increases to 26%.
- The child birth after the myomectomy decreases the chance of another myoma drastically.

TREATMENT PLAN

The treatment plan for the management depends on multiple factors which are following:
- The age of the patient
- Desire to preserve fertility
- Ovarian reserve
- Fibroid's position, for example, myoma indenting the endometrial cavity will have to be removed
- Tubal patency and location of fibroids in relation to tubes
- Type of fibroids—subserous, submucous, and intramural
- Future plan in terms of conception and immediate goals.

CONCLUSION

Though fibroids are most common benign tumor of reproductive age group, its course is not unpredictable and majority shrink over the course of time, especially menopause. Only important thing is proper counseling of the woman and taking her into confidence about its progression so that she does not undergo unnecessary hysterectomy or lose her sleep over it. At the same time, she also has to understand the importance of surgical interventions, if and when needed, especially in cases of submucosal fibroids distorting the uterine cavity and posing a threat over her reproductive potential and physical well-being.

BIBLIOGRAPHY

1. Ghant M, Sengoba K, Mendoza G, et al. Seeking the truth: a qualitative assessment of women's experiences seeking and obtaining knowledge of uterine fibroids. Fertil Steril. 2015;104(3):e155.
2. Lee HJ, Norwitz ER, Shaw J. Contemporary management of fibroids in pregnancy. Rev Obstet Gynecol. 2010;3(1):20-7.
3. Martin-Merino E, Wallander MA, Andersson S, et al. The reporting and diagnosis of uterine fibroids in the UK: An observational study. Gynecol Surg. 2015;12(3):165-77.
4. Practice Committee of ASRM in Collaboration with the Society of Reproductive Surgeons. Myoma and reproduction. Fertil Steril. 2008;90(5):S125-30.
5. Pritts EA, Vanness DJ, Berek JS, et al. The prevalence of occult leiomyosarcoma at surgery for presumed uterine fibroids: a meta-analysis. Gynecol Surg. 2015;12:165.
6. Shavell VI, Thakur M, Sawant A, et al. Adverse obstetric outcomes associated with sonographically identified large uterine fibroids. Fertil Steril. 2012;97(1):107-10.
7. Simms-Stewart D, Fletcher H. Counselling patients with uterine fibroids: a review of the management and complications. Obstet Gynecol Int. 2012;2012:539365.

23
Holistic Approach to Fibroids
Gunjan Gupta

INTRODUCTION

Holistic health is actually an approach to life. Rather than focusing on illness or specific parts of the body, this ancient approach to health considers the whole person and how he or she interacts with his or her environment. It emphasizes the connection of mind, body, and spirit.

When I started working on this chapter, I thought there is no holistic approach to fibroids, but actually there is a scientific basis to treatment to fibroids holistically.

WAYS TO REDUCE FIBROIDS

What leads to fibroids?

Estrogen

Translated, this means that increases in estrogen production and decreases in estrogen elimination lead to fibroids.

Therefore, the scientific basis for an integrative treatment plan involves:
- Enhancing estrogen elimination
- Normalizing estrogen production
- Decreasing inflammation and dysglycemia
- Reducing as many life stressors as possible.

Conventional treatment may also involve inducing a medical menopause to reduce estrogen levels, which is not an effective long-term solution because the drug is approved only for 6 months of use fibroid may regain original size.

Enhancing Estrogen Elimination

Ensuring adequate estrogen elimination is fundamental to any integrative approach to managing them.

Estrogen is eliminated through phase I and II liver detoxification, a process by which estrogen is dissolved in bile and excreted into the gut to leave the body via stool. Thus, it should be clear that impaired detoxification (phase I or II) or impaired elimination from the gut should be identified and corrected as part of any strategy to improve estrogen elimination.

Phase-I detoxification:
Hydroxylation: Addition of a hydroxyl group to 1 of 3 carbons on the estrogen ring, at the 2, 4, or 16 position.

Through hydroxylation, estrogen is dissolved in bile and thereby excreted hydroxylation is dependent on:
- *Genetic*: Cytochrome P450 estrogen detoxification enzyme systems
- *Lifestyle factors*: Physical exercise improves hydroxylation
- *Nutrition*:
  - Flax seeds
  - Omega-3 essential fatty acid sources
  - Cruciferous vegetables containing indole-3-carbinol increase the hydroxylation.

Phase-II detoxification:

Glucuronidation: Conjugation of other compounds to enable the estrogen molecule to be excreted in bile.

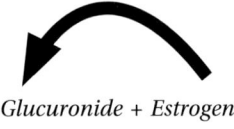

Glucuronide + Estrogen

Excretion through the bile into the gut
=
Estrogen glucuronide

Impaired glucuronidation occurs most commonly when unhealthy gut flora secretes an enzyme called beta-glucuronidase. This enzyme cleaves the glucuronide molecule from estrogen and allows the estrogen that was supposed to be eliminated in stool to be reabsorbed systemically via enterohepatic recirculation.

Key points to remember:
Glucuronidation can be improved through:
- Low animal fat diet
- Supplementation with probiotics and calcium-D-glucarate
- Eliminating constipation and ensuring regular bowel movements
- Detoxification by consumption of artichoke, broccoli, green tea, garlic, pomegranate, shallots, and watercress, as well as adequate protein intake.

Normalizing Estrogen Production

Estrogen production can be normalized by:
- Decreasing aromatase activity
- Decreasing adipose tissue
- Decreasing insulin levels
- Increasing sex hormone-binding globulin (SHBG) levels.

The basic principles for estrogen production are as follows:
- All estrogens made in the body is produced by the enzyme aromatase.
- Aromatase is present and active in adipose tissue; therefore, adipose tissue produces estrogen. Fibroids have high levels of aromatase activity, which is stimulated by prostaglandin E2 (PGE2).

- Certain pesticides (e.g. atrazine) stimulate aromatase.
- Insulin stimulates aromatase.
- Estrogen is transported throughout the body in an inactive form and bound to SHBG.
- In order for estrogen to bind to its receptor and have an estrogenic effect, it must be free (unbound).
- Insulin decreases SHBG, leading to more unbound estrogen.

All fat cells (adipocytes) contain aromatase and produce estrogen; we will now discuss the additional qualities of adipocytes that support the growth of fibroids. If the adipocyte is too full of fat, it will produce less of the hormone adiponectin. This leads to decreased insulin sensitivity and higher circulating insulin levels because adiponectin causes insulin sensitivity. As stated previously, insulin decreases SHBG and, therefore, increases free estrogen. Thus, a body filled with full adipocytes leads to even higher free estrogen levels. Second, in addition to secreting adiponectin, adipocytes secrete proinflammatory cytokines (such as PGE2 and others), making obesity a proinflammatory state. Inflammation is important to our discussion of fibroids because PGE2 stimulates aromatase and causing increased production of estrogen. Interestingly, estrogen itself stimulates the proinflammatory enzyme cyclooxygenase (COX-1 and COX-2), causing the production of PGE2, which in turn stimulates aromatase to make more estrogen in a kind of "feed forward" cycle. Third, it is important to note that not all adipocytes are equally metabolically active. The adipocytes surrounding the internal organs of the abdomen and pelvis (visceral adipocyte) are the most metabolically active. Therefore, a trip to the plastic surgeon for liposuction will do nothing to improve the proinflammatory, estrogenic effects of the "apple" phenotype because liposuction does not remove the visceral adipose tissue. The only solution is weight loss and exercise (Flowchart 23.1) [This is not such a concern for the "pear" phenotype that has weight (fat) around the hips, which is not a metabolically active fat].

Key points to remember:
- Visceral fat increases estrogen (increases aromatase).
- Estrogen causes inflammation (stimulates COX-1 and COX-2).
- Inflammation increases estrogen (stimulates aromatase).
- Visceral fat also increases inflammation (produces proinflammatory cytokines).
- Insulin increases total and free estrogen (lowers SHBG).

Decreasing Inflammation and Dysglycemia

Suggestive ways to decrease inflammation and dysglycemia are:
- Maintaining a healthy weight (through proper eating and exercise and, if necessary, weight loss).
- Decrease inflammation [through eating a pescatarian diet and supplementing with omega-3 essential fatty acids (EFAs), bromelain, curcumin, and quercetin].

Normalizing insulin and glucose dynamics:
Insulin and glucose dynamics can be normalized by:
- Low-glycemic index diet
- Micronutrients such as alpha-lipoic acid, cinnamon, chromium, and vanadium.

Increasing SHBG:
Sex hormone-binding globulin can be increased by:
- Lowering insulin levels
- Supplementing with flax or other EFA.

182 Fibroids

Flowchart 23.1: How obesity impacts estrogen production leading to fibroids?

```
                    Obesity–visceral fat (VAT) is most metabolically active
                                            │
                                            ▼
                              Increased fat in adipocytes
                       ┌────────────────────┴────────────────────┐
                       ▼                                         ▼
              Decreased adiponectin              Increase proinflammatory  ◄──┐
                       │                              cytokines (PGE2)        │
            ┌──────────┴──────────┐                        │                  │
            ▼                     ▼                        ▼                  │
     Decreased insulin     Higher circulating       Increased aromatase    Feed
        sensitivity          insulin levels                │               forward
            └─────────┬───────────┘                        │                cycle
                      ▼                                    │                  │
              Decreased SHBG                               │                  │
                      └─────────────────┬─────────────────┘                   │
                                        ▼                                     │
                              Increased estrogen                              │
                                        │                                     │
                                        ▼                                     │
                     Increased proinflammatory cyclooxygenase ────────────────┘
                              (COX-1 and COX-2)
```

(SHBG: Sex hormone-binding capacity)

Reducing as Many Life Stressors as Possible

While it is extremely critical to address the above three factors for reduction of fibroids, it is equally important to manage the other external life stress factors that include:
- *Environmental and nutritional sources of estrogens to be avoided*:
  - Avoid pesticides and plastics and estrogens are routinely added during the farming of poultry.
  - *Go organic*: Use organic spring or filtered water; organic beef, chicken, and fat-free dairy products.
  - Add cold-water fish to the diet for the EFAs.
- *Impact of stress and emotional and spiritual health*:
  - Stress is known to cause an increase in proinflammatory cytokines.
  - I have witnessed in my own clinical practice the direct impact that emotional and spiritual issues—such as childbearing conflicts, lack of creative self-expression, sexual issues, unresolved anger, and severe self-criticism—have on these illnesses in my patients.
- *Herbs for fibroids*: How do herbs help?
  - Astringent helps to control menstrual-related bleeding
  - Diuretic properties or a suitable detoxing agent
  - Balancing hormonal levels
  - Anti-inflammatory properties.

Which herbs help in reduction of fibroids?
- *Dandelion*: Detoxes the liver, kidneys, and blood due to its diuretic properties and pulls estrogen out of the system. It is widely used in teas and the leaves added to food as a flavor enhancer and even taken in pill form.

- *Vitex/chasteberry*: Herbal remedy for uterine fibroids that relieves feminine problems including uterine growths, premenstrual syndrome (PMS), and other hormone-related issues. Taking approximately 25 drops of this as a tincture at least three times per day will help to control the production of fibroid-producing estrogen. The properties in Vitex work to slow the growth of the fibroids while helping to bring hormonal levels under control.
- *Ginger*: Soak a towel in hot ginger water and place this hot compress on the belly at least twice per day to help to shrink uterine fibroids. It is effective at minimizing pain as well. Get the benefits of the anti-inflammatory properties of ginger by drinking ginger root tea a few times per day.
- *Bladderwrack*: This seaweed contains iodine, which is useful for thyroid problems and, therefore, helpful in balancing hormones. Making a tea from this herb and drinking it at least three times per day is the recommended dosage for shrinking fibroids. Add one or two teaspoons of the seaweed to a cup of hot water to create the infusion. Some people also take bladderwrack in tablet form three times daily.
- *False unicorn root*: This multipurpose root not only helps to shrink fibroids, it is great in treating other feminine problems such as ovarian cysts and even infertility.
  - *Acupuncture*: Usually a last resort as far as natural remedies for uterine fibroids are concerned.
  - Sitz bath—for symptomatic relief of fibroids.
  - *Aromatherapy*: The essential oils of ginger, rose, and marjoram are greatly beneficial.

CONCLUSION

It has been discussed how fibroids can all be addressed by a holistic treatment plan that focuses on normalizing estrogen production and then optimally metabolizing it. There are ways to reduce inflammation, optimize blood sugar metabolism, and body composition.

In addition, there is importance of reducing stress, resolving conflicts, and addressing spiritual issues through meditation and yoga.

But amidst all of the above, the most critical aspect of holistic approach lies within the control of practitioner.

Doctors should be able to spend time in their rush hours for counseling the patients.

The magical balance and key differentiator to holistic treatment would hence depend on how the causality between physical problems and emotional issues will unfold, so that the healing can truly begin and is sustainable in long-term. At the same time, the importance and place of allopathic treatment cannot be neglected. A judicious approach with both allopathic and holistic will be boon for the patients.

BIBLIOGRAPHY

1. Bland J, Jones D. Chapter 32: Hormonal and neuroendocrine imbalances. In: Quinn S, Jones D (Eds). Textbook of Functional Medicine. Gig Harbor, WA: Institute for Functional Medicine; 2005. p. 581.
2. Bradlow HL, Davis DL, Lin G, et al. Effects of pesticides on the ratio of 16 alpha/2-hydroxyestrone: a biologic marker of breast cancer risk. Environ Health Perspect. 1995;103(Suppl 7):147-50.
3. Cordain L, Eaton SB, Sebastian A, et al. Origins and evolution of the Western diet: health implications for the 21st century. Am J Clin Nutr. 2005;81(2):341-54.
4. Cordain L, Watkins BA, Florant GL, et al. Fatty acid analysis of wild ruminant tissues: Evolutionary implications for reducing diet-related chronic disease. Eur J Clin Nutr. 2002;56(3):181-91.
5. Gaspani L, Limiroli E, Ferrario P, et al. In vivo and in vitro effects of bromelain on PGE(2) and SP concentrations in the inflammatory exudate in rats. Pharmacology. 2002;65(2):83-6.
6. Kabat GC, O'Leary ES, Gammon MD, et al. Estrogen metabolism and breast cancer. Epidemiology. 2006;17(1):80-8.

7. Libby P. Chapter 18: Biology of inflammation. In: Quinn S, Jones D (Eds). Textbook of Functional Medicine. Gig Harbor, WA: Institute for Functional Medicine; 2005. p. 203.
8. Libby P. Chapter 27: Clinical approaches to immune imbalance and inflammation. In: Quinn S, Jones D (Eds). Textbook of Functional Medicine. Gig Harbor, WA: Institute for Functional Medicine; 2005. p. 405.
9. Michnovicz JJ, Adlercreutz H, Bradlow HL. Changes in levels of urinary estrogen metabolites after oral indole-3-carbinol treatment in humans. J Natl Cancer Inst. 1997;89(10):718-20.
10. Quinn S, Jones D. Textbook of Functional Medicine. Gig Harbor, WA: Institute for Functional Medicine; 2005.
11. Trepel F. Dietary fibre: more than a matter of dietetics. II. Preventative and therapeutic uses [article in German].Wien Klin Wochenschr. 2004;116(15-16):511-22.
12. Walaszek Z, Szemraj J, Narog M, et al. Metabolism, uptake, and excretion of a D-glucaric acid salt and its potential use in cancer prevention. Cancer Detect Prev. 1997;21(2):178-90.
13. Yun AJ, Lee PY, Doux JD. Are we eating more than we think? Illegitimate signaling and xenohormesis as participants in the pathogenesis of obesity. Med Hypotheses. 2006;67(1):36-40.
14. Zavadova E, Desser L, Mohr T. Stimulation of reactive oxygen species production and cytotoxicity in human neutrophils in vitro and after oral administration of a polyenzyme preparation. Cancer Biother. 1995;10(2):147-52.

24
Uterine Fibroid in a Nutshell

Ruchika Garg

INTRODUCTION

Uterine fibroid (UF) (leiomyoma or myoma) is a slowly growing benign smooth muscle tumor. These are the most frequently seen tumors of the female reproductive system. Approximately, 25% of women after the age of 35 years harbor UF. Since histologic confirmation of the clinical diagnosis is not necessary in most cases, and there is both growth and regression of fibroids, asymptomatic UFs can usually be followed without any intervention.

Prophylactic therapy to avoid potential future complications from myomas or their treatment is not recommended. Possible exceptions include women with significant submucosal leiomyomas who are contemplating pregnancy and women with ureteral compression leading to moderate or severe hydronephrosis. In these women, prophylactic treatment may prevent miscarriage or urinary tract obstruction.

For those with symptomatic UF, several treatment options are available. The type of treatment depends on the age, desire for future fertility, previous obstetrical performance, and location and the size of the myoma.

DIAGNOSTIC MODALITIES FOR UTERINE FIBROIDS

Fibroids may be detected for the first time during a routine *bimanual pelvic examination*.

For symptomatic women, consideration of medical therapy, noninvasive procedures, or surgery often depends on an accurate assessment of the *size, number, and position of the fibroids*.

Following investigation techniques may be used for the above purpose:
- Ultrasonography:
    - Most readily available
    - Least costly technique to differentiate fibroid from any other pelvic pathology
    - Reasonably reliable for evaluation of uterine volume less than 375 cc and containing four or fewer fibroids.
    - Appearance of fibroid on sonography:
        - Symmetrical
        - Well defined
        - Hypoechoic
        - Heterogeneous masses.
- *Hysteroscopy*—used for the diagnosis of submucosal fibroids.
- *Hysterosalpingography*
- *Sonohysterography*
- *Laparoscopy*

- *Magnetic resonance imaging (MRI)*:
  - MRI is the best investigation modality for the diagnosis of submucosal fibroids.
  - It allows evaluation of the number, size, and position of the submucous, intramural, and subserosal fibroid and evaluates their proximity to the bladder, rectum, and endometrial cavity.
  - MRI helps to define what can be expected at the time of surgery and might help the surgeon to avoid missing fibroids during the surgery.
  - For women who wish to preserve fertility, MRI to document location and position relative to the endomyometrium may be helpful prior to hysterscopic, laparoscopic, or abdominal myomectomy.

MANAGEMENT OF UTERINE FIBROIDS

Medical Therapy

Medical therapy provides symptomatic relief, however, it may not prevent the growth of the fibroids and recurrence of symptoms may occur as soon as the medical therapy is discontinued.

Medical therapy prevents complications associated with surgery and permits uterine preservation.

Aims of Medical Therapy

- To provide symptomatic relief to the patient.
- To reduce the size of the fibroid.
- To improve the hematological status of the patient.

Following are the various options available for the medical management of the patient with UF.

Nonhormonal Treatment

Nonsteroidal anti-inflammatory drugs (NSAIDs) and antifibrinolytics are the nonhormonal alternatives used for treatment of UFs. *NSAIDs* are commonly prescribed for the management of AUB, especially in cases with no identified organic pathology.

Tranexamic acid is also commonly prescribed to the patients with fibroids presenting with menorrhagia. It may provide symptomatic relief but has no role in altering the size of the fibroids.

Although there is a lack of high-quality evidence, nonhormonal treatments are commonly used for symptomatic control during an acute UF-related uterine bleeding episode.

Hormonal Treatment

Oral contraceptives: Combined oral contraceptive pills and progesterone-only pills are effective for relief from heavy bleeding and painful menses. Furthermore, estrogen and progesterone may promote the growth of uterine myoma.

Long-acting progesterone: Administration of medroxyprogesterone acetate (Depo-Provera, 150 mg/month) for 6 months decreased uterine bleeding in 30–70% of patients.
- The volume of the fibroid also reduced.
- However, the effect is temporary and it is not as effective as gonadotropin-releasing hormone agonists (GnRHa).

Levonorgestrel-releasing intrauterine contraceptive device (IUD): The addition of L-norgestrel to the IUD is associated with a reduction in the amount and duration of menstrual blood loss.

It is a reasonable treatment for selected women with fibroid-associated menorrhagia.

However, those with intrauterine lesion such as submucous fibroid or with uterine size of more than 12 weeks' gestational size are not good candidates.

Furthermore, the IUD expulsion rate in these patients is high (12%).

Antiprogestin (mifepristone, RU 486): Mifepristone (RU 486) is a derivative of norethindrone that has both antiprogesterone and antiglucocorticoid activities. In the endometrium, it exerts an antiestrogenic effect.

Morales et al. reported that *mifepristone (25 mg daily for 3 months)* resulted in 50% decrease in the size of uterine myoma. Compared to GnRH agonists, its use is associated with less hypoestrogenic side effects.

Selective progesterone receptor modulator (SPRM): SPRM is a new class of progesterone receptor modulators available with brand name of *Ulipristal* and *Asoprisnil*.

They exert tissue-selective progesterone agonist, antagonist, or mixed agonist/antagonist effects on various tissues including the endometrium.

Ulipristal acetate is given in *daily doses of 5 mg or 10 mg for a period of 12 weeks*.

It effectively controls bleeding and pain, reduces fibroid volume, and restores quality of life in patients with symptomatic fibroids.

Selective estrogen receptor modulator (SERM): *Raloxifene* and *Ormeloxifene* are one of the SERMs that have been evaluated in women with UFs.

In postmenopausal women, it reduces the volume of the fibroid. *Ormeloxifene is given as 60 mg orally twice a week for first 12 weeks, followed by once a week for another 12 weeks.*

However, due to the spontaneous shrinkage in myoma after menopause, it might not be relevant clinically.

Aromatase inhibitors: Aromatase inhibitors inhibit the conversion of androgen to estrogen. In theory, the reduction in estrogen level might be beneficial for UF.

Bulun et al. administered aromatase inhibitor, *fadrozole* to a woman with urinary retention secondary to a large fibroid. The fibroid volume decreased 71% in 8 weeks.

Gestrinone: Gestrinone is a derivative of ethynyl nortestosterone with antiestrogen and antiprogesterone properties.

A few studies have shown that gestrinone treatment leads to a reduction in UF of up to 40%.

Unfortunately, it is associated with significant androgenic side effects.

Androgenic steroids (danazol): Danazol has multiple effects at different levels of the hypothalamic-pituitary-ovarian axis by binding to intracellular steroid receptors for androgens, progesterone, and glucocorticoids.

It reduces the volume of fibroids (average 23.6%) and improves uterine bleeding.

However, its use is limited by the side effects of acne, hirsutism, and weight gain.

GnRH agonist: GnRH agonist is the most effective and widely used medical treatment of uterine myomas.

It causes a hypoestrogenic state leading to 35% shrinkage of the myoma and 61% decrease in uterine volume.

Obese women show less diminution in uterine volume, probably because of the availability of extragonadal estradiol.

As other medical treatments in reproductive aged women, the uterine size gradually returns to its pretreatment size following discontinuation of GnRH agonist.

Its use in perimenopausal women is more advantageous.

It is hoped that during or immediately after GnRH agonist treatment, natural menopause ensues, thus reducing the probability of myoma regrowth.

For preoperative treatment before laparoscopic myomectomy or hysterectomy, most surgeons will use a *3-month course of GnRH agonist.*

Reduction in the size of myoma and decrease in its vascularity facilitate the procedure.

Prior to hysteroscopic procedure, a single dose of GnRH agonist is usually given *4 weeks* before the procedure.

Side effects of GnRH agonist are:
- Hot flashes
- Vaginal dryness
- Headaches
- Depression
- Hair loss
- Musculoskeletal stiffness and discomfort
- A slight decrease in bone mineral density can occur after long-term treatment of more than 6 months.

Gonadotropin-releasing hormone antagonist (GnRH-ag): GnRH antagonist acts by competitive binding of the GnRH receptors. Unlike GnRH agonist, its treatment is not associated with an initial *"flare-up" phenomenon.*

This leads to a *faster effect* than that with GnRH agonist.

In spite of this advantage, GnRH antagonist is not widely used for UF due to the requirement of daily treatment.

If longer-acting GnRH antagonist becomes available, preoperative treatment with GnRH antagonist would be preferable.

Radiological Therapy

Uterine fibroid embolization (UFE): UFE has become one of the main treatments of UF.

Uterine artery embolization (UAE) is contraindicated in patients who want future fertility.

Candidates for treatment with UAE include those who have symptoms bothersome enough to warrant hysterectomy or myomectomy.

Contraindications to treatment of fibroids with UAE include:
- Women with active genital infection
- Genital tract malignancy
- Diminished immune status
- Severe vascular disease limiting access to uterine arteries
- Contrast allergy
- Impaired renal function.

Magnetic resonance imaging (MRI)-guided focused ultrasound: Latest technique to treat UF is the use of a high-intensity focused ultrasound (HIFU).

The basic principle behind this technique is that ultrasound energy can be focused to create sufficient heat at a focal point, so that the protein is denatured and cell death occurs.

This technique is contraindicated in women wishing future fertility.

However, volume reduction with this treatment is small and recurrence rate is high.

In addition, the treatment is associated with side effects including full thickness burns of the abdominal wall.

MRI-directed cryotherapy: Another MR-controlled treatment of fibroid is MRI-directed cryotherapy. Initial report revealed a 65% volume reduction.

Surgical Therapy

Indications for surgical management of fibroid include:
- Persistent abnormal uterine bleeding
- Pelvic pain
- Pressure symptoms
- Rapidly enlarging fibroid
- Recurrent pregnancy loss.

Myomectomy

The standard surgical treatment for women who have large UFs and wish to retain their fertility is myomectomy.

Submucous myomectomy is performed by hysteroscopy, whereas intramural or subserous myoma by laparoscopy or laparotomy.

Laparoscopic myomectomy is associated with lower operating times but reduced operative blood loss, less postoperative decline in hemoglobin levels and reduced postoperative pain.

Laparoscopic Myolysis

Myoma coagulation or myolysis has been advocated.

However, this treatment is associated with adhesion formation and possible uterine rupture in pregnancy.

Most gynecologists have abandoned myolysis.

Myolysis is *not recommended for the women who wish future fertility*.

Laparoscopic Uterine Artery Occlusion

Realizing the efficacy of UFE, gynecologists have started to occlude the *uterine arteries as well as it leads to* decreased uterine bleeding and less pressure symptoms.

The main disadvantages of laparoscopic uterine artery occlusion are that:
- It requires general anesthesia
- It is invasive
- It requires a skilled laparoscopic surgeon.

Hysterectomy

Hysterectomy is a definitive treatment of UF and advanced laparoscopic surgeons perform hysterectomy by laparoscopy. Many studies have shown the safety and efficacy of laparoscopic hysterectomy. It could be performed in an outpatient setting with reduced hospital costs. However, laparoscopic hysterectomy requires special skills and training.

CONCLUSION

Myomas are most frequently found tumors of female genital tract. Diagnosis is clinical and ultrasound is helpful in confirmation, specially trans vaginal. Treatment is not surgical in all cases. Medical management is helpful in most cases specially in controlling symptoms. Drugs can only reduce the size of fibroid on temporary basis. In refractory cases and in cases of large fibroids surgery is required. Surgery can be myomectomy or hysterectomy according to the need of patient.

BIBLIOGRAPHY

1. Baakdah H, Tulandi T. Uterine fibroid embolization. Clin Obstet Gynecol. 2005;48:361-8.
2. Bernard G, Darai E, Poncelet C, et al. Fertility after hysteroscopic myomectomy. Eur J Obstet Gynecol Reprod Biol. 2000;88:85-90.
3. Brown WW III, Coddington CC III. Expectant and medical management of uterine fibroids. In: Tulandi T (Ed). Uterine Fibroids: Embolization and Other Treatments. London: Cambridge University Press; 2003.
4. Bulun SE, Imir G, Utsunomiya H, et al. Aromatase in endometriosis and uterine leiomyomata. J Steroid Biochem Mol Biol. 2005;95:57-62.
5. Chan AH, Fujimoto VY, Moore DE, et al. An image-guided high intensity focused ultrasound device for uterine fibroids treatment. Med Physics. 2002;29:2611-20.
6. Chrisman HB, Saker MB, Ryu RK, et al. The impact of uterine fibroid embolization on resumption of menses and ovarian function. J Vasc Intervent Radiol. 2000;11:699-703.
7. Chwalisz K. Therapeutic potential for the selective progesterone receptor modulator asoprisnil in the treatment of leiomyomata. Sem Reprod Med. 2004;22:113-9.
8. Cowan BD. Myomectomy and MRI-directed cryotherapy. Sem Reprod Med. 2004;22:143-8.
9. Dubuisson JB, Fauconnier A, Chapron C, et al. Reproductive outcome after laparoscopic myomectomy in infertile women. J Reprod Med. 2000;45:23-30.
10. Eisinger SH. Twelve-month safety and efficacy of low-dose mifepristone for uterine myomas. J Min Inv Gynecol. 2005;12:227-33.
11. Flierman PA, Oberyé JJ, van der Hulst VP, et al. Rapid reduction of leiomyoma volume during treatment with the GnRH antagonist ganirelix. BJOG. 2005;112:638-42.
12. Goldfarb HA. Myoma coagulation (myolysis). Obstet Gynecol Clin North Am. 2000;30:421-7.
13. Gutmann JN, Corson SL. GnRH agonist therapy before myomectomy or hysterectomy. J Min Inv Gynecol. 2005;12:529-37.
14. Johnson N, Fletcher H, Reid M. Depot medroxyprogesterone acetate (DMPA) therapy for uterine myomata prior to surgery. Int J Gynaecol Obstet. 2004;85:174-6.
15. La Marca A, Giulini S, Vito G, et al. Gestrinone in the treatment of uterine leiomyomata: effects on uterine blood supply. Fertil Steril. 2004;82:1694-6.
16. Lichtinger M, Hallson L, Calvo P, et al. Laparoscopic uterine artery occlusion for symptomatic leiomyomas. J Am Assoc Gynecol Laparos. 2002;9:191.
17. Mercorio F, De Simone R, Di Spiezio Sardo A, et al. The effect of a levonorgestrel-releasing intrauterine device in the treatment of myoma-related menorrhagia. Contraception. 2003;67:277-80.
18. Morales AJ, Kettel LM, Murphy AA. Mifepristone: clinical application in general gynecology. Clin Obstet Gynecol. 1996;39:451-60.
19. Murphy A, Morales A, Kettel M, et al. Regression of uterine leiomyomata to anti-progesterone RU 486: does response effect. Fertil Steril. 1995;64:187.
20. Palomba S. Long-term effectiveness and safety of GnRH agonist plus raloxifene administration in women with uterine leiomyomas. Hum Reprod. 2004;6:1308-14.
21. Pron G, Bennett J, Common A, et al. Technical results and effects of operator experience on uterine artery embolization for fibroids: The Ontario Uterine Fibroid Embolization Trial. J Vasc Intervent Radiol. 2003;14:545-54.
22. Pron G, Bennett J, Common A, et al. The Ontario Uterine Fibroid Embolization Trial. Part 2. Uterine fibroid reduction and symptom relief after uterine artery embolization for fibroids. Fertil Steril. 2003;79:120-7.
23. Pron G, Cohen M, Soucie J, et al. The Ontario Uterine Fibroid Embolization Trial. Part 1. Baseline patient characteristics, fibroid burden, and impact on life. Fertil Steril. 2003;79:112-9.
24. Sarmini OR, Lefholz K, Froeschke HP. A comparison of laparoscopic supracervical hysterectomy and total abdominal hysterectomy outcomes. J Min Inv Gynecol. 2005;12:121-4.
25. Seidman DS, Nezhat CH, Nezhat F, et al. Laparoscopic management of uterine myoma. In: Tulandi T (Ed). Uterine Fibroids: Embolization and Other Treatments. London: Cambridge University Press; 2003.
26. Tulandi T. Uterine Fibroids: Embolization and Other Treatments. London: Cambridge University Press; 2003.
27. Venkatachalam S, Bagratee JS, Moodley J. Medical management of uterine fibroids with medroxyprogesterone acetate (Depo Provera): a pilot study. J Obstet Gynaecol. 2004;24:798-800.
28. Walker CL. Role of hormonal and reproductive factors in the etiology and treatment of uterine leiomyoma. Recent Prog Hormone Res. 2002;57:277-94.

25

Case Scenarios

Diksha Goswami Sharma, Anita Kant

INTRODUCTION

Fibroids are the most common benign tumors in women, faced throughout the lifespan. These can have varied presentations, which pose a diagnostic and clinical dilemma for the treating doctor. Here, we discuss different clinical scenarios and their ideal management strategies.

CASE 1: INTRAMURAL FIBROID WITH SUBFERTILITY

History

Mrs PG 35-year-old and her husband 38 years presented with inability to conceive for last 7 years. She had no significant medical or surgical history. They had normal coital frequency and had been undergoing treatment for last 3 years.

The couple had been taking treatment for subfertility for last 3 years and had undergone two cycles of intrauterine insemination (IUI) and one cycle of in vitro fertilization (IVF). IVF cycle was done 3 months back in which three good quality embryos were transferred with negative result.

Menstrual History

She had regular 28-day cycles with heavy flow and occasional history of mid-cycle spotting, no dysmenorrhea.

Investigations

- *Anti-Mullerian hormone (AMH)*: 2 ng/mL
- *Semen analysis*: 45 million/65% motility/20%
- *Transvaginal ultrasonography*: Uterus found to be enlarged 94 mm × 71 mm × 85 mm with two intramural fibroids, 56 mm × 65 mm anterior wall abutting the cavity and 44 mm × 35 mm posterior wall 8 mm from cavity.
- *Sonohysterogram done*: Sizes of fibroids were confirmed; anterior fibroid was close to cavity and pushing endometrium anteriorly and posterior fibroid was away from cavity. Cavity did not distend well.

Diagnosis

Thirty-six years, primary infertility, previous failed two cycles IUI and one cycle IVF, with two intramural big fibroids.

Management

In view of intramural fibroid more than 5 cm in size, which was very close to uterine cavity and past history of implantation failure, decision for myomectomy was made after discussing pros and cons with the couple. The lady was posted for laparoscopic myomectomy. Hysteroscopy was performed first; there was no intracavity component of the fibroid. A horizontal incision was made on the anterior wall fibroid after instillation of dilute vasopressin, which was then enucleated. Similarly, posterior wall fibroid was enucleated through a separate incision. Uterine bed was sutured well in layers (Fig. 25.1) ensuring hemostasis and fibroid was removed by in bag morcellation. Cavity was not entered during the procedure.

Postoperative period was uneventful. Repeat transvaginal sonohysterogram (TVS) was done 3 months later and showed normal cavity. The couple underwent second IVF cycle subsequently; antagonist protocol and conceived. The pregnancy was uneventful and planned lower segment cesarean section (LSCS) done at 38 weeks, delivering a 2.7 kg female baby.

Discussion

While evidence shows that submucosal and intramural fibroids that protrude into the endometrial cavity have been associated with decreased pregnancy and implantation rates (IRs) after IVF, the effect of fibroids not distorting the uterine cavity remains poorly understood with studies yielding conflicting results. Recent systematic review by Sunkara et al. 2010 demonstrated that noncavity distorting intramural fibroids reduce the live birth rate by 21% and the clinical pregnancy rate (PR) by 15% per IVF cycle. This may be explained by altered uterine vascular perfusion, myometrial contractility, endometrial function, gamete migration, or myometrial/endometrial gene expression. Also, it is not clear whether myomectomy

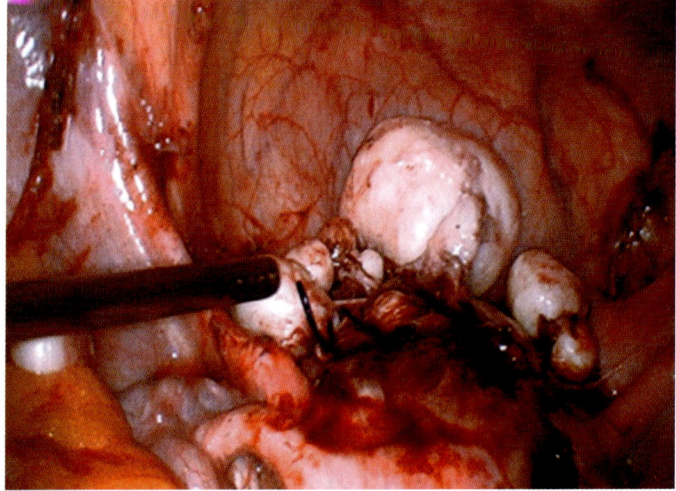

Fig. 25.1: After myomectomy suture line on posterior uterine surface.

improves IVF outcome in such patients. Cochrane review concludes that there is insufficient evidence regarding effect of myomectomy on reproductive outcomes.

Benecke et al. have suggested that surgical approach in patients with a history of previous failed attempts in case of intramural myomata more than 2 cm in diameter is warranted, if all other factors have been evaluated.

Thus, it is challenging to manage such women; however, decision was also based on the fibroid size and location. Studies have demonstrated negative impact on implantation by fibroids more than 4 cm and less than 4 mm from cavity.

During myomectomy, precautions to minimize blood loss should be adopted. Also, there is consensus regarding cautious use of morcellation in order to prevent seeding of specimen within the cavity or port site and it is advisable to use intraperitoneal isolation bags.

In case, endometrial cavity has been breeched pregnancy should be planned after 6 months and, if not, treatment can begin after 3 months of surgery allowing for adequate healing.

CASE 2: BROAD LIGAMENT FIBROID

History

Mrs HK 31-year-old nullipara married for 2 years presented with heaviness and pain in lower abdomen.
- *Menstrual cycles*: Regular, last for 3–4 days with average flow
- General examination normal
- On per abdomen examination—no mass or lump palpable
- On pelvic examination, adnexal mass of about 14 weeks size, restricted mobility, and firm in consistency.

Investigations

- On ultrasound, a well-defined and mixed echogenic lesion measuring 13 cm × 8 cm × 8 cm was seen posterior to bladder pushing the uterus anterolaterally toward the left side. There was mild hydroureteronephrosis in the right kidney likely due to ureteric obstruction by the right adnexal mass.

The right ovary was not seen separate from the mass. Left ovary was normal. On magnetic resonance imaging (MRI) of abdomen and pelvis, a large mixed density abdominopelvic lesion was seen with thick internal septations and solid components.
- *Cancer antigen (CA) 125*: 25 (normal range).

Management

With a provisional diagnosis of adnexal mass, the patient was taken up for an exploratory laparotomy. Preoperatively, an urologist opinion was taken and ureteric stent was inserted.

Pfannenstiel incision was given. Intraoperatively, pelvic mass arising from broad ligament of size approximately 14 cm was seen, arising from the right side of the uterus pushing the uterus laterally, right ovary, and right Fallopian tube stretched and adherent over the mass. As the tumor was distorting the pelvic anatomy, careful dissection was done to prevent ureteric injuries. Then the broad ligament was opened showing a large broad ligament fibroid (14 cm in diameter) attached to the lower uterine segment and with a thin stalk measuring about 4 cm. Keeping the age of the patient and to conserve reproductive function, decision for myomectomy was taken, fibroid was dissected and removed, and complete hemostasis in the pedicle was achieved using the bipolar cautery. The anterior leaf of the broad ligament was sutured. Postoperative period was uneventful. Histopathology confirmed the diagnosis.

Discussion

The broad ligament is the most common extrauterine site for the occurrence of leiomyoma but with a very (<1%) low incidence rate. Because of its overall low incidence rate, it poses both clinical and radiological difficulty in differentiating with an ovarian tumor.

In the broad ligaments, the fibroid can be of two types—(1) true broad ligament fibroid, which can arise from smooth muscle of round ligament, tubo-ovarian ligament or smooth muscle of uterine artery or ovarian vessels; (2) false broad ligament fibroid, which arises from lateral wall of uterus or cervix.

Our case was a false broad ligament fibroid, which arose out from uterus and grew within the folds of broad ligament. These broad ligament fibroids can achieve enormous size and generally present with pressure symptom like bladder and bowel dysfunction.

Myomectomy in such cases poses intraoperative challenges such as excessive bleeding and ureteric injury or late complications such as pelvic hematoma and infection. During surgery, one should be careful about the ureteric course and surrounding organs, especially in this critical area where the myoma is in close proximity to the ureter and the uterine vessels.

Choice of route of surgery depends on myoma size and surgical expertise. Although minimally invasive surgery has known advantages over open surgery, including shorter hospital stay, quicker recovery, less blood loss, and fewer postoperative adhesions, most of the myomectomies are done abdominally due to the complexity and the necessity of extensive suturing for the desired multilayered uterine closure.

CASE 3: PERIMENOPAUSAL BIG FIBROID WITH ABNORMAL UTERINE BLEEDING

History

Mrs SS, 49-year-old P2L2 both normal deliveries presented with abdominal pain and heavy bleeding during periods for last 2 years. She had history of hypertension, on treatment.

Menstrual cycles: Patient had short cycles 20–22 days with prolonged bleeding for 7–8 days with clots.

Examination

- Patient was overweight with body mass index (BMI): 31
- Pallor present
- Abdomen examination revealed a nontender and solid mass of 20-week uterus size with restricted mobility. Lower border of the mass could not be felt.
- On pelvic examination, cervix was pulled up, mass of 18–20-week size with side-to-side mobility, uterus could not be felt separately, symptom is suggestive of uterine mass.

Investigations

- Hemoglobin: 7 g/dL
- *Coagulation profile*: Within normal limit
- *Transvaginal and transabdominal ultrasound*: A large well-defined hypoechoic intramural mass lesion seen in the anterior wall of uterus (10.5 cm × 9.3 cm × 8.1 cm) displacing endometrial cavity posteriorly. Two more lesions in posterior wall 55 mm × 46 mm and 66 mm × 45 mm with subserous component.

Diagnosis

A 49-year-old/P2L2 with multiple fibroid uterus, menorrhagia, and anemia.

Management

- After considering patients age, completion of the family, long duration of symptoms, and large size of fibroid, decision of hysterectomy was taken. Patient opted for laparoscopic route after discussing pros and cons.
- Endometrial aspiration was done preoperatively to rule out any malignant changes.
- In view of anemia, intravenous iron therapy was administered and patient was given injection leuprolide depot 3.75 mg, which was repeated 4 weeks later. Repeat hemoglobin increased to 10.5 gm%.
- After anesthetic clearance, patient was posted for total laparoscopic hysterectomy (TLH). TLH was done with abdominal morcellation.
- Postoperative stay uneventful and patient was discharged on 4th day.

Discussion

- Treatment of patients with fibroid uterus must always be individualized based on considerations such as the presence and severity of symptoms, size, and location of fibroids, patient's desire for definitive treatment and the desire to preserve reproductive function.
- In patients presenting with heavy menstrual bleeding, medical management or conservative surgical approaches can be tried initially depending on above factors and discussion with patient.
- However, hysterectomy is the most effective and definitive surgical option and was chosen by family after counseling.
- The surgical approach can be via laparoscopy or open surgery, which is usually preferred in the case of very large uteri depending on surgical skill.
- Nowadays, improvements in minimally invasive techniques have increased the number of patients who undergo laparoscopic hysterectomy.
- Complications such as hemorrhage, bladder, and ureteric injuries are directly or indirectly related to the method of securing the vascular pedicles and can occur in both abdominal and laparoscopic hysterectomies.
- Obesity is a relative contraindication to laparoscopy because it presents a major difficulty in establishing pneumoperitoneum and anesthesiological difficulties with the Trendelenburg position in these women.
- Main concerns during laparoscopic hysterectomy in large uterus are poor access and exposure and can be overcome by few modifications in hysterectomy technique like placement of the optical trocar supraumbilically and use of myoma screw for manipulation.
- Due to large size of the uterus, there is distortion of normal anatomy, especially the ureters and the uterine vessels and careful dissection of pedicles should be done to avoid ureteric injuries. Myomectomy may be done prior to the hysterectomy so as to create space for the procedure.

CASE 4: SOLITARY INTRAMURAL FIBROID

History

- Age—33 years, married for 6 years presented with menorrhagia and severe abdominal pain.
- Parity—one child, normal vaginal delivery, 4 years back, and not planning for conception.
- No history of medical illness, not on any medication.

Examination
- On pelvic examination, uterus was enlarged to about 8–10-week size of a pregnant uterus. No adnexal mass palpable.
- On ultrasound, an intramural fibroid about 8 cm in size was seen.

Management
- Considering age and parity of the patient pros and cons of available options; medical, surgical, and magnetic resonance-guided focused ultrasound (MRgFUS) treatment were discussed with the patient. Since there was a solitary intramural fibroid and no contraindications for MRgFUS, patient opted for MRgFUS.
- The patient was referred for MRI screening to evaluate her suitability for the MRgFUS treatment. MRI showed a single large intramural fibroid in the posterior myometrium measuring 7.0 cm × 5.6 cm × 7.2 cm (craniocaudal × AP × transverse) with a volume of 145 cc on T2-weighted image (T2WI). Intensity of the fibroid relative to the uterine wall was hyperintense on T2WIs.
- Patient was posted for MRgFUS, procedure was performed under sedation after filling bladder with saline, and patient was discharged next day.
- She returned to work 3 days later. Follow-up of the patient showed 60% relief of symptoms after 6 months; and on MRI, nonperfused volume was 30%.

Discussion
- Magnetic resonance-guided focused ultrasound surgery offers a noninvasive day care and approved method for treating uterine fibroids, especially for women who wish to retain their fertility. It works on the principle of using focused ultrasound waves to generate and maintain high temperatures within the targeted fibroid, resulting in protein denaturation and coagulative necrosis.
- While choosing suitable candidates, one needs to consider fibroid type and location, number, position relative to adjacent anatomical structures, and the presence of coexistent pelvic disease.
- Exclusion criteria are women with pacemakers, morbid obese women, contraindications to MRI, massive abdominal scarring, uterine size more than 24 weeks, pedunculated fibroids, nonenhancing fibroids, and heavily calcified fibroids.
- Reported side effects with this technique include skin burns, inflammation of the fat and underlying abdominal wall musculature;[16] and rarely, damage to adjacent organs, such as bowel perforation.
- In various clinical trials, MRgFUS resulted in significant relief of uterine fibroid symptoms.
- Rabinovici et al. recently reported on all pregnancies that occurred after MRgFUS at all sites worldwide. There were 54 reported pregnancies in 51 women. The live birth rate was 41% with a significant number of ongoing pregnancies.

CASE 5: PERIMENOPAUSAL SYMPTOMATIC FIBROID

History
- Mrs R, 44-year-old, presented with menorrhagia since last 3 months. She had three normal vaginal deliveries and last childbirth 10 years ago.
- Presented with complaint of increased bleeding during periods lasting for 10–15 days and lower abdominal pain from past 1 year.
- No history of medical illness and not on any medication.

Examination

- On pelvic examination, uterus was enlarged to about 8–10-week size, side-to-side mobility is present.
- On ultrasound, one anterior wall intramural fibroid of about 5 cm × 4 cm and other posterior wall small (2 × 1 × 1) submucosal fibroid were seen.
- Sonohysterogram findings were confirmed.

Diagnosis

P3L3 44 years menorrhagia with submucous and intramural fibroids.

Management

- Since the patient was premenopausal but symptomatic, and not desirous of surgical intervention trial of medical treatment was discussed. Alternatives in this category of women include gonadotropin-releasing hormone (GnRH) analogs, progesterone receptor modulators like mifepristone and ulipristal, danazol, and levonorgestrel intrauterine system (LNG-IUS). After weighing all the issues, the patient opted for trial of ulipristal acetate (UPA). She was prescribed 5 mg ulipristal daily for 3 months.
- Significant reduction in symptoms was seen in the patient with decreased menstrual bleeding as early as 1 month of the treatment. Amenorrhea was achieved after 15 days of therapy. Repeat TVS after 3 months demonstrated reduction in size of intramural fibroid to 3 cm and submucous fibroid to 0.5 cm. The beneficial effects of drug were maintained 6 months after stopping treatment.

Discussion

- In the perimenopausal symptomatic women with fibroids, medical management is a good alternative and trial should be considered before any surgical therapy.
- Choice is usually governed by the extent and severity of symptoms, size, number, and location of myomas, risk of malignancy, and proximity to menopause. As demonstrated in above scenario, with use of ulipristal for 3 months, surgery could be avoided and patient had good relief of symptoms.
- Armamentarium of agents for use include GnRH analogs, danazol, and progesterone antagonist like mifepristone. Ulipristal was preferred, as it is faster acting and more prolonged effects, along with a better tolerability and safety profile.
- Ulipristal acetate is an oral selective progesterone-receptor modulator, and characterized by a tissue-specific partial progesterone antagonist effect. In uterine fibroids, estrogen and progesterone receptors are expressed at higher levels than in normal myometrium.
- Now abundant emerging data has shown ulipristal to be faster than GnRH analogs in reducing the fibroid-associated bleeding, improving hemoglobin, and significant reduction in the size of fibroids, which lasts for at least 6 months after the end of the treatment.
- Repeat treatment courses can also be prescribed for women with larger fibroids after a gap. Endometrium treated with short-term UPA shows reversible changes, which are included in the range of histologic alterations induced by selective progesterone receptor modulators (SPRMs) in general and the endometrial thickness is restored to baseline levels after treatment discontinuation.
- GnRH agonists were not preferred due to significant side effect profile (e.g. hot flashes, vaginal dryness, bone demineralization) and also the beneficial effects on fibroid volume revert early after completion of course.

- Although LNG-IUS can also cause dramatic reduction in menstrual flow in women with fibroids, there have been no randomized controlled trials (RCTs) of its use in these women, in whom rates of expulsion of the device appear to be high.
- Although this patient showed 70% relief in symptoms, but patient should always be informed regarding need of surgery in case of nonresolution of the symptoms.

CASE 6: INFERTILITY WITH SUBMUCOUS FIBROID

History

Mrs R, 32-year-old, married for 5 years, presented with menorrhagia since last 3 months and was trying for second child last 1½ years.
- Menstrual cycles are regular and last for 8–10 days with heavy flow and passage of clots.
- *Obstetric history*: One child, normal vaginal delivery 3 years back.
- No history of medical illness and not on any medication.

Examination

On pelvic examination, uterus was enlarged to about 6-week size with no tenderness.

Investigations

Transvaginal ultrasound and sonosalpingography demonstrated hypoechoic broad-based lesion 3.3 cm × 2.6 cm subendometrial in location in lower part of uterine cavity submucous fibroid.

3D scan: Confirmed submucous fibroid located completely within cavity arising from anterior wall located in lower part of cavity, Lasmar score—2.

Diagnosis

P1L1 secondary infertility and submucous fibroid.

Management

Since the lady was symptomatic and trying for conception, they were counseled for myomectomy. On the basis of 3D scan findings, decision for hysteroscopic myomectomy was taken. On hysteroscopy, submucous fibroid of approximately 3 cm × 2.5 cm was seen arising from lower part of anterior wall, and lying totally in the cavity. Hysteroscopic myomectomy could be performed completely in a single sitting using resectoscope. Procedure was uneventful. Intraoperative intrauterine contraceptive device (IUCD) was inserted to prevent postoperative adhesion formation. In the postoperative period, cyclical estrogen and progesterone therapy were given and endometrial thickness was assessed. The intrauterine device was removed after 1 month and couple conceived spontaneously 3 months later.

Discussion

- Several studies have shown that submucous fibroids are associated with infertility, probably as a result of decreased implantation by disrupting the endometrial blood supply, affecting nidation, and sustenance of early embryo. Pritts et al. concluded that all pregnancy outcomes were negatively affected by presence of submucous fibroids and myomectomy improved the clinical pregnancy rates when compared to controls with fibroids.

- STEP-W/Lasmar scoring system for fibroids classifies submucous fibroids on basis of size, topography, penetration into cavity, extension of the base, and lateral wall involvement. Fibroids with score less than 4 are amenable to low complexity hysteroscopy, while those with score 5–6 usually need a two-stage procedure. Hysteroscopy is not recommended for fibroids with a score more than 7. In such fibroids, abdominal myomectomy or a combined approach is preferable.
- Electrosurgical loop electrodes using bipolar technology and also vaporizing electrode are being used for doing hysteroscopic myomectomy. Now, hysteroscopic morcellators are also available, which reduce the operating time but more data is needed on the efficacy and safety.
- Hysteroscopic myomectomy involves complications like fluid imbalance, hyponatremia, and intraoperative excessive bleeding; and a written consent should be obtained after discussion.
- The incidence of intrauterine adhesions after hysteroscopic myomectomy has been shown to be around 7.5%. Postoperative adjuvant therapy including estrogen therapy for 4–8 weeks or insertion of an intrauterine device/pediatric Foley catheter postoperatively have all been used to prevent further adhesion development. However, there is scant evidence to support the use of these postoperative therapies.

CASE 7: YOUNG GIRL WITH SYMPTOMATIC FIBROID

History
- A young unmarried girl, Miss N, 18-year-old, presented with heavy bleeding during periods since 4 months and continuous bleeding last 20 days
- Associated with pain in lower abdomen
- No history of any medical ailment or medication
- *Menstrual history*: Menarche 14 years, past cycles were regular and lasted for 4–5 days with average flow and no dysmenorrhea

Examination
- She was anemic.
- P/A no mass palpable, uterus not felt.

Investigations
- Hemoglobin 9 g/dL, coagulation profile was normal.
- Ultrasound examination revealed a 6 cm × 6 cm × 5.5 cm hypoechoic lesions in the posterior wall uterus symptoms of is suggestive of intramural fibroid. Endometrium 7-mm thick and bilateral ovaries being normal.

Diagnosis
An 18-year-old unmarried with symptomatic intramural fibroid uterus.

Management
- In view of patient's age, symptoms, and size of fibroid, parents were counseled about possibility of trial of medical management with option of surgical treatment in the form of myomectomy, if medical management fails. Initially, she was prescribed antifibrinolytics (tranexamic acid) at maximum permissible dose for 2 months with some relief of symptoms followed by oral combined contraceptive pills for 3 months.

- Patient reported only 25% improvement in symptoms with above therapy; and after discussion, she was switched to UPA 5 mg daily once following which her bleeding stopped in 6 days. As patient was anemic, so oral iron therapy was started. At the end of 6 months of treatment, on ultrasound, the fibroid size had decreased to 5 × 4 × 4.5 size. Her menstrual cycle resumed within 25 days of stopping the UPA. For the last 6 months, her cycles are regular and flow has been average since then.

Discussion

In this case, conservative management was desirous mode of treatment. Medical treatments may decrease symptoms potentially related to fibroids. Although most of them are not capable of treating the tumor itself and lead to marked decreases in fibroid volume, symptomatic control may still be achieved in many patients, who may prefer treating their conditions medically rather than resorting to invasive procedures. Various medical agents have been used for treatment of fibroids. GnRH analogs are not preferred in young women because of potential to cause bone loss.

Ulipristal is an SPRM has been successful to reach amenorrhea in 70–80% of women, with a faster median onset of 4 days to reach it and less adverse effects when compared to GnRH analogs.

G Lo Monte et al. reported that UPA ensures prompt symptom relief, significant reduction in uterine bleeding by day 8 of starting the medicine and is safe and also reduces the size of fibroid. Levens et al. report when given in a daily dose of 5 or 10 mg, it there was 92% reduction in the amount of bleeding when compared to placebo where the reduction of bleeding was 19%. Besides this, the size of the fibroid may also decrease. In the PEARL I and II trials in Europe where women received 5 mg or 10 mg per day of UPA when given for 13 weeks, uterine bleeding was controlled in 91%. They also reported that both these doses (5 mg or 10 mg) were not inferior to once monthly dose of leuprolide acetate in controlling bleeding. Hot flushes are less likely to occur with UPA and effect on bones can also be avoided.

Avendos et al. in a study also concluded that UPA can be a useful treatment to control emergency cases where fibroid-related abnormal uterine bleeding is there.

To conclude, UPA seems to be a viable option for controlling bleeding and pain associated with fibroids.

CASE 8: CERVICAL FIBROID

History

- Mrs R 49 years married presented with pain in lower abdomen and backache
- Menstrual cycles are regular and last 3–4 days
- *Obstetric history*: P2L2, both normal vaginal delivery
- No history of medical illness and not on any medication.

Examination

On pelvic examination, uterus enlarged to 8–10 weeks with bulge felt through left fornix.

Investigations

Ultrasonographic examination revealed a hypoechoic intramural mass of 8 cm × 7 cm in the cervical region extending toward left pelvic wall symptom of myoma with mild left hydronephrosis.

Diagnosis

P2L2 with lateral cervical fibroid.

Management

Due to the advanced age and as family was complete, couple were counseled for hysterectomy. They were posted for TLH after complete preoperative workup and fitness for surgery. Preoperative ureteric stent was placed by urologist. During surgery, supraumbilical trocar was placed and myoma screw was used from lateral port to manipulate the uterus. On laparoscopy, a 9 cm × 7 cm mass was seen arising from cervical region extending to left lateral wall, displacing bladder upwards. For ease of procedure and to delineate anatomy well, myomectomy of the cervical fibroid was done after bilateral uterine artery ligation. The broad ligament was opened with an anterior approach and a transverse incision was made on the myoma using a harmonic scalpel. Rest of the TLH was done in usual steps. Specimen sent for histopathology confirmed presence of big cervical fibroid. Postoperative stay was uneventful and patient was discharged after 2 days.

Discussion

Fibroids arising from cervix are rare tumors accounting for 2% of all fibroids. Lateral cervical fibroid, starting on the side of the cervix, burrows out into the broad ligament and expands it. TLH is currently accepted as a safe, efficient way to manage benign uterine pathology, and is an acceptable alternative to standard abdominal hysterectomy. Relationship of the cervical fibroid to the ureter is important.

Wherever the ureter and uterine artery may be in relation to the fibroid, they will always be extracapsular. The knowledge of this fact can turn potentially dangerous procedure into a relatively safe operation. An additional difficulty may be the introduction of conventional manipulators during TLH where a myoma screw with additional port may be utilized to manipulate the uterus. Steps of surgery differ according to the type and location, either anterior or posterior. The optical trocar should be placed supraumbilically to facilitate proper visualization. The use of myoma spiral increases the mobility of the uterus and frequent changes in its positioning can help access to all pedicles. Prior identification of the ureters with either retroperitoneal dissection or preprocedure cystoscopic ureteric stenting may be of help in selected cases of very large cervical myomas with lateral projection. In cases of anterior myomas, prior bladder dissection helps in reaching the uterines.

A reasonable option is to perform myomectomy and correct the distortion of the anatomy before proceeding to the hysterectomy in selected cases. Surgical difficulties associated with these cases are poor access to the operative field, difficulty in suturing the repairs, increased blood loss, and distortion of the anatomy of the vital neighboring structures in the pelvic cavity.

Thus, with the accuracy to identify vital structures, appropriate case selection and surgeon's skill TLH can be a reasonable mode of treatment for cervical fibroid in such cases.

CASE 9: PREGNANCY WITH FIBROID

History

Mrs S, a 30-year-old primigravida 32 weeks of pregnancy, presented in emergency severe pain in abdomen.
- Booked elsewhere fully immunized, no illness in past and no drug allergies too.

Examination

Blood pressure and vitals were normal.

Perabdominal examination: Uterus was large for gestational age, tense, and tenderness was present in the suprapubic region with no contractions observed. Fetal heart was regular.

Investigations

Ultrasonography: Single live fetus with normal growth parameters and a 7 cm × 6 cm × 5 cm size solid hypoechoic lesion fibroid in the lower part of uterus, with anechoic cystic areas.

Management

- Patient was advised bed rest and analgesics and responded well to conservative management. Antenatal steroids were given.
- After discharge, she returned 2 weeks later with premature rupture of membranes and established labor at 35 weeks' gestation, which did not respond to tocolytics. Fetus was in breech position, so she was taken up for LSCS and two units of packed red blood cells (PRBCs) were cross-matched before procedure. Intraoperatively, the fibroid was present in the lower segment on the left side and the incision was made through the fibroid at the left end. After delivery of fetus and placenta, myoma was enucleated, myoma bed sutured and included in the stitch line only. Active prophylactic measures for postpartum hemorrhage were employed in form of intramuscular carboprost and per rectal misoprostol.
- Postoperative period was uneventful with average blood loss.

Discussion

The incidence of uterine myomas varies from 0.3% to 7.2% during pregnancy. These tumors respond differently in individual women and may grow, regress, or remain unchanged in size during pregnancy. Fibroids during pregnancy rarely leads to complications like pain in abdomen and fever, which can be managed conservatively.

Fibroids sometimes grow fast during pregnancy and outgrow their blood supply leading to red degeneration as in the presented case.

In past, it was recommended that myomectomy during cesarean section should be avoided, as it leads to severe hemorrhage, necessitating hysterectomy. But in recent times, concept has changed and many studies have conducted to support it. Retrospective cohort study done by Ashley et al. concluded that myomectomy during cesarean delivery does not appear to result in an increased risk of intrapartum or short-term postpartum morbidity. Myomectomy during caesarean section have advantages because uterus in the postpartum phase is better adapted physiologically to control hemorrhage. As contractions and retractions of the muscles occur, the blood vessels are closed. Also, the onset of vascular changes for clot formation in placental bed helps in stopping the bleeding, hence have the above advantages. Several authors have published their results on myomectomy during cesarean section and now this procedure is not considered as dangerous and is no more taboo.

Decision for cesarean myomectomy should take into consideration location of the fibroid as serosal and pedunculated fibroids poses less danger while intramural myomectomy in fibroids obstructing the lower uterine segment, fundal myomas located proximal to the Fallopian tubes, and cornual myomas should be avoided. Several recent studies have described techniques, which can minimize blood loss at cesarean myomectomy, including uterine tourniquet, clamps, and electrocautery. Meticulous attention to hemostasis with enucleation using

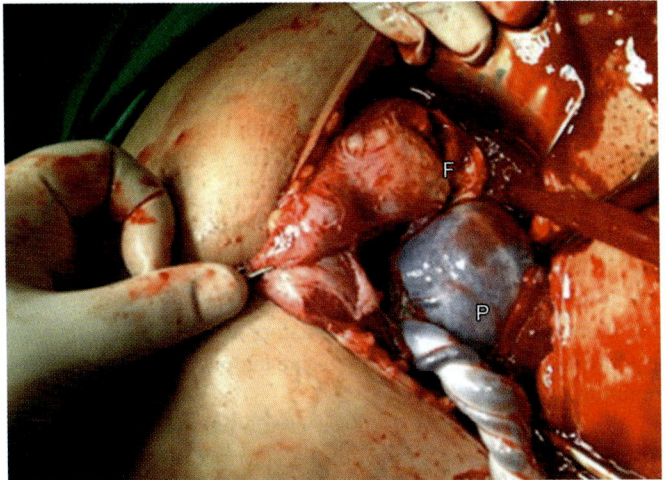

Fig. 25.2: Lower segment cesarean section (LSCS) in a case of fibroid. (P: Placenta with cord; F: Fibroid)

sharp dissection with Metzenbaum scissors and adequate approximation of the myometrium and all dead spaces to prevent hematoma formation can increase the safety of the procedure (Fig. 25.2).

CASE 10: PEDUNCULATED SUBSEROUS FIBROID

History
A 35-year-old lady presented to the emergency with lower abdominal pain for 2 days with increased intensity over last few hours. She had been prescribed analgesics by some local doctor with no relief.

Examination
She had tachycardia. Per abdominally there was deep tenderness and rebound tenderness in the left lower quadrant.

Investigations
- Total leukocyte count was 9,500 cells/L.
- *Transvaginal sonography*: Uterus was deviated to right with hypoechoic solid mass 7 cm × 6 cm in left adnexa separated from uterus; suggestive of subserosal fibroid.
- *Magnetic resonance imaging*—revealed a pelvic mass 6.7 cm × 7.2 cm × 4 cm connected to posterior wall of uterus with some ascites. Bilateral ovaries were visualized separately and normal.

Management
On the basis of the imaging findings and escalation of symptoms, provisional diagnosis of subserosal fibroid with degeneration or torsion was made. Antibiotics and analgesics were prescribed and patient was kept fasting.

As there was no relief in symptoms, decision for laparoscopy was taken. Laparoscopy revealed a bluish subserosal leiomyoma, approximately 7 cm in size, with pedicle twisted twice on the posterior surface of the uterus. Bilateral ovaries and Fallopian tubes were grossly normal and there was approximately 15 mL of ascites. Laparoscopic myomectomy was performed uneventfully. Histopathology was consistent with fibroid with areas of hemorrhage and infarction. Postoperative course was uneventful, and she was discharged from the hospital 3 days after the operation.

Discussion

If any patient with a leiomyoma experiences acute abdominal pain, differential diagnoses include appendicitis, gastroenteritis, pelvic inflammatory disease, and torsion of ovarian cyst. Even when the acute complication is due to uterine leiomyoma, the pain can be caused by secondary degeneration or torsion.

Torsion is usually seen in pedunculated subserous fibroids with thin and long stalks. Torsion in subserous fibroid might be difficult to diagnose preoperatively by imaging and is usually suspected when color Doppler shows twisted pedicle. Bloch et al. reported that the diagnosis of torsion of pedunculated leiomyoma could be established by MRI but in the ultrasound pedicle of a subserous leiomyoma can be very thin, which is frequently invisible.

In addition to the difficult preoperative diagnosis, a delayed diagnosis may result in ischemic necrosis and continuous abdominal pain, which in turn could lead to peritonitis. While myomectomy is treatment of choice in younger women desirous of future fertility, in older women with complete family hysterectomy can be considered. Katsumori et al. described uterine artery embolization for the treatment of pedunculated leiomyoma.

Early diagnosis and prompt management are keys to a successful outcome in these cases.

BIBLIOGRAPHY

Case 1

1. Benecke C, Kruger TF, Siebert TI, et al. Effect of fibroids on fertility in patients undergoing assisted reproduction; a structured literature review. Gynecol Obstet Invest. 2005;59:225-30.
2. Oliveira FG, Abdelmassih VG, Diamond MP, et al. Impact of subserosal and intramural uterine fibroids that do not distort the endometrial cavity on the outcome of in vitro fertilization-intracytoplasmic sperm injection. Fertil Steril. 2004;81(3):582-7.
3. Somigliana E, Vercellini P, Daguati R, et al. Fibroids and female reproduction: a critical analysis of the evidence. Hum Reprod Update., 2007;13(5):465-76.
4. Sunkara SK, Khairy M, El-Toukhy T, et al. The effect of intramural fibroids without uterine cavity involvement on the outcome of IVF treatment: a systematic review and meta-analysis. Hum Reprod. 2010;25(2):418-29.

Case 2

1. Goel N, Laddad M. Rare case of giant broad ligament fibroid with cervical fibroid mimicking ovarian tumour: interesting case report. Int J Rec Trends Sci Technol. 2014;10(2):208-9.
2. Low SC, Chong CL. A case of cystic leiomyoma mimicking an ovarian malignancy. Ann Acad Med Singapore. 2004;33:371-4.
3. Malik R, Agarwal GA. Large cystic degenerating broad ligament leiomyoma masquerading as ovarian malignancy! JCR. 2015;5:486-9.
4. Parker WH. Uterine Myoma: An Overview of Development, Clinical Features and Management. Obstet Gynecol. 2005;105:216-7.

Case 3

1. Eltabbakh GH, Piver MS, Hempling RE, et al. Laparoscopic surgery in obese women. Obstet Gynecol. 1999;94:704-8.
2. Lumsden MA, Wallace EM. Clinical presentation of uterine fibroids. Baillieres Clin Obstet Gynaecol. 1998;12:177-95.
3. Schmandt RE, Iglesias DA, Co NN, et al. Understanding obesity and endometrial cancer risk: opportunities for prevention. Am J Obstet Gynecol. 2011;205:518-52.
4. Sinha R, Sundaram M, Lakhotia S, et al. Total laparoscopic hysterectomy for large uterus. J Gynecol Endosc Surg. 2009;1(1):34-9.

Case 4

1. Fennessy FM, Tempany CM. A review of magnetic resonance imaging-guided focused ultrasound surgery of uterine fibroids. Top Magn Reson Imaging. 2006;17(3):173-9.
2. Rabinovici J, Inbar Y, Eylon SC, et al. Pregnancy and live birth after focused ultrasound surgery for symptomatic focal adenomyosis: a case report. Hum Reprod. 2006;21:1255-9.
3. So MJ, McDannold N, Fennessy FM. Evaluation of the impact of body mass and abdominal fat on MR-guided focused ultrasound surgery for uterine fibroids. Proc Int Soc Magn Reson Med. 2005;13:2141.
4. Ter Haar G. Wood and Loomis: the physical and biological effects of high frequency sound waves of great intensity. Phil Mag. 1927;4:7-14.
5. Yoon SW, Lee C, Cha SH, et al. Patient selection guidelines in MR-guided focused ultrasound surgery of uterine fibroids: a pictorial guide to relevant findings in screening pelvic MRI. Eur Radiol. 2008;18:2997.

Case 5

1. Donnez J, Tatarchuk TF, Bouchard P, et al. PEARL I Study Group. Ulipristal acetate versus placebo for fibroid treatment before surgery. N Engl J Med. 2012;366(5):409-20.
2. Donnez J, Vivancos BH, Kudela M, et al. A randomized, placebo-controlled, dose-ranging trial comparing fulvestrant with goserelin in premenopausal patients with uterine fibroids awaiting hysterectomy. Fertil Steril. 2003;79:1380-9.
3. Rackow BW, Arici A. Options for medical treatment of myomas. Obstet Gynecol Clin North Am. 2006;33:97-113.
4. Sammartino PS, Di Carlo C, Affinoto P, et al. Effects of raloxifene treatment on uterine leiomyomas in postmenopausal women. Fertil Steril. 2001;76:38-43.
5. Steinauer J, Pritts EA, Jackson R, et al. Systematic review of mifepristone for the treatment of uterine leiomyomata. Obstet Gynecol. 2004;103:1331-6.

Case 6

1. Lasmar RB, Lasmar BP, Celeste RK, et al. A new system to classify submucous myomas: a Brazilian multicenter study. J Minim Invasive Gynecol. 2012;19(5):575-80.
2. Li C, Dai Z, Gong Y, et al. A systematic review and meta-analysis of randomized controlled trials comparing hysteroscopic morcellation with resectoscopy for patients with endometrial lesions. Int J Gynaecol Obstet. 2017;136(1):6-12.
3. Parazzini F, Tozzi L, Bianchi S. Pregnancy outcome and uterine fibroids. Best Pract Res Clin Obstet Gynaecol. 2016;34:74-84.
4. Pritts EA, Parker WH, Olive DL. Fibroids and infertility: an updated systematic review of the evidence. Fertil Steril. 2009;91(4):1215-23.
5. Touboul C, Fernandez H, Deffieux X, et al. Uterine synechiae after bipolar hysteroscopic resection of submucosal myomas in patients with infertility. Fertil Steril. 2009;92:1690-3.

Case 7

1. Donnez J, Tomeszewski J, Vazquez F, et al. PEARL II study group ulipristal versus leuprolide acetate for uterine fibroids. N Engl J Med. 2012;366(5):421-32.
2. Donnez J, Vazquez F, Tomaszewski J, et al. Long-term treatment of uterine fibroids with ulipristal acetate. Fert Steril. 2014;101(6):1565-73.
3. Levens ED, Potlog-Naheri C, Armstrong AY, et al. CDB-2914 for uterine leiomyomata treatment: a randomized controlled trial. Obstet Gynecol. 2008;111:1129-36.
4. Lo Monte G, Piva I, Graziano A, Engl B, et al. Ulipristal acetate prior to in vitro fertilization in a female patient affected by uterine fibroid: a case report. Eur Rev Med Pharmacol Sci. 2016;20:2002-207.

Case 8

1. Kaur AP, Saini AS, Kaur D, et al. Huge cervical fibroid: unusual presentation. J Obstet Gynaecol India. 2002;52(1):164.
2. Matsuoka S, Kikuchi I, Kitade M, et al. Strategy for laparoscopic cervical myomectomy. J Minim Invasive Gynecol. 2010;17:301-5.
3. Patel P, Banker M, Munshi S, et al. Handling cervical myomas. J Gynecol Endosc Surg. 2011;2(1):30-2.

Case 9

1. Adesiyun AG, Ojabo A. Fertility and obstetric outcome after caesarean myomectomy. J Obstet Gynaecol. 2008;28(7):710-2.
2. Kwawukume EY. Myomectomy during cesarean section. Int J Gynecol Obstet. 2002;76:183-4.
3. Laughlin SK, Baird DD, Savitz DA, et al. Prevalence of uterine myomas in the first trimester of pregnancy: an ultrasound screening study. Obstet Gynecol. 2009;113(3):630.
4. Roman AS, Tabsh KM. Myomectomy at time of cesarean delivery: a retrospective cohort study. BMC Pregnancy Childbirth 2004;4:14.

Case 10

1. Dua A, Fishwick K, Deverashetty B. Uterine torsion in pregnancy: a review. Int J Gynecol Obstet. 2006;6(1).
2. Foissac R, Sautot-Vial N, Birtwisle L, et al. Torsion of a huge pedunculated uterine leiomyoma. Am J Surg. 2011;201:e43-5.
3. Katsumori T, Akazawa K, Mihara T. Uterine artery embolization for pedunculated subserosal fibroids. AJR Am J Roentgenol. 2005;184(2):399-402.
4. Marcotte-Bloch C, Novellas S, Buratti MS, et al. Torsion of a uterine leiomyoma: MRI features. Clin Imaging. 2007;31(5):360-2.
5. Nicholson WK, Coulson CC, McCoy MC, et al. Pelvic magnetic resonance imaging in the evaluation of uterine torsion. Obstet Gynecol. 1995;85(5 Pt 2):888-90.

Perplexing Situations with Fibroids

Poonam Goyal

INTRODUCTION

It is incredible how after decades of experience an innocent tumor like fibroid surprises you. As we have already discussed in earlier chapters of the book that fibroid disease has a very wide spectrum of presentation, still there are situations that are weird.

PARASITIC FIBROID

Fibroid can be:
1. Primary parasitic
2. Secondary parasitic

A fibroid can become parasitic and can confuse clinician. By definition parasite means an organism that lives off or in another organism, obtaining nourishment and protection while offering no benefit in return.

Sometimes a subserosal fibroid can have an elongated peduncle and grows to large size; in a way it starts hanging and with time the peduncle gets elongated and thinned out. This large tumor stabilizes itself on some extrauterine organ and gradually develops vascular connections with that abdominal organ. With time that primary stalk shrinks becomes avascular and breaks down. Thus, tumor starts enjoying his new found space and blood supply grows. It is called primary parasitic fibroid. This now looks like a growth of another organ having no relation with uterus. Only histopath can determine final diagnosis. Though very few primary parasitic fibroids have been reported in literature but still a clinician should be aware of the possibility and existence of such condition. Case has been reported from India as well.

There are secondary parasitic fibroids also which start from bits and pieces of morcellated fibroid. Some bits may fall and remain in peritoneal cavity after morcellation or in the process of lap-myomectomy some parts are by mistake left behind in abdomen. These gradually find their nourishment in some other organ; becoming parasite. USG in these patients will be normal for uterus size. Only histopath will confirm diagnosis.

UNEXPECTED COLLAPSE OF PATIENT

Another such situation is when the fibroid becomes unusually vascular and large blood vessels are seen at surface and periphery. With further growth of tumor there is extreme stretching of surface vessels and veins can rupture leading to sudden hemoperitoneum. Patient will present with sudden collapse or acute abdomen. When such a patient presents it causes a lot of diagnostic dilemma. Most of the times diagnosis is intraoperative. There will be anaemia, shock and ruptured blood vessels on the surface of subserosal myoma. All over world less than 100 cases have been reported and in only 2% of cases preoperative diagnosis was possible.

CONCLUSION

A clinician must be prepared for almost anything when dealing with fibroid disease.

BIBLIOGRAPHY

1. Dahiya K, Walecha N. Uterine Leiomyoma presenting with hemoperitoneum. JSAFOG. 2013;5:33-4.
2. Danikas D, Theodorou SJ, Kotrotsios J, et al. Hemoperitoneum from spontaneous bleeding of uterine leiomyoma. Am Surg. 1999;65:1180-2.
3. Drutman J, Fruechte DM. Hemoperitoneum due to traumatic avulsion of pedunculated uterine leiomyoma. AJR Am J Roentgenol. 1992;158:1410.
4. Mandal D, Dattaray C, Roy S. Spontaneous parasitic leiomyoma: A rare Clinical Experience. JSAFOG. 2013;5:85-6.
5. Ritchie AC. Boyd Textbook of Pathology. Philadelphia: Lea and Febiger; 1990.
6. Robins SL, Cotran RS, Kumar V. Pathologic basis of disease, 3rd edition. Philadelphia: WB Saunders; 1985.
7. Sinha R, Sundaram M, Lakhotia S, et al. Parasitic Myoma after morcellation. J Gynecol Endosop Surg. 2009;1:113-5.
8. Sule AZ. Traumatic rupture of uterine fibroid: An uncommon cause of post traumatic hemoperitoneum. West Afr J Med. 2000;19:158-9.

Counseling in a Patient of Fibroid

27

Poonam Goyal

INTRODUCTION

Counseling is an art, which as a clinician, we all must learn. It is important part of treatment for patients suffering from chronic problems. Patients with fibroid disease may have no symptom at all or she may have debilitating problem because of severe anemia. They may go to quacks for cure just to avoid surgery. They may be depressed and anxious, which affects their quality of life. Most of them are unaware that allopathy has also come up with nonsurgical options.

COUNSELING IN A PATIENT OF FIBROID

It is the duty of the treating gynecologist to spare few minutes to understand patient's problem, her needs, her psyche, and then give her treatment options. Clinician being a professional knows about the disease and treatment modalities, but she is the sufferer, so her concern must be respected.

We need to give her the best as a medical person fully understanding the patient's perspective. Treatment can be surgical, medical, or simple wait and watch. Proper consent should be there.

Ten very important counseling tips are:
1. Incidence of fibroid disease is very rampant. One out of four women is suffering from it. So, we as a doctor must reassure her so that she has confidence in us.
2. She should be explained that there is no defined cause of disease and no fixed clinical presentation and thus there is no blanket treatment, it is according to the symptoms and presentation.
3. Take some time to explain to her in case she does not require any treatment or intervention. If you fail to do so, she will land in someone else's clinic for hysterectomy.
4. In patients having fibroid disease with infertility, she should be encouraged to bear pregnancy especially if fibroids are not disturbing the endometrial cavity.
5. If she is pregnant and has coexisting fibroid disease, explain her the extra care she needs and counsel her about institutional delivery.
6. The disease progress being slow follow-up is advised yearly in a nonsymptomatic patient.
7. While giving medical treatment, patient should be explained in detail that we are addressing her bleeding problem. No medical treatment can make the fibroid disappear from the scene, only shrinkage occurs and it may again resort to same size later. Pros and cons all should be clear in her mind and what is the aim of treatment. In other words, judicious use of medical treatment should be done. Every Tom, Dick, and Harry is not for this.

8. Surgery, if required, it should be done in experienced hands. Proper consent is mandatory prior to surgery. If myomectomy done in infertility cases, treatment for infertility should be started after 3 months of surgery. Myomectomy is now considered to be a safe procedure.
9. In poor surgical risk cases, newer modalities like uterine artery embolism (UAE) and magnetic resonance-guided focused ultrasound (MRgFUS).
10. Malignancy should be ruled out prior to starting any medical management or surgery. Thus, treatment is individualized and clinician–patient bonding is important.

CONCLUSION

Thus, treatment is individualized and clinician-patient bonding is important. Counseling is an art which is must learn for all in this current situation of strained patient doctor relationship. Patient should have realistic expectations from the treatment and treatment should be on the basis of recommended guidelines.

BIBLIOGRAPHY

1. Ghant M, Sengoba K, Mendoza G, et al. Seeking the truth: a qualitative assessment of women's experiences seeking and obtaining knowledge of uterine fibroids. Fertil Steril. 2015;104(3):e155.
2. Lee HJ, Norwitz ER, Shaw J. Contemporary management of fibroids in pregnancy. Rev Obstet Gynecol. 2010;3(1):20-7.
3. Martin-Merino E, Wallander MA, Andersson S, et al. The reporting and diagnosis of uterine fibroids in the UK: An observational study. BMC Women Health. 2016;16:45.
4. Practice committee of ASRM in collaboration with the Society of Reproductive Surgeons. Myomas and reproductive function. Fertil Steril. 2008;90(5 Suppl):s125-30.
5. Pritts EA, Vanness DJ, Berek JS, et al. The prevalence of occult leiomyosarcoma at surgery for presumed uterine fibroids: a meta-analysis. Gynecol Surg. 2015;12:165-77.
6. Shavell VI, Thakur M, Sawant A, et al. Adverse obstetric outcomes associated with sonographically identified large uterine fibroids. Fertil Steril. 2012;97(1):107-10.
7. Simms-Stewart D, Fletcher H. Counselling patients with uterine fibroids: A review of the management and complications. Obstet Gynecol Int. 2012;2012:539365.

Emerging and Hopeful Strategies toward Nonsurgical Management of Fibroids

28

Narendra Malhotra, Manpreet Sharma, Shemi Bansal, Poonam Goyal, Jaideep Malhotra

INTRODUCTION

Fibroids are the most common benign tumors seen in women of reproductive age group. Adolescent girls also present with symptomatic and asymptomatic fibroids.

Fibroids are tumors of the uterine myometrium smooth muscles and contain muscles plus collagen, fibronectin, and proteoglycan.

Many women will show nonsymptomatic presence of fibroids of various sizes—single or multiple, which are detected in routine screenings by ultrasound.

Symptoms of fibroids are dependent on their size and location and vary from menstrual irregularities to pressure symptoms.

CLINICAL MANAGEMENT

About 40% of women with fibroids present with heavy menstrual bleeding and will seek treatment.

The treatment mainly is operative, depending on age and fertility, it may be myomectomy or hysterectomy.

Operative treatments have a great impact on the uterine strength and integrity resulting in revels of adhesions inside and outside the uterus.

Medical Treatments (Chapter 13)

Among the medical treatment available are:
- Gonadotropin-releasing hormone (GnRH) agonists (depot injection)
- Selective progesterone receptor modulators (SPRMs) (5 mg ulipristal acetate)
- Mifepristone 10 mg/25 mg (SPRM)
- GnRH antagonists
- Vaginal delivery of GnRH analogs (under trial)
- Progesterone receptor modulators (PRMs)
- Aromatase inhibitions
- Selective estrogen receptor modulators (SERMs)
- Oral antagonists (three types under trial).

Medical treatment of fibroids has been discussed in detail in Chapter 13.

Emerging New Treatments

Newer nonsurgical treatment of fibroids has been discussed in Chapter 14.
To enumerate these are:
- Uterine artery embolization
- Magnetic resonance-guided focused ultrasound (MRgFUS)
- Transvaginal uterine artery occlusion
- Endometrial ablation (Chapter 7).

Emerging and Hopeful Strategies as per FIGO Classification (Fig. 28.1)

Fibroid types range from 0 to 8 (drawing adapted from Munro et al. FIGO classification, 2011):
- 0 = Pedunculated, intracavitary
- 1 = Submucosal, less than 50% intramural
- 2 = Submucosal, more than or equal to 50% intramural
- 3 = Contact with endometrium, 100% intramural
- 4 = Intramural
- 5 = Subserosal, more than or equal to 50% intramural
- 6 = Subserosal, less than 50% intramural
- 7 = Subserosal, pedunculated
- 8 = Other (e.g. cervical, parasitic).

When two numbers are given separated by a hyphen, the first refers to the relationship with the endometrium, while the second refers to the relationship with the serosa (see example below).

2-5 = Submucosal and subserosal, each with less than half of its diameter in the endometrial and peritoneal cavity, respectively.

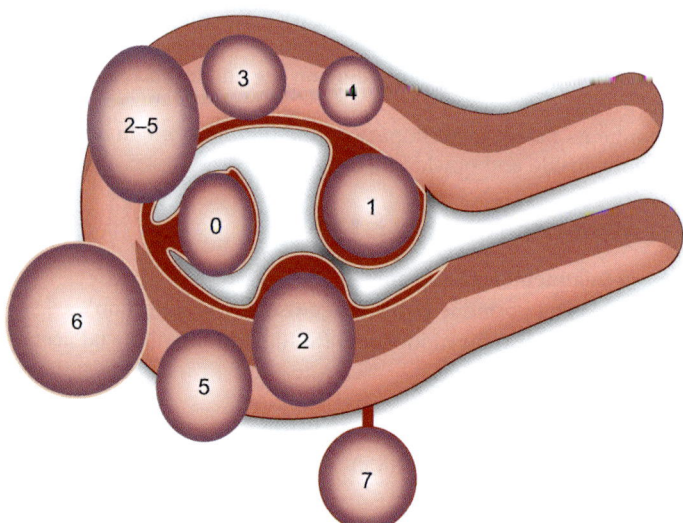

Fig. 28.1: International Federation of Gynecology and Obstetrics (FIGO) classification according to Munro et al. (2011).
Source: Adapted from Munro MG, Critchley HO, Broder MS, et al. FIGO classification system (PALM-COEIN) for causes of abnormal uterine bleeding in nongravid women of reproductive age. Int J Gynaecol Obstet. 2011;113(1):3-13.

Management Strategies

- *Management of Type 0 myoma (Fig. 28.2)*
- *Management of Type 1 myoma (Fig. 28.3)*
- *Management of Type 2 myoma (Fig. 28.4).*

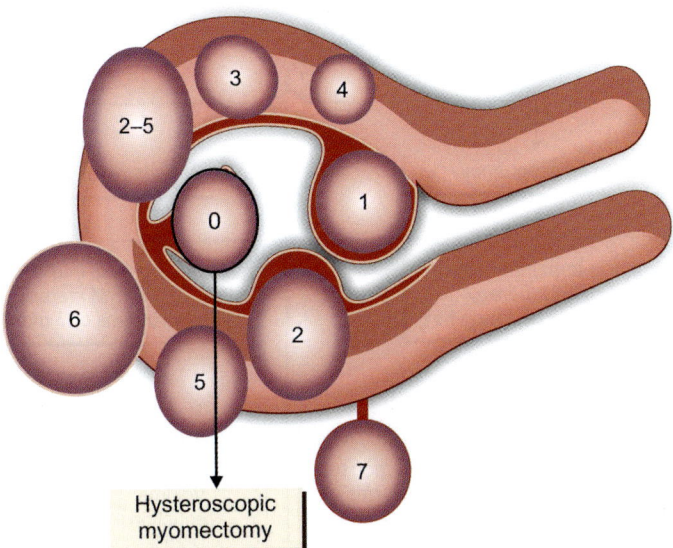

Fig. 28.2: Management of Type 0 myomas.

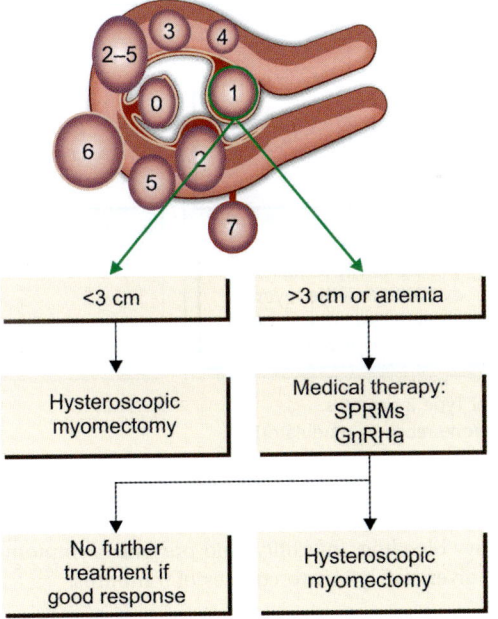

Fig. 28.3: Management of Type 1 myomas.
(GnRHa: Gonadotropin-releasing hormone agonists; SPRMs: Selective progesterone receptor modulators).

214 Fibroids

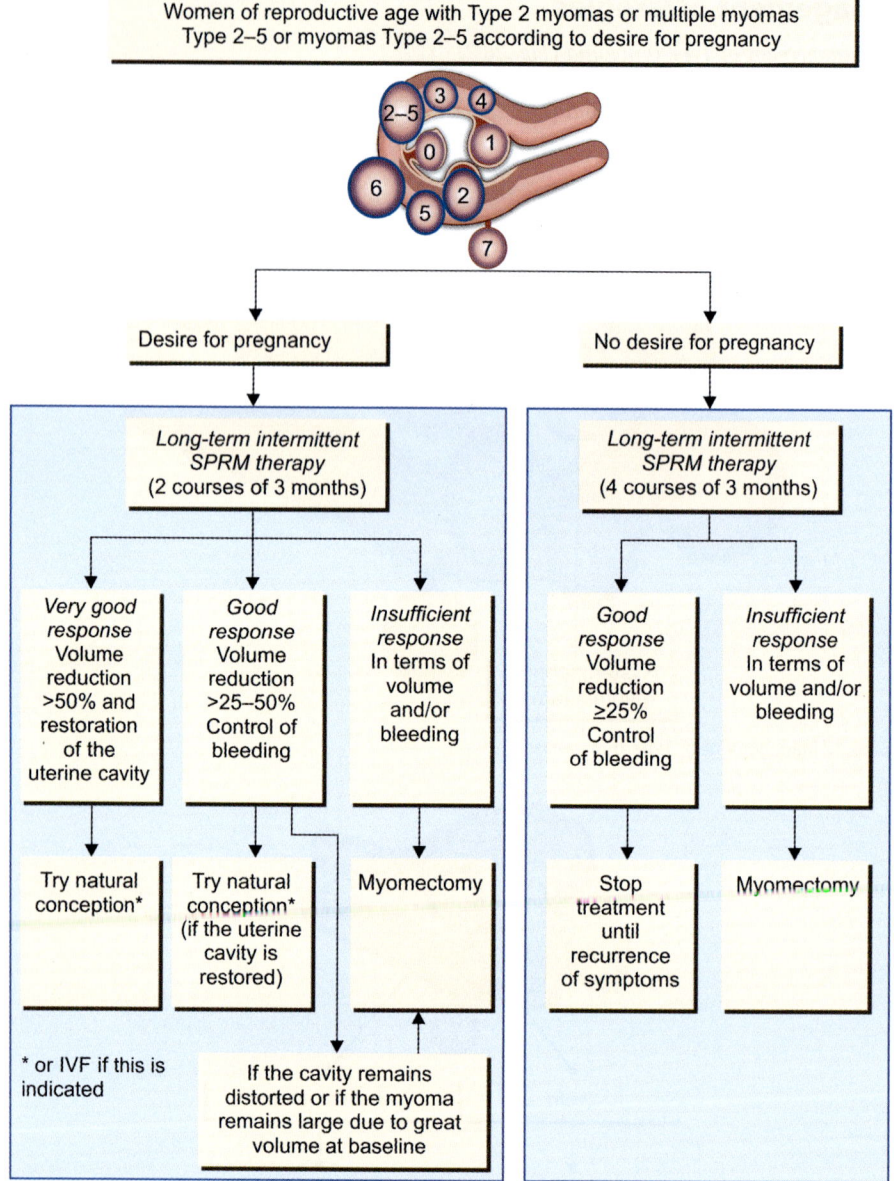

Fig. 28.4: Management of Type 2 myomas.
(SPRM: Selective progesterone receptor modulator).

Medical management of fibroids with SPRMs is a good alternative to treat the symptoms due to fibroids like heavy bleeding, infertility, and presence symptoms.

The SPRMs can be given safely in two courses of 3 months.

With two courses, we can expect:
- Fifty percent decrease in volume of the fibroids and if this patient is for infertility treatment can be allowed to conceive if cavity becomes normal.

- Size reduction of fibroid occurs, but cavity is still distorted and now laparoscopic or hysteroscopic surgery can be undertaken for myomectomy.
- There may be no reduction or response to medical treatment with ulipristal such patients will need surgery, if symptomatic.

Future Perspectives and Hopeful Strategies

While ulipristal has shown great promise in managing fibroids, further trials are on for safety (hepatotoxicity) and future trials for use as preventive strategies in women who are genetically prone to have fibroids and to prevent recurrences after surgery.

CONCLUSION

Selective progesterone receptor modulators have shown promise in significant reduction of size and symptoms of fibroids.

The need of medical treatments and newer strategies is requirement of the day.

Selective progesterone receptor modulators can be used as adjunct to surgery and/or alternative to surgery for fibroids.

BIBLIOGRAPHY

1. Bestel E, Donnez J. The potential of selective progesterone receptor modulators for the treatment of uterine fibroids. Expert Rev Endocrinol Metab. 2014;9:79-92.
2. Donnez J, Arriagada P, Donnez O, et al. Emerging treatment options for uterine fibroids. Expert Opin Emerg Drugs. 2018;23(1):17-23.
3. Donnez J, Dolmans MM. Uterine fibroid management: from the present to the future. Hum Reprod Update. 2016;22:665-86.
4. Donnez J, Donnez O, Matule D, et al. Long-term medical management of uterine fibroids with ulipristal acetate. Fertil Steril. 2016;105:165-73.
5. Donnez J, Tomaszewski J, Vázquez F, et al.; PEARL II Study Group. Ulipristal acetate versus leuprolide acetate for uterine fibroids. N Engl J Med. 2012;366:421-2.
6. Donnez J, Vázquez F, Tomaszewski J, et al.; PEARL III and PEARL III Extension Study Group. Long-term treatment of uterine fibroids with ulipristal acetate. Fertil Steril. 2014;101:1565-73.
7. Kim J, Sefton EC. The role of progesterone signaling in the pathogenesis of uterine leiomyoma. Mol Cell Endocrinol. 2012;358:223-31.
8. Lumsden MA, Hamoodi I, Gupta J, et al. Fibroids: diagnosis and management. BMJ. 2015;351:h4887.
9. Munro MG, Critchley HO, Broder MS, et al. FIGO classification system (PALM-COEIN) for causes of abnormal uterine bleeding in nongravid women of reproductive age. Int J Gynaecol Obstet. 2011;113(1):3-13.
10. Stewart EA. Clinical practice. Uterine fibroids. N Engl J Med. 2015;372(17):1646-55.

Ulipristal: Experience in Few Cases

Poonam Goyal

CASE 1: LARGE FIBROID IN ADOLESCENT AGE GROUP/MENORRHAGIA/ANEMIA

History

Miss PJ, 18-year-old:
- *Chief complaints*: She presented with heavy menses for last 6 months, feeling of tiredness and not able to concentrate in studies.
- *Past history*: She had no significant medical or surgical history. She took treatment from local doctor in the form of some syrup.
- *Menstrual history*: She had regular 28-day cycles with heavy flow for 7–8 days since 6–7 months with history of midcycle spotting, dysmenorrhea for past two to three cycles.

Investigations

- *Complete blood count (CBC)*: Hemoglobin (Hb) 5.6 gm%, microcytic hypochromic
- *Liver function test (LFT)*: Normal
- *Kidney function test (KFT)*: Normal
- *Thyroid-stimulating hormone (TSH)*: Normal
- Serum iron study showed iron deficiency
- *Serum ferritin*: 3 ng/mL
- *Prolactin*: Normal
- *Transabdominal ultrasound:* Uterus found to be enlarged 64 × 71 × 81 mm³ with intramural fibroid, 76 × 45 mm² anterior wall abutting the cavity. Upper abdomen scan showed normal findings.

Diagnosis

Severe anemia with abnormal uterine bleeding (AUB)/cause intramural fibroid, touching endometrium.

Management

Patient admitted for transfusion of packed cells. Two units were given, it was uneventful. Two doses of injection isomaltose 2 injection 100 mg/mL IV in 100 mL of normal saline. Total 4 injections option of medical management or surgical management (myomectomy) discussed with patient and her parents. Pros and cons of both the methods explained.

Patient and parents opted for trial of medical management because being unmarried they were very reluctant for operation. Ulipristal acetate was given in a dose 5 mg/day for 3 months. Oral hematinics, iron pyrophosphate 4 tablets/day were also started simultaneously.

In follow-up after 3 months, patient had relief in symptoms. Hemoglobin was 9.6 gm%. Ultrasound showed shrinkage in fibroid size 50 × 42 mm^2 and also fibroid margin was 6 mm away from endometrial lining. After a gap of 1 month, another 3 months of ulipristal given. USG after that showed fibroid size 42 × 36 mm^2, 9 mm from endometrium. Hb was 11 gm%.

Follow-up

Oral iron preparation continued and patient advised 6 monthly ultrasound follow-up for the 1st year and then yearly for 2 years. Patient was also advised to contact in case of menorrhagia.

CASE 2: INTRAMURAL FIBROIDS IN REPRODUCTIVE AGE GROUP

History

Mrs PJ, 25-year-old, presented with heavy menses for last 4–5 months. She had no significant medical or surgical history.

Obstetrical History

P1L1A0 3 years back uneventful vaginal delivery. Only using barrier contraception.

Menstrual History

She had regular 30-day cycles with 3–4 days normal flow, but for past 4–5 months history of heavy flow for 7–8 days and history of postmenstrual spotting in last cycle, dysmenorrhea also present.

Investigations

- *CBC*: Hb 10.5 gm%, erythrocyte sedimentation rate (ESR) 28, counts, etc. are normal.
- *TSH*: 4.9
- LFT—normal
- KFT—normal
- Prolactin—normal
- *Transvaginal USG*: Uterus found to be enlarged 95 × 71 × 80 mm^3 with intramural fibroid, 36 × 45 mm^2 in posterior myometrium. Another small myoma seen in anterior wall of 20 × 19 mm^2, both away from cavity. Endometrium normal 9 mm.
- *Endometrial biopsy (EB)*: Histopathology examination (HPE) shows normal secretory endometrium.

Diagnosis

Mild anemia with AUB cause intramural fibroids.

Management

Patient given option of medical management to which she willingly agreed. Pros and cons of medical method discussed, including chances of conception and pregnancy complications with fibroid.

Patient opted for trial of medical management. Ulipristal acetate was given in a dose 5 mg/day for 3 months, and drug was given daily at the same time. She was amenorrheic for 3 months. In follow-up after 3 months, patient had relief in symptoms. Ultrasound showed shrinkage in fibroid size 33 × 24 mm² and also other fibroid could not be imaged on USG.

Follow-up

Patient advised 6 monthly ultrasound follow-up for the 1st year and then yearly for 2 years. Patient was also advised to plan early for conception.

CASE 3: INTRAMURAL FIBROIDS IN REPRODUCTIVE AGE GROUP

History

Mrs AG, 35-year-old, presented with primary infertility for 10 years. Couple was on barrier contraception for first 2 years of marriage. She had open myomectomy 3 years back. It was followed by one cycle in vitro fertilization (IVF) 2 years back, indication being male factor. This cycle was failure. She remained well for sometime but developed heavy menses for last 7–8 months. At present keen to conceive. She was diagnosed to be having fibroid and poor ovarian reserve. Patient had been advised another surgery for fibroid before undergoing another IVF cycle.

Obstetrical History

G0P0A0 married for 12 years.

Past History

She had a large intramural myoma for which open myomectomy was done 3 years back. She had IVF 2 years back indication being male factor sperm count 5 million 10% motility, 3% normal morphology, and two cycle intrauterine insemination (IUI) failure.

Menstrual History

She had regular 30-day cycles with 2–3 days normal flow, but for past 7–8 months history of heavy flow for 7–8 days no history of postmenstrual spotting but dysmenorrhea present.

Investigations

- *CBC*: Hb 11.5 gm%, ESR 28, counts, etc. are normal
- *TSH*: 0.85
- LFT—normal
- KFT—normal
- Prolactin—normal
- Anti-Müllerian hormone (AMH) 1.65
- *Transvaginal USG*: Uterus found to be enlarged 98 × 70 × 80 mm³ with intramural fibroid, 62 × 42 mm² in posterior myometrium. Two small seedling myomas seen in anterior wall of 20 × 19 mm² and 18 × 17 mm² both away from cavity. The larger myoma seen to be indenting endometrium in fundal part.

Diagnosis

Primary infertility with intramural fibroid indenting endometrium, postmyomectomy, poor ovarian reserve, and one cycle IVF failure with severe oligoasthenoteratozoospermia (OAT).

Management

Since patient was reluctant for second surgery, she was given option of medical management to which she willingly agreed. Pros and cons of medical method discussed, including pregnancy complications with fibroid.

Patient opted for trial of medical management. Ulipristal acetate was given in a dose 5 mg/day for 3 months, and drug was given daily at the same time. She was amenorrheic for 3 months. In follow-up after 3 months, her ultrasound showed shrinkage in fibroid size 44 × 34 mm^2 and now there was no indentation on endometrium. Diagnostic hysteroscopy confirmed smooth cavity. She was taken for IVF after 6 weeks. Antagonist protocol, stimulation done with 300 IU of human menopausal gonadotropin (hMG) injection for 11 days. We retrieved 8-M2 oocytes. Intracytoplasmic sperm injection (ICSI) done of good-quality oocyte with poor quality sperm. Only six oocytes fertilized and four cleaved. There were three grade I and one grade II embryos. Embryo transfer done on day 3 with three grade I embryos. She conceived and had dichorionic diamniotic (DCDA) twins one of which stopped growing at 6–7 weeks of gestation. She continued as singleton pregnancy and delivered a healthy female baby by lower segment Cesarean section (LSCS) at 34 weeks of gestation because of ruptured membranes. Fibroids left as such not removed during surgery.

Follow-up

Patient advised 6 monthly ultrasound follow-up for the 1st year and then yearly for 2 years.

CASE 4: SUBMUCOUS FIBROIDS IN PERIMENOPAUSAL AGE GROUP

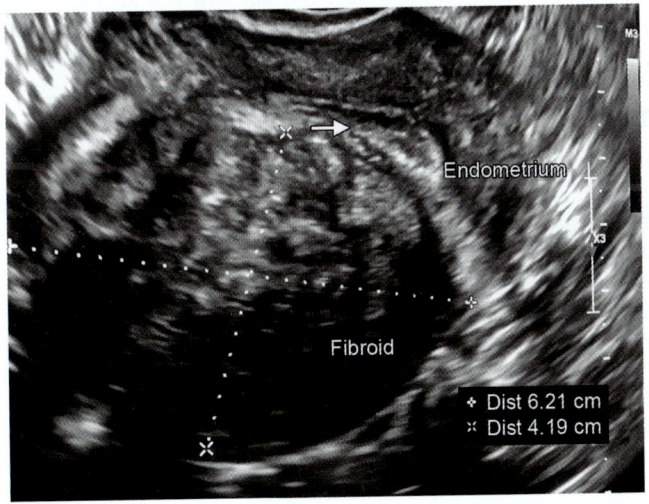

Fig. 29.1: Posterior wall myoma abutting endometrium.

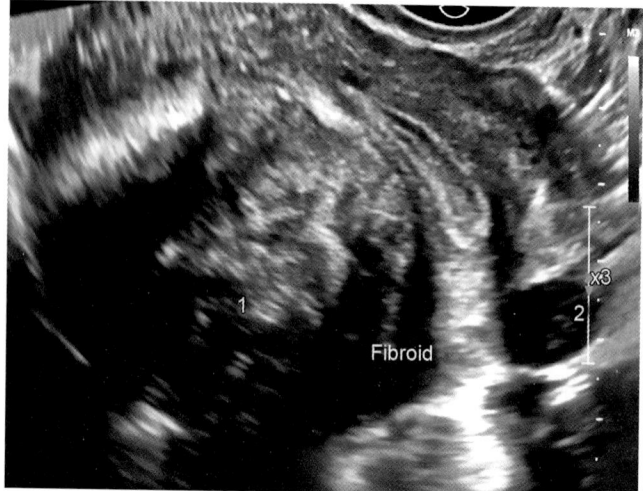

Fig. 29.2: Large posterior wall myoma (1) not disturbing the cavity. Small seedling myoma (2).

History

Mrs NG, 50-year-old, presented with menorrhagia for 7–8 months.

Obstetrical History

G2P2A0, married for 23 years. LCB 19 years back, both VD.

Past History

History of chronic renal disease and known case of bronchial asthma.

Menstrual History

She had regular 30-day cycles with 2–3 days normal flow but for past 7–8 months history of heavy flow for 7–8 days, no history of postmenstrual spotting, history of dysmenorrhea present.

Investigations

- *CBC*: Hb 11.2 gm%, ESR 28, counts, etc. are normal
- *TSH*: 0.85
- LFT—normal
- KFT—serum creatinine 2.8, blood urea 80
- X-ray chest—normal
- Pulmonary function tests (PFTs) were deranged
- Cardiac evaluation with electrocardiography (ECG) and echocardiography (ECHO) was normal.
- Pap smear—normal
- *EB Histopath report*: secretory and no atypia
- *Transvaginal USG*: Uterus found to be enlarged 94 × 71 × 85 mm^3 with submucous/intramural fibroid, 30 × 28 mm^2 in posterior myometrium. Fibroid was less than 50% in the cavity mainly it was intramural.

Diagnosis

Abnormal uterine bleeding, perimenopausal, cause intramural/submucosal fibroid with chronic renal disease and bronchial asthma.

Management

Since patient was high risk for surgery, she was given option of medical management to which she willingly agreed. Pros and cons of medical method discussed.

Patient opted for trial of medical management. Ulipristal acetate was given in a dose 5 mg/day for 3 months; drug was given daily at the same time. She had irregular spotting for 1 month then she became amenorrheic. In follow-up after 3 months, her ultrasound did not much shrinkage in fibroid size 28 × 25 mm^2, but it had become mainly intramural.

Follow-up

Medicine was stopped and patient was followed up after another 3 months, she remained amenorrheic, fibroid size was the same. On further follow-up, patient went into menopause. Patient was advised 6 monthly check-up for next 2 years.

BIBLIOGRAPHY

1. Donnez J, Dolmans MM. Uterine fibroid management: from the present to the future. Hum Reprod Update. 2016;22(6):665-86.
2. Kalampokas T, Kamath M, Boutas I, et al. Ulipristal acetate for uterine fibroids: a systematic review and meta-analysis. Gynecol Endocrinol. 2016;32(2):91-6.
3. Schreiber CA, Barnhart K. Ulipristal acetate (UPA) is a selective progesterone receptor modulator approved for use as an emergency contraceptive in the United States and Europe and for preoperative treatment of uterine myomas. Side Effects Drugs Ann. 2017;39:417-26.
4. Stewart EA. Clinical practice. Uterine fibroids. N Engl J Med. 2015;372(17):1646-55.

Fibroid Management Guidelines

Kavita Agarwal

INTRODUCTION

Uterine fibroids (myomas and leiomyomas) are benign smooth muscle tumors found in intramural, submucosal, and subserosal region of the uterus. They are often asymptomatic but can be associated with heavy menstrual bleeding and pressure symptoms.

DIAGNOSIS

The working party of New Zealand guidelines group[1] states that transvaginal ultrasound and transvaginal sonohysterogram are more accurate than hysteroscopy in diagnosing uterine fibroids. However, transabdominal ultrasound should be considered in women with uterus size more than 12 weeks. Magnetic resonance imaging (MRI) should be considered to know more about location and size of fibroids but not as an initial diagnostic test. CT scan is not recommended for assessment of fibroids. According to American Association of Gynecologic Laparoscopists (AAGL) practice guidelines, for submucous fibroids, hysteroscopy, saline infusion sonography, and MRI are all highly sensitive and specific compared to hysterosalpingography and ultrasound. Diagnostic hysteroscopy can be avoided in 40% cases by considering transvaginal sonohysterography prior to hysteroscopy for diagnosis of submucous fibroids.

TREATMENT

Society of Obstetricians and Gynecologists of Canada Clinical Practice Guidelines on Treatment of Fibroids

Fibroids in Pregnancy

Additional maternal and fetal surveillance is required. Concern about possible complications is not an indication for myomectomy in pregnancy.

Asymptomatic Fibroids

No treatment is required where the uterine size is less than 16 weeks. Reassure the woman as there is no evidence of major concern about malignancy. The incidence of leiomyosarcoma has been estimated to be around 0.22–0.49%. 3–7% of untreated fibroids regress over 6 months to 3 years.

Indication for hysterectomy in asymptomatic woman is enlarging fibroid after menopause without hormone replacement therapy, as it raises risk of leiomyosarcoma.

Symptomatic Fibroids

Individualize treatment based on symptomatology, desire of woman to preserve fertility and uterus, and expertise of surgeon.

Medical Treatment

- *Medical treatment for fibroids with abnormal uterine bleeding (AUB)*: Effective treatment includes levonorgestrel intrauterine system (LNG-IUS), gonadotropin-releasing hormone (GnRH) analogs, selective progesterone receptor modulators, oral contraceptives, progestins, and danazol.
- *Medical treatment for fibroids with bulk symptoms*: Treatment includes GnRH analogs and selective progesterone receptor modulators. However, fibroids will return to pretherapy size within 6 months of stopping the therapy.

Surgical Treatment

Preoperative anemia should be corrected by using GnRH analogs and selective progesterone receptor modulators.

1. *Women who want to preserve fertility (conservative surgical management)*:
   - Myomectomy is the option but carries potential for further intervention. Consider use of vasopressin, bupivacaine, epinephrine, pericervical tourniquet, misoprostol, or gelatin–thrombin matrix to reduce blood loss.
   - Myomectomy by laparotomy, laparoscopy, or hysteroscopy should be planned on mapping location, size, and number of fibroids with imaging. MRI helps in diagnosing the relationship of leiomyoma with myometrium and serosa.

   Delivery after myomectomy: Although there is limited data and cesarean delivery is recommended, if endometrial cavity is entered during myomectomy. However, uterine scar integrity and rupture depend on total extent of defect, absence of multilayer closure in intramural myomas, excessive use of electrosurgical repair, and time period between myomectomy and subsequent pregnancy. Hence, treatment should be individualized for each patient.

   Submucous fibroids: Hysteroscopic myomectomy is the first line of management.

   AAGL practice guideline for the diagnosis and management of submucous leiomyomas:
   - Hysteroscopic removal can be done in types 0, I, and II, up to 4–5 cm in diameter. Risk of uterine perforation and excessive fluid absorption are increased, if there is less than 5 mm thickness between fibroid and uterine serosa. If three or more myomas then abdominal approach may be considered. Cervical preparation with prostaglandins before hysteroscopic myomectomy minimizes trauma.
   - Postoperative bleeding can be managed by prostaglandin F2α (PGF2α) or balloon tamponade. Hysteroscopic adhesiolysis should be considered in woman with postmyomectomy intrauterine synechiae.
   - *Submucous fibroid with infertility*: Removal improves pregnancy rate.
   - *Morcellation*: According to society of gynecologic oncology, the use of power morcellator is contraindicated in documented/suspected malignancy. Food and Drug Administration (FDA) discourages its use during hysterectomy/myomectomy.

2. *Women who want to conserve uterus but not fertility*:
   - Ablative and embolic therapies are appropriate for those not desirous of fertility. Endometrial ablation is most suitable in type 2 leiomyomas with AUB. Also, ablation can be added to hysteroscopic myomectomy when fertility is not desired.
   - Uterine artery embolization (UAE) has been shown to be effective and has longest track record but can have impact on fecundity and pregnancy.

RCOG[15] and NICE guidelines on uterine artery embolization for fibroids:
- Uterine artery embolization is a less invasive alternative to hysterectomy/myomectomy/medical management. It offers shorter recovery time and preservation of uterus. UAE is efficacious in AUB with fibroids in short and medium term (up to 5 years).
- It has no major safety concerns. Symptoms may return and patient may require hysterectomy. Effects of AUB on fertility are uncertain. Treatment of fibroids in women who wish or might wish to become pregnant should be offered UAE only after discussion and informed consent. The procedure is contraindicated in cases of pregnancy, pelvic infection, or doubt about benign pathology.
- Royal College of Obstetricians and Gynecologists (RCOG) recommends appropriate diagnosis by MRI before the procedure. The procedure should be undertaken only by a competent radiologist with adequate training.
- MRI-guided transcutaneous focused ultrasound treatment for fibroids has promising results but lack long-term data.

NICE guidance on MRI-guided transcutaneous focused ultrasound for uterine fibroids:
- Efficacy of MRI-guided transcutaneous focused ultrasound is adequate for short term. Further treatment may be required. There are associated complications like sciatic nerve palsy, skin burns, bowel injuries but evidence on safety is adequate to support the use of this procedure. Effect on fertility and subsequent pregnancy is uncertain.

3. *Women who want to neither preserve fertility nor conserve uterus*: Hysterectomy by least invasive approach is most effective, definitive treatment with high level of satisfaction.

CONCLUSION

To conclude, these guidelines include Canadian clinical practice guidelines and guidance from New Zealand on management of uterine leiomyomas. Also included is AAGL practice report on diagnosis and management of submucous leiomyomas, RCOG recommendations on UAE, National Institute for Health and Care Excellence (NICE) guidance on UAE and MRI-guided transcutaneous focused ultrasound.

BIBLIOGRAPHY

1. American Association of Gynecologic Laparoscopists (AAGL); Advancing Minimally Invasive Gynecology Worldwide. AAGL practice report: practice guidelines for the diagnosis and management of submucous leiomyomas. J Minim Invasive Gynecol. 2012;19:152-71.
2. Ang WC, Farrell E, Vollenhoven B. Effect of hormone replacement therapies and selective estrogen receptor modulators in postmenopausal women with uterine leiomyomas: a systematic review. Climacteric. 2001;4:284-92.
3. College National des Gynécologues et Obstétriciens Français (CNGOF). Actualisation de la prise en charge des myomes [Myoma management recommendations]. J Gynecol Obstet Biol Reprod. 2011;40:693-708.
4. DeWaay DJ, Syrop CH, Nygaard IE, et al. Natural history of uterine polyps and leiomyomata. Obstet Gynecol. 2002;100:3-7.
5. Farquhar C, Arroll B, Ekeroma A, et al. An evidence-based guideline for the management of uterine fibroids. Aust N Z J Obstet Gynaecol. 2001;41:125-40.
6. Food and Drug Administration. (2014). Quantitative assessment of the prevalence of unsuspected uterine sarcoma in women undergoing treatment of uterine fibroids: summary and key findings. [online] Available from http://www.fda.gov/downloads/MedicalDevices/Safety/AlertsandNotices/UCM393589.pdf. [Accessed June, 2018].
7. Friedman AJ, Haas ST. Should uterine size be an indication for surgical intervention in women with myomas? Am J Obstet Gynecol. 1993;168 (3 Pt 10):751-5.

8. Leibsohn S, d'Ablaing G, Mishell DR Jr., et al. Leiomyosarcoma in a series of hysterectomies performed for presumed uterine leiomyomas. Am J Obstet Gynecol. 1990;162:968-74; discussion 974-6.
9. Loffer FD. Improving results of hysteroscopic submucosal myomectomy for menorrhagia by concomitant endometrial ablation. J Min Invas Gynecol. 2005;12:254-60.
10. National Institute for Health and Clinical Excellence. (2011). Magnetic resonance image-guided transcutaneous focused ultrasound for uterine fibroids. NICE Interventional procedure guidance IPG 413. [online] Available from https://www.nice.org.uk/guidance/ipg413. [Accessed June, 2018]
11. National Institute of Health and Care Excellence. (2010). Uterine artery embolisation for fibroids. NICE Interventional procedure guidance IPG 367. [online] Available from https://www.nice.org.uk/guidance/IPG367. [Accessed June, 2018].
12. Parker WH, Fu YS, Berek JS. Uterine sarcoma in patients operated on for presumed leiomyoma and rapidly growing leiomyoma. Obstet Gynecol. 1994;83:414-8.
13. Royal college of obstetricians and Gynaecologists. Clinical recommendations on the use of uterine artery embolisation (UAE) in the management of fibroids, 3rd edition. London: RCOG; 2013.
14. Society of Gynecologic Oncology. (2013). SGO position statement: morcellation. [online] Available from https://www.sgo.org/newsroom/position-statements-2/morcellation. [Accessed June, 2018].
15. Vilos GA, Allaire C, Laberge PY, et al. SOGC clinical practice guideline. The management of uterine leiomyomas. J Obstet Gynaecol Can. 2015;37(2):157-78.
16. Wamsteker K, Emanuel MH, de Kruif JH. Transcervical hysteroscopic resection of submucous fibroids for abnormal uterine bleeding: results regarding the degree of intramural extension. Obstet Gynecol. 1993;82:736-40.
17. Weber AM, Mitchinson AR, Gidwani GP, et al. Uterine myomas and factors associated with hysterectomy in premenopausal women. Am J Obstet Gynecol. 1997;176:1213-7.

Index

Page numbers followed by *b* refer to box, *f* refer to figure, *fc* refer to flowchart, and *t* refer to table.

A

Abdomen
   acute 19
   for hemostasis before closing, inspecting 91*f*
   lower 144
Abdominal cavity 103*f*
Abdominal examination 14*f*
Abdominal hysterectomy, total 177
Abdominal mass 146
   occupying left hypogastrium 127*f*
Abdominal pain, lower 13
Acrochordons 155
Adenomyosis 7, 9*f*, 21, 79, 123
Adenomyotic tissue 163
Adherent placenta cesarean section 46
Adipocytes 181
Adiponectin 181
Adnexal mass, diagnosis of 193
American Association of Gynecologic Laparoscopists 85, 92, 97, 222
American College of Obstetricians and Gynecologist 97
Androgen receptor 164
Androgenic steroids 187
Anemia 75, 216
   postpartum 175
   severe 216
Angiofibromas 155
Antenatal complications 27
Antiadhesion barriers 94
Antifibrinolytic agents 33
Anti-inflammatory drugs 145
Anti-müllerian hormone 175, 191
Antiprogestin 57, 132, 187
Antiprogestogen 39
Antiretroviral therapy 41
Antral follicle count 175
Appendicitis 204
Aromatase inhibitor 39, 64, 114, 132, 167, 187
Arousal 139
Artery embolization 97
Asoprisnil 114, 164
Association of Fibroids and Infertility 75
Atrazine 181
Atypia 110
Automatic tissue extraction 104

B

Bacterial collagenase, purified 169
Bag morcellation, contained in 128
Bag with atraumatic graspers 100*f*
Bag with single tooth grasper 101*f*
Barbed suture, stitching with 82*f*
Birt-Hogg-Dubé syndrome 155, 155*f*
Bladder
   injury 93
   obstruction, chronic 148
Bladderwrack 183
Bleeding 42, 146
   during myomectomy 84
   issues, regression of 115
Blenching fibroid 84*f*
Blood
   pressure 84
   supply, inadequate 36
Bone demineralization 197
Bonney's myomectomy clamp 83
Bowel injury 93
Bridging vascular sign 19, 32
Bulky uterus with adenomyosis 15*f*
Bupivacaine 84

C

Cabergoline 114
Calcareous degeneration 6
Carboprost 85
Cardiac failure 89

Cell
　　growth, regulation of 109
　　proliferation 166
　　structures 109
Cellular leiomyoma 126
Cervical fibroid 147, 150, 200, 201
　　large 148f
　　operative management of 147
Cervix 18
Cesarean delivery 47
Chasteberry 183
Chromosomal abnormalities 135
Clinical pregnancy rate 192
Clostridium histolyticum 169
　　collagenase, injection of 170f
Collapse of patient, unexpected 207
Combined oral contraceptives 114
Complete blood count 216
Cytokines 135

D

Danazol 39, 132, 187, 223
Dandelion 182
Depomedroxyprogesterone acetate 64
Depression 139, 188
Detoxes 182
Detoxification, phase-I 179
Dietary supplements 165
Disseminated peritoneal leiomyomatosis 158
Doppler ultrasonography 147
Doppler ultrasound 16
　　enabled transvaginal clamp 120
Drug
　　current status of 113
　　facts about research on 113
　　newer 64
Dysglycemia 181
Dysmenorrhea 26, 106, 139, 146
　　prevalence of 57
Dyspareunia 139, 140, 146
Dystocia 43

E

Early pregnancy 42
　　loss 25, 27
Elagolix 165
Electrolyte imbalance 89

Electromechanical morcellation 96
Emotional and spiritual health, stress and 182
Endo bag
　　piecemeal removal from 86f
　　plastic 86f
Endocrine neoplasia type 1, multiple 156
Endometrial ablation 56, 117, 212
Endometrial biopsy 217
Endometrial carcinoma 7, 10f
Endometrial cavity 53
Endometrial curettage 21
Endometrial hemostasis 61
Endometrial hyperplasia 7, 9f, 173
Endometrial myomectomy, technique of 45
Endometrial polyp 9f
Endometrial stromal sarcoma 7, 103, 126
Endometriosis 79, 139
Endometrium 113, 117, 219
Epigallocatechin gallate 165
Estrogen 64, 70, 135, 179
　　dependence 2
　　dependent tumors 41
　　elimination, enhancing 179
　　environmental sources of 182
　　glucuronide 180
　　nutritional sources of 182
　　production, normalizing 180
　　receptor 164
　　　　modulator, selective 39, 63, 64, 71, 108, 114, 132, 165, 166f, 187
　　therapy, cyclical 198
Ethinyl-testosterone 132
Ethisterone 132
European Society of Gastrointestinal
　　Endoscopy 85

F

Fadrozole 39
Female reproductive system 185
Female sexual dysfunction 139
　　cause of 139, 141
　　cycle of 140, 141fc
Fertility 174
　　after myomectomy 38
　　implications on future 34
　　preservation of 62
　　reduce 36

Index **229**

Fertility-preserving strategy 59
Fetal growth restriction and malformations 43
Fibrofolliculomas 155
Fibroid 1, 13, 16, 19, 22, 24, 31, 36, 41, 46, 49, 74, 79, 126, 139-141, 161, 163, 170*f*, 172, 174, 203*f*, 211, 215, 219
    ablation, vizablate system during 169*f*
    affect sex life 139
    after myomectomy 26*f*
    alone 74
    and fertility 36, 175*fc*
    and gastrointestinal symptoms 143
    and in vitro fertilization outcome 37
    and infertility 36
    and sexual dysfunction 139
    artery embolization 72
    associations, rare 28
    asymptomatic 211
    broad ligament 193
    capsule around 3*f*
    cases of large 44
    cells 91
    cervical 143
    classification of atypical 152
    clinical effects of 75*b*
    comparison of surgeries for 80*t*
    counseling of 209
    degeneration of 42, 75
    diagnosed, number of 162
    diagnosis of 13, 144, 176*fc*
    differential diagnosis in 7*t*
    distorted by 27
    during pregnancy, diagnosis of 41
    enlarging 222
    epidemiology 24
    evaluation of 172
    growth rate of 173*f*
    herbs for 182
    holistic approach to 179
    in adolescent age group, large 216
    in adolescent girl, management of 31
    in menopausal woman, management of 69
    in postmenopausal woman, management of 70*fc*
    in pregnancy 41, 43, 175, 222
    infection of 42
    infertility
        associated with 75
        with submucous 198
    intramural 143
    location of 37, 49
    magnetic resonance imaging of 55*f*
    management guidelines 222
    management of 56*fc*, 211
    manifestations of symptomatic 140*fc*
    medical management of 106
    medical treatment of 108*fc*, 144, 223
    morcellation of 98, 103*f*, 104*f*
        controversies regarding 96
    multiple 173
    new occurrence of 130
    newer nonsurgical treatment options for 117
    nonsurgical
        newer options 145
        treatment of 41
    nonsymptomatic presence of 211
    number of 32, 39
    occurrence of 130
    on pregnancy, effects of 42, 43*f*
    on sexual dysfunction 141
    on transabdominal scan 52*f*
    on USG with increased peripheral vascularity 29*f*
    pedunculated 20
    pedunculated large 42
    perimenopausal big 194
    perplexing situations with 207
    polyp 13
    presence of 71
    presentation of 25*f*, 176*fc*
    primary parasitic 207
    progressions of 170
    pseudocervical 13
    reassuring with 172
    recurrence of 130
        incidence of 130
    reduce 179
    reduction of 182
    registry 119
    regrowth 79
    removal of 65
    resectable with hysteroscope 123
    retroplacental 43

230 Fibroids

secondary changes in 6
secondary parasitic 207
shrinkage 109
size of 69, 115
small 31, 77
stepwise slow enucleation of 82*f*
submucosal 143
subserosal 143
   symptomatic 59
subserous and intramural 58
surface, incision on 82*f*
surgical management of 79, 145
surgical treatment of 41
symptomatic 74, 139, 141, 211, 223
   treatment 145
symptoms of 146, 176*fc*
treatment for 39, 64, 113, 144, 222
treatment outcomes in 130
types of 16, 36, 143
understanding 1
using hysteroscopy, location of 55*f*
volume 43
with menorrhagia 176
world of 161
Fibroid and malignancy 126
   management 128
   proposed alternatives 128
   role of imaging 127
Fibroid and pregnancy 75
   outcome 39
Fibroid disease
   clinical spectrum of 24
   patients with 209
Fibroid in perimenopausal
   age 177*fc*
   group 177
   women 61
      management of 62*fc*
Fibroid on transvaginal
   sonography 16*f*
   USG, posterior wall 51*f*
Fibroid syndrome
   atypical 152, 152*fc*
   rare 24
Fibroid tumors 12
   symptoms related to 13
Fibroleiomyoma 1
Fibroma 1

Fibromyoma 1
Fibrous tissue, tumors of 24
Fimbrial cyst, small 11*f*
Fine-needle aspiration cytology 106
Fluorodeoxyglucose 127
Follicle-stimulating hormone 56, 109
Food and Drug Administration 96, 135
Fundal right cornual fibroid after vasopressin injection 82*f*

G

Gastroenteritis 204
Gastrointestinal symptoms 143
Genetic predisposition 2
Genitourinary dysfunction 146
Gentle tissue handling 94
Gestrinone 132, 187
Ginger 183
Gonadotropin-releasing hormone 56, 62, 63, 70, 107, 108, 133, 144, 166, 211
   agonist 39, 64, 107, 109, 131, 187, 213
      role of 109
      side effects of 188
      use of 135
   analogs 33, 56, 223
      pretreatment with 132
   antagonist 109, 133, 165, 188
      disadvantages of 109
      side effects 107
Gravid uterus, comparing with 143
Green tea extract 165, 167*f*
Growth factor-beta, transforming 109
Gynecological ailments 139
Gynecological symptoms 24, 26
Gynecological tumors 74
   benign 94

H

Haematocrit, postoperative 109
Haemoglobin, postoperative 109
Hair loss 188
Halt ablation system 168, 169*f*
Headaches 188
Hematogenous dissemination 128
Hemorrhage 93
   intraoperative 45
   postpartum 25, 44, 175
   risk of postpartum 44

Hepatotoxicity 215
Hereditary leiomyomatosis 158
High-intensity focused ultrasound 34, 188
Hormone replacement therapy 65, 69, 72
Hostile endometrial environment 36
Hot flashes 197
Human chorionic gonadotropin 7
Human menopausal gonadotropin 219
Hyaline degeneration 6
Hydronephrosis 148
Hydroxylation 179
Hypermenorrhea 39
Hyperplasia 113
   atypical 113
Hypointense lesion 127*f*
Hysterectomy 65, 74, 92, 94, 98, 119, 126, 189
   abdominal 92
   crude rate of 134
   indication for 222
   subtotal 141
   total 141
Hysteroscopic myomectomy 58, 85, 134
   complications 89
Hysteroscopic resection 133
   advantages of 87
Hysteroscopy 19, 53, 64
   lesions on 55*f*
   ultrasound-guided 20

I

In vitro fertilization
   cycle of 191, 218
   results after myomectomy 38
   treatment 37
Infection 75
Infertility 20, 36, 61, 106, 146
   treatment for 41
   unexplained 133
Infrequent fibroid
   classification of 152
   syndrome 152
Infundibulopelvic ligament 83, 84
Insulin and glucose dynamics, normalizing 181
Intermenstrual bleeding 61, 75
International Federation of Gynecology and Obstetrics 53*b*
   classification 212*f*

Intraclinical myomatous nuclei, small 131
Intralesional drug delivering systems 167
Intramural fibroid 37, 38, 192
   cause 217
   in reproductive age group 217, 218
   pushing endometrial cavity, posterior wall 53*f*
   with subfertility 191
Intramural myoma, adverse effect of 174
Intranatal complications 28
Intraoperative adjuncts 93
Intrauterine
   contraceptive device 198
   growth restriction 39
   insemination, cycles of 191
Intravenous leiomyomatosis 126, 153
Intravenous pyelogram 176
Invasive prenatal testing, difficulty in 43

K

Kidney function test 216

L

Labor
   and puerperium 43
   dystocia 47
      cause 43
   preterm 25, 43, 47
Lap myomectomy, stepwise 90*f*
Laparoscopic approach 132
Laparoscopic hysterectomy 58, 96
   complications of 93
   total 177
Laparoscopic morcellation 104
Laparoscopic myolysis 189
Laparoscopic myomectomy 58, 91
   advantages 91
   complications 92
   in intramural fibroid, steps of 83*f*
   specimen morcellation 91
Laparoscopic uterine artery occlusion 189
Laparoscopy 20, 21*f*, 65, 135
   hemostatic options at 91
   over laparotomy, advantages of 58
   robotic-assisted 92
Laparotomy 65, 134, 135
Leiomyofibroma 1

Leiomyoma 1f, 13, 17, 18, 61, 74, 79, 126, 146, 153, 161, 185, 194, 222, 223
  atypical 126
  benign 58, 126, 128
  location of 162
  presumed 103
Leiomyomata 97, 109, 134
  after myomectomy, risk of recurrence of 134
Leiomyomatosis peritonealis disseminata 126
Leiomyosarcoma 7, 65, 126, 173, 177
  detection of 127t
  risk of 222
Letrozole 64
Leukorrhea 146
Levonorgestrel intrauterine system 62, 63, 110, 114, 144, 163, 176, 223
Levonorgestrel-releasing intrauterine contraceptive device 186
Libido, decreased 140
Ligament leiomyoma 150
Ligand-agonist binds 112f
Liver function test 216
Lower abdomen, heaviness in 28
Lower segment cesarean section 192
  in case of fibroid 203f
Luteinizing hormone 109

M

Magnetic resonance imaging 7, 18f, 32, 52, 174
  guided focused ultrasound 70, 71, 133
  on fertility, effects of 124
  surgery 65
Magnetic resonance-guided focused ultrasound 62, 121
  contraindications of 123t
  procedure for 122f
Malignancy, risk of 34, 58, 65, 135
Malpresentation 47
Masses, benign 106
Maternal and fetal well-being 44
Matrix metalloproteinases 164
Medical diseases 139
Medical management, counseling before 107
Medical therapy, selection of women for 106
Medroxyprogesterone acetate 33

Menorrhagia 39, 49, 75, 146, 216
  and menstrual irregularities 139
  mild 106
Menstrual bleeding
  heavy 26, 49, 166
  profuse 26
  treatment options for heavy 166f
Menstrual disturbances 8
Menstrual history 220
Menstrual symptoms 75
Mesodermal tumor, mixed 7
Metastasizing fibroid, benign 152
Metastasizing leiomyoma, benign 126, 152, 154f
Meticulous hemostasis 94
Metrorrhagia 26, 49
Mifepristone 32, 39, 110, 163
  emergence of 111
Minilaparotomy 65, 128
Minimal invasive surgery, recurrence after 133
Minimally invasive technique 63, 64
Miscarriage 43
  increased risk of 46
Misoprostol 93
Mitotic activity, low or nil 110
Morcellation done under vision 101f
Morcellation techniques, modified 128
Muscle
  tissue 143
  tumors, smooth 126
Musculoskeletal stiffness 188
Myofibroma 1
Myohyperplasia 21
Myolysis 174
Myoma 1, 24, 75, 79, 135, 161f, 185, 189, 222
  abutting endometrium, posterior wall 219f
  after surgery, newer 178
  cells 107
  complications of 6
  conservative treatment for 74
  development 161
  differential diagnosis of 6
  distribution of 5f
  in adolescent 173
    girl 174fc
  in body of uterus, distribution of 4

in unmarried girl 173
large 58, 85, 88f, 126, 218
    posterior wall 220f
location of 197
management
    of type 0 213f
    of type 1 213f
    of type 2 214f
multiple 85
number of 130,
on open myomectomy, multiple 88f
rapid growing 126
shrinkage of 77
types of 13

Myomata
    family predisposition to 135
    individual 135
    number of 131
    preoperative detection of 132

Myomatous nuclei
    perioperatively 131
    preoperatively 131

Myomectomy 33, 38, 65, 74, 81, 94, 97, 120, 126, 130, 131, 134, 174, 189, 210, 216
    abdominal 134, 135
    after 135
    and pregnancy outcome 39
    by hysteroscopy 134
    by laparoscopy 134
    by laparotomy 134
    complications of 59
    conventional 141
    delivery after 223
    during cesarean section 44
    during pregnancy 44
    effectiveness of 38
    hemostasis during 81
    parity after 132
    series of 132
    suture line, after 192f

Myometrial contractility 192
Myometrial disease 131
Myometrial stretching 28
Myometrial-cultured cells 64
Myometrium 117, 223
    meticulous palpation of 131
    normal 110

N

National Institute for Health and Care Excellence 224
Necrotic tissue, excision of 94
Neurological disorders, absence of 148
Newer conservative methods 34
Nonmenstrual abdominal pain 57
Nonpeptide 165
Nonperfusion volume 122
Nonsteroidal anti-inflammatory drugs 33, 63, 70, 186

O

Obstetrical history 218, 200, 220
Obstetrical symptoms 24, 27
Obstructed labor 43
Occult malignancy, dissemination of 97
Oligoasthenoteratozoospermia, severe 219
Open myomectomy, steps of 87f
Oral contraceptive 186, 223
    pills 33, 163, 166
Oral progesterones 176
Orally active gonadotropin-releasing hormone antagonist 165
Orgasm 139
Ormeloxifene 187
Ovarian cancer 7, 10f
Ovarian cyst, torsion of 204
Ovarian mass 79
Ovarian tumor 21
Oxidized regenerated cellulose 94

P

Packed cells 216
Pain 61, 146
Parasitic fibroid 207
Parasitic myoma 6
Pedunculated subserous fibroid 203
Pelvic
    congestion 29
    discomfort 146
    disease, coexistent 196
    endometriosis 20
    examination 14, 51
        bimanual 14f, 185
    inflammatory disease 123, 204

pain 13, 20, 74
  chronic 140
  in fibroids 61
  pressure 57
  tumors in women 130
Perifollicular fibromas 155
Perimenopausal status 63
Perimenopausal symptomatic fibroid 196
Peritoneal cavity 102
Peritoneal leiomyomatosis, diffuse 153
Placenta
  abruption 47
  adherent and retained 44
Plastic bag, strong 99*f*
Pneumothorax 156
Polymenorrhea 49
Polymeric membrane 167
Postcoital bleeding 140
Post-gadolinium administration 19
Postmenopausal
  fibroids 72
  women 58
Postmyomectomy 219
Postnatal complications 28
Pregnancy 21
  after high-intensity focused ultrasound 46
  after myomectomy 45
  after uterine artery embolization 46
  common symptom in 47
  complications during 75
  late 43
  on fibroid
    disease, effect of 28, 41
    effects of 42*fc*
  wastage 146
  with fibroid disease 11*f*, 201
Premenopausal women 63
Pressure effects 28
Pressure symptoms 24, 29, 61, 106
  relief of 115
Preterm premature rupture of membranes 25
Progesterone 70, 135
  long-acting 132, 186
  pills 163
  therapy, cyclical 198
Progesterone receptor 41, 110, 112*f*, 164
  ligands 112*f*
  modulator 110, 164*f*, 165
    action of 111*f*
    advantages of 164
    selective 34, 57, 62, 64, 108, 111, 132, 163, 187, 197, 211, 213, 214, 223
  selective 63
Progestin 33, 57, 63, 64, 167, 223
Proinflammatory cytokines 181
Proinflammatory enzyme cyclooxygenase 181
Prolactin 216
Prophylactic therapy 185
Pulmonary and cerebral edema 89
Pulmonary manifestation 156

Q

Quality of life, impact on 77

R

Racial predominance 2
Radiofrequency
  ablation system 168
  cryomyolysis 65
Raloxifene 39, 63, 70, 132
Randomized controlled trial 119*t*, 164
Recurrent pregnancy loss 25
Renal cell cancer 158
Renal tumor 156
Reoperation and hysterectomy, role of 134
Reproductive problems 24, 26
Residual myomatous nuclei, growth of small 135
Resveratrol 166
Routes of surgery, comparison of 80*t*
Rubber-shod clamps 83

S

Saline infusion
  sonography 17*f*, 51
  of fibroids 54*f*
  sonohysterography 16, 17, 176
Saline injection 17
Salpingo-oophorectomy, bilateral 62, 128, 177

Sarcoma
  dissemination 103
  undifferentiated 126
Scar with intercede, covering 86f
Secrete proinflammatory cytokines 181
Semen analysis 191
Serum
  ferritin 216
  lactate dehydrogenase 127
Sex hormone-binding capacity 182
Sex pain disorders 139
Sexual abuse, history of 139
Sexual desire in women, decreased 139
Sexual dysfunction 139, 141
  woman suffering from 140
Sexual functioning 141
Shear wave elasticity imaging 163
Society of Obstetricians and Gynaecologists 81, 222
Solitary intramural fibroid 195
Sonosalpingography 51
Spasmodic dysmenorrhea 61, 75
Spontaneous miscarriage 47
Stress urinary incontinence 149
Submucous fibroid 13, 36, 38, 43, 53b, 223, 198
  cavity-distorting 37
  classification of 54f
  diagnosis of 222
  in perimenopausal age group 219
  on hysteroscopy 20f
  resection for 46
  with infertility 223
Submucous leiomyomas
  diagnosis of 85, 223
  management of 85, 223
Submucous myomectomy 85
Subserosal fibroids 18, 37
  in hysterectomy specimen, multiple 25f
  multiple small 11f
  on laparoscopy 5f
Suprapubic ultrasound investigation 131
Supraumbilical trocar 201
Surgery and routes, types of 80
Surgery, planning of 79
Surgical procedure, property of 131
Symptomatic fibroid
  treatment for 141
  young girl with 199
Symptomatic intracavitary fibroids,
  management of 58

Symptomatic submucous fibroids, treatment of 59
Symptomatic uterine fibroids
  presumed 96
  treatment for 94
Synthetic vasopressin, use of 94

T

Take-home message 104
Tamoxifen 63
Telapristone acetate 163
Thyroid-stimulating hormone 216
Tibolone 70
Tissue
  disruption 97
  inhibitors of metalloproteinases 164
  retrieval 97
Torsion 6, 42
Tranexamic acid 33, 63, 84
Transabdominal sonography 174, 177
Transabdominal ultrasonography 148f
Transabdominal ultrasound 216
Transcervical resectoscopic myomectomy 85
Transformation, malignant 77
Transient ischemia 120
  causes 117
Transvaginal
  sonography 51, 176, 177
  sonohysterogram 192
  ultrasonography 191, 218
  uterine artery occlusion 117, 212
Trichodiscomas 155
Triptorelin 64
Tubo-ovarian mass 21
Tumor
  benign 61
  degeneration in central part of 3f

U

Ulipristal acetate 34, 111, 163, 187, 219
  chemical structure of 112
  structure of 112f
Ultrasonography 33, 175–177
Ultrasound 32
Upper abdomen 144
Ureteric injury 93
Urinary incontinence 149
  mixed 149
Urinary retention 147

Urinary symptoms 75
Urinary tract symptoms, lower 146, 149
Urine, acute retention of 148
US Food and Drug Administration 92, 106
Uterine artery embolism 210
Uterine artery embolization 18, 34, 46, 58,
        64, 74, 117, 119, 119f, 119t, 120, 121t,
        130, 133, 174, 212, 223
    advantages 118
    and myomectomy 120t
    complications 119
    contraindications 118
    disadvantages 118
    effects of 120
    for fibroids 224
    in women 141
    indications 118
    mode of action 117
    pretreatment 118
    procedure 118
Uterine artery occlusion 121
    transvaginal temporary 120, 121f
Uterine bleeding
    abnormal 25, 26, 49, 61, 62, 69, 74, 79,
        106, 174, 175, 194, 216, 221, 223
        clinical presentation in 49
        pain and pressure symptoms 74
    causes of abnormal 53b
    conservative treatment for abnormal 74
    diagnosis of abnormal 50fc
    with fibroids, management of abnormal 49
Uterine cavity 20
Uterine dehiscence 59
Uterine fibroid 2, 18, 27, 58, 61, 74, 94,
        111f, 126, 133, 146, 164f, 166f, 174,
        185, 222
    color Doppler of 54f
    development of 161
    diagnostic modalities for 185
    distribution of 5fc
    embolization 56, 71, 188
    on fertility 120
    in nutshell 185
    large 150
    management of 66, 76f, 186
        hormonal treatment 186
        medical therapy 186
        nonhormonal treatment 186
    surgeries 57
    symptomatic 65, 97
    symptoms of 143
    tissue 121

    treatment of 74, 111f, 130, 154f
    ultrasound for 224
Uterine leiomyoma 49, 126, 149, 204
    management of 81, 224
    treatment of women with 81
Uterine leiomyomatosis, diffuse 153
Uterine leiomyosarcoma, risk for 97
Uterine masses 17
Uterine morcellation 92
Uterine muscle, laparoscopic closure of 91
Uterine musculature, tumors of 22
Uterine myoma 31, 130
    asymptomatic 98
Uterine sarcoma 7, 10f, 103, 126, 127
Uterine serosa 85
Uterine smooth muscle tumor 154, 155f
Uterine stone 161, 161f
Uterine surface, posterior 192f
Uterine surgery 124
Uterine tissue
    benign 98
    malignant 98
    normal 163
Uterine vascular perfusion 192
Uterine volume 109
Uterus 62
    conserve 223
    inversion of 8
    morcellation of 98
    normal sized 148f

V

Vaginal bleeding, undiagnosed 123
Vaginal delivery 124
Vaginal dryness 109, 188, 197
Vaginal hysterectomy 93
    complications 93
    prerequisites 93
Vaginal morcellation 128
Vaginismus 139
Vascular control systems 120
Vasopressin 94
Vilaprisan 164
Vitamin D3 165
    structure of 167f
Vitex 183
Vizablate treatment device 168f
von Hippel-Lindau disease 157
    differential diagnosis 157
    prognosis 158
    signs and symptoms 157
    treatment 157